D0864538

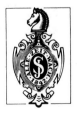

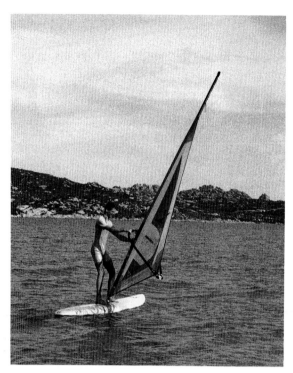

A dream fulfilled – 10 years after his accident R. B. learns to windsurf. (See Chapter 3 – A Case in Point)

Patricia M. Davies

Starting Again

Early Rehabilitation After Traumatic
Brain Injury or Other Severe Brain Lesion

Foreword by David Butler

With 286 Figures
in 605 Separate Illustrations

Springer-Verlag
Berlin Heidelberg New York London Paris Tokyo
Hong Kong Barcelona Budapest

Patricia M. Davies, MCSP., Dip. Phys. Ed.
Switzerland

Photographs: Rainer Gierig, D-82362 Weilheim, Germany

1st edn. 1994, corrected printing 1998

ISBN 3-540-55934-5 Springer-Verlag Berlin Heidelberg New York
ISBN 0-387-55934-5 Springer-Verlag New York Berlin Heidelberg

Library of Congress Cataloging-in-Publication Data
Davies, Patricia M. Starting again : early rehabilitation after traumatic brain injury or other
severe brain lesion / Patricia M. Davies ; foreword by David Butler.   p. cm.
Includes bibliographical references and index.
ISBN 3-540-55934-5 (alk. paper). – ISBN 0-387-55934-5 (alk. paper)
1. Brain damage–Patients–Rehabilitation.   I. Title.
[DNLM: 1. Brain Injuries–rehabilitation.   2. Head Injuries,
Closed–rehabilitation.   WL 354 D257s 1994]
RC387.5.D38   1994   617.4'8103–dc20
DNLM/DLC   for Library of Congress   94-9131

© Springer-Verlag Berlin Heidelberg 1994
Printed in Germany

Cover: H. Lopka, Ilvesheim
Typesetting: Mitterweger Werksatz GmbH, Plankstadt bei Heidelberg
SPIN: 10658716   21/3133 - 5 4 3 2 1 0 - Printed on acid-free paper

This book is dedicated to Evi Schuster, whose courage and determination in the face of such suffering inspired me to put pen to paper in the first place, and to William Casey, whose unending bravery, courtesy and humour despite the many setbacks spurred me on to complete the manuscript The dedication embraces also the families of Evi, William and the many others like them, for caring enough to keep on helping and not give up when the going is hard. Their love and care is a continuous inspiration. For them I include these words from the lovely song, *The Rose*.

When the night has been too lonely
And the road has been too long,
And you think that love is only
For the lucky and the strong;
Just remember in the winter
far beneath the bitter snows
Lies the seed that with the sun's love
In the spring becomes the rose.

AMANDA MCBROOM 1977

Foreword

What does *"Starting Again"* mean to the many different people this book reaches out to? This positive title may draw the reader to enquire why an immensely experienced physiotherapist is considering starting again. Perhaps it challenges patients to rethink their own limitations, or therapists to reconsider their own management strategies. Does it refer to a change in life for head-injured patients and their carers, or does it hint at a fresh approach to old problems?

Since *"Steps to Follow"* and *"Right in the Middle"*, Pat Davies has not been idle. She has remained aware of what may be new and worthwhile in therapy around the world, incorporated it into her own vast experience and taken ideas, concepts and techniques back to her patients to test their clinical validity. This is, therefore, not a pedestrian text but one brimming with new ideas for immediate use. That in itself should be a message of hope for all involved in the consequences of head injury. The future will always hold new and better management strategies, the understanding of the nature and consequences of head injury will improve, and thus there should never be limits placed on what patients can achieve.

Reduced to its simplicity and presented in modern day thinking, the nervous system is a neural network. It requires input for output, yet it possesses a delicate, powerful, inherent feedback system so it can drive itself optimally, test itself out, learn and adapt. Tragically, many therapists and doctors look solely at the output of the system, forgetting the input, and neglect the fact that the nervous system is continually seeking feedback. This is manifest in treatments aimed predominantly at improving motor control and ranges of movement, where quality of movement and aiming at specific individual goals are sometimes missed and which at worst, consist of management from crisis to crisis, rather than prevention.

Pat Davies presents a balanced view. She acknowledges and teaches skilled task-specific motor control, but she also focuses on the importance of input to the nervous system, for example, the quality of touch, minimisation of fear, maintenance of dignity during treatment, the importance of enthusiasm and the removal of painful stimuli. It follows that this book, as in all of Pat Davies' books, respects the circumstances peculiar to each individual.

"Starting Again" is refreshing because of the awareness it evokes about non-neural tissues. There are other structures that may need treatment and the cause of some signs and symptoms may not be totally in the head. One unique aspect of this text is that it integrates the examination and treatment of abnormal mechanics in neural tissues. The clinical application of these concepts to head-injured patients is logical and clinically valid, highlighted by some excellent photographic examples. While the primary functions of the nervous system are encoding, relaying and decoding impulses, the nervous system must be free to glide and stretch during movement to allow this. This contribution to therapy is an example of the way Pat Davies' writing bridges the gap between orthopaedically and neurologically based physiotherapists. Another example is her suggestion to make the neck mobile and painfree, easing facial pain to enhance orofacial rehabilitation.

"Starting Again" is aimed at real everyday problem solving – ranging from less expensive options for shoe alterations to where to start initiating treatment on a maltreated patient who has lain supine for the majority of time post head injury. Readers should take time to observe the many clear photographs and note the handling of patients by the therapists. Skilled patient handling and positioning does not require great strength, numerous assistants and years of experience. It is a combination of preplanning, patient and therapist positioning, patience, a basic knowledge of underlying pathological processes, communication skills and a desire to help. You do not have to be a Pat Davies to perform the techniques, utilise her wealth of experience, explore her rationales. She rightly takes on the responsibility of arming all her readers with the information, understanding, handling and positioning skills which should be available to all those who have suffered head injury and those who care for them.

The real strength of the writing, photography and compilation that make up *"Starting Again"* is that it can be shared among all who are associated with those who suffer serious injury to their nervous system. This eloquent yet simple text cuts across medical boundaries, it enhances teamwork, it demystifies the effects of head injury, and it gives new hope for all.

Adelaide, 1994   DAVID BUTLER

Preface

It is a sad fact but true that every year, many thousands of young, active people sustain a severe head injury and a great number of others will have similar problems as a result of equally devastating nontraumatic brain lesions. Alone from head trauma, in the region of 150 000 patients are admitted to British hospitals each year (Jorinet 1976), while in the United States the figure is well over 400 000, an occurrence of approximately 200 cases per year per 100 000 population (Cope and Hall 1982). A significant proportion of these people who have had the misfortune to suffer acquired brain damage will need prolonged and intensive rehabilitation in order to have the chance to rebuild their shattered lives.

Unfortunately, the treatment which brain-damaged patients receive in the acute care stage and later when they no longer require intensive care is often far from ideal. Due to the course which my professional life has taken, I have been able to observe a vast number of patients in a great variety of hospitals and rehabilitation centres in different countries. I have also been privileged to treat many who came for help to overcome particular difficulties at different stages of their rehabilitation or been consulted to advise on vexing problems confronting individual patients and their therapists. Through my observations it has become clear that certain problems keep recurring and that the reasons for the difficulties are relatively homogeneous. The experience has shown me that there is an urgent need for change, not only in the actual treatment itself, but also in the way in which the patients as individuals are regarded.

In an age of enormous advances in other areas of medicine and health care, it would seem only fair that a more successful treatment concept should likewise be made available for victims of traumatic and other brain injuries. Not only is later rehabilitation seriously impeded by inadequate treatment in the primary stages, but failure to prevent secondary complications can lead to permanent loss of function. The additional suffering for the patient, the expense involved in overcoming avoidable complications and the increased length of the overall rehabilitation period make a new approach imperative. It should also be remembered that, no matter how good the treatment, premature culmination of therapy will mean that goals which would otherwise have been possible are never attained. With treatment, improvement in functions has been noted to continue for several years post trauma. (Scherzer 1988)

My determination to find an improved way of treating brain-injured patients started many years ago when I was primarily engaged in treating patients with spinal cord injuries in a paraplegic centre. Attached to the hospital was a chronic section where numbers of brain-damaged patients were hospitalized on a long-term or permanent basis and received a limited amount of physiotherapy as well. Looking down at the terribly distorted form of a young man who had sustained a brain injury in an accident involving fireworks, I could not but compare his hopeless, neglected condition to that of the patients in the spinal injuries unit who were receiving such intensive, informed and up-to-date care. My immediate thoughts were, "There just has to be a better way", but at the time I was powerless to help. Even in the literature there was no mention of how to overcome the problems or prevent them in the first place

Since then, unprecedented good fortune has allowed me to meet personally, work together with and learn from such well-known experts in the field of physiotherapy, rehabilitation, and related topics as Maggie Knott, Bertie Bobath, Sir Ludwig Gutmann, Dr Wilhelm Zinn, Geoff Maitland, Susanne Klein-Vogelbach, David Butler, Felicie Affolter, Kay Coombes, Margaret Rood, Susanne Naville, Trudy Schoop, Leo Gold and Samy Molcho. I should like to share what I have learned from them and from many others perhaps less known, who have in turn shared their knowledge and expertise with me. I have, therefore, written this book in the hope that it will be of help to all those involved in the treatment and care of brain-damaged patients.

Within the limitations inevitably imposed by the condensed form of a book, I have included what I consider to be essential treatment measures for all patients who have suffered a brain injury severe enough to cause loss of consciousness and the ability to function normally. I have also described how secondary complications can be overcome so that they no longer stand in the way of progress. Apart from the therapeutic activities and treatment concept presented in the book, during 30 years of working with neurologically impaired patients, I have come to realize that other factors make a world of difference to achieving a successful outcome. I should like to pass on some thoughts about these factors as well.

The enthusiasm of the staff caring for the patient is an important factor particularly if his progress is slow and working with him fraught with frustrating difficulties. Many years ago I came across the following quotation which inspired me then and still seems so appropriate today:

You can do anything if you have
enthusiasm. Enthusiasm is the yeast
that makes your hopes rise to the stars.
Enthusiasm is the sparkle in your eyes,
the swing in your gait, the grip of your
hand, the irresistible surge of will and
energy to execute your ideas.
Enthusiasts are fighters. They have
fortitude. They have staying qualities.
Enthusiasm is at the bottom of all
progress. With it, there is accomplishment.
Without it, there are only alibis.   *Henry Ford*

Indeed such "alibis" can often lead to the patient missing out on his treatment. It may be tempting to say that he was too tired to perform, too ill to be stood up with support or that we could not find someone to assist with lifting him out of bed when in fact we ourselves made too little effort for some reason or another.

A positive approach right from the start can contribute greatly to the success of the treatment. I find it helpful when I first start treating a patient to picture him walking out of the hospital unaided one day, well-dressed and waving goodbye with a smile, even if things look bleak during the early days following his admission. Should a patient not survive the initial trauma or sadly never regain consciousness, nothing will have been lost by the active intervention, but so much gained. All too often I am told that things went so wrong because everyone thought that the patient would not survive for long. Statistical studies concerning prognosis can also lead to negative attitudes, but statistics are not about individuals, and there have been many surprising exceptions. It has been wisely pointed out that the clinician's attitude may influence the recovery to the extent that cessation of recovery after 6 months, a widely held belief, may possibly in fact be the result of a self-fulfilling prophesy (Bach-y-Rita 1981).

The patient is a person not a "head injury" and should be treated with the same respect afforded him before the accident. He should on no account be regarded as a second-class citizen, as sometimes unfortunately happens with an adverse affect on the standard of rehabilitation he receives. He should be addressed by name in a way appropriate to his age and standing as he would have been before his injury and not be automatically called "Bill" or "Joe" by all and sundry. Care should be taken with the patient's appearance because it can help to preserve his dignity and encourage his family and the staff as well. If his hair is washed and brushed, his nails clean and trimmed, and if he is dressed in his own freshly laundered clothes instead of being left to lie or sit in a backless hospital nightdress, not only will the patient feel better but others will react to him differently too.

A team approach is essential for optimal management and it is important that all members of the team work together in harmony and are in agreement as to the type of treatment. Good communication within the team is, therefore, essential, and adequate in-service instruction required to make cooperation possible. "Preaching without the 'P'" (Gold 1990) is the key to sharing knowledge and teaching new methods without encountering resistance or resentment.

Brain damage is a family affair (Lezac 1988) and the patient's relatives must therefore become an integral part of the team, When the going is difficult for the staff, it is all too easy to blame our failures on the relatives for being difficult, meddlesome and interfering (Schmidbauer 1978). In fact, they are only deeply concerned and, if given adequate instruction and encouraged to help in more therapeutic ways, they can be invaluable supporters. It is of no use to send them out of the treatment area with the excuse that the patient works better if his wife or mother is not present, because in the end it is the close family who will be the carers when he is discharged from hospital. "Successful work with the brain-injured patient almost automatically includes successful work with the family (Johnson and Higgins 1987).

The right treatment really does make a difference, and it is irresponsible to suggest otherwise. It is most important for those who work with the patient to be convinced of this fact so that they are not disheartened by sceptical remarks and contradictory publications. Very few prognostic studies have mentioned the type of active therapy employed or included in the results that therapy had a positive effect on the results. However, in animal studies it has been convincingly shown that intensive therapy and stimulation made a big difference. The importance of physical therapy to avoid contractures that would mask spontaneous recovery in brain. damaged monkeys has been reported by Travis and Woolsey (1956) who were thus able to demonstrate considerable return of function following extensive neocortical damage. As a result of such therapy, a totally decorticated monkey learned to right itself, get to its feet unaided, sit, stand and walk alone. Rehabilitation studies undertaken with brain-injured rats have provided strong evidence that an enriched environment, comparable to a rehabilitation programme, promotes overall recovery of function (Schwartz 1964; Rosenzweig 1980). Even if the enriched conditions were only available for two hours a day, the effect proved to be equally positive (Rosenzweig et al. 1969). Many human studies close by suggesting that controlled trials are necessary before it can be shown that therapy makes any difference, but I believe that we cannot ethically withhold treatment until such time as experiments have been completed. Far too many control groups in the form of great numbers of untreated or inadequately treated patients already exist in many places. As Kesselring (1992) so rightly explains, though the effectiveness of rehabilitation, unlike other forms of therapy, cannot be evaluated in a double-blind study, the fact should not deter us from continuing in the field. "After all", he points out with some humour, "we would not deprive our children of the possibility of a school education just because it has never been proved in a double-blind study that it is of some use!"

In the end "the goal is the best possible for the patient and not who is right" (Gold 1990).

The book is intended to be of practical help to all members of the rehabilitation team, which includes the patient's relatives as well. It is his relatives who bear the responsibility of making many decisions concerning the future and who are required to give permission for any interventions and so it is most important for them to be well-informed. I have, therefore, tried to use language that can be easily comprehended and have included numerous illustrations of patients, both young and older, in different stages of rehabilitation, from the intensive care unit to learning to dress and climb stairs. To provide a theoretical, scientific background, I have, however, gone more deeply into some of the more complex problems associated with brain damage with references from up-to-date literature. It is my earnest wish that therapists, doctors and nurses will really be able to use the book as a practical guide for their clinical work and find it helpful when treating their patients.

In the text the therapist, nurse or assistant is referred to as "she" and the patient as "he" although in the figure captions the correct personal pronoun has been used.

Switzerland   PAT DAVIES

Acknowledgements

Many people have helped to make this book a reality, people from many different parts of the world. Some may not even have been aware that they were helping when, through a case history they told, an argument they presented or a discussion they look part in, a new idea took form or another treatment possibility was explored. Certainly all who have attended courses, lectures or seminars which I have given have played an important role, their interest and enthusiasm showing me that the information which is presented in the book was urgently needed. I thank all those people who wittingly or unwittingly stimulated me to develop my thoughts and put them into words. My special thanks go to all who have helped in more concrete ways and I beg forgiveness if I have forgotten to mention anyone by name.

Because it cannot be easy to live with someone who is writing a book, with papers scattered everywhere and little time for sharing the burden of household chores, first and foremost I should like to thank my friend and partner, Gisela Rolf, for her unstinting support during the production years. Even more important than the practical help in daily life were the stimulating discussions and exchanged ideas made possible by virtue of her expert knowledge and clinical expertise, the shared patients and her own therapeutic discoveries,

Words can never express my gratitude to Max Schuster nor my appreciation of his incredible achievement in setting up a facility where patients with severe brain damage could be given the chance of returning to a worthwhile life again. I thank him for inviting me to advise on the treatment concept for the centre and for providing a situation where the concept could be put into practice and proved workable before appearing in book form. Max is an inspiration to all because he made the words of the famous Nike advertisement, "Just do it" a reality.

My thanks go to Karen Nielsen in the Therapy Centre Burgau who gave so unstintingly of her time, energy and knowledge to assist me in producing the book. Not only did she provide the location for the photography, but she always found exactly the right patients to demonstrate each activity or problem, and with much personal effort ensured that everything ran smoothly and according to plan. I should also like to express my appreciation for the cooperation of all those members of the Burgau staff who helped so willingly. A special thanks to Dr Wolfgang Schlaegel who agreed to be photographed while performing PEG's and applying serial casting, and for his help with patients, X-rays and permission forms. Another centre which deserves special mention is the SUVA Rehabilitation Centre, Bellikon, where invaluable assistance was given to me. I am deeply indebted to Violette Meili who sought out such excellent patients for the photographs and convinced all to agree to being published for the sake of the book. Her efficient organisation greatly facilitated the whole proceedings, and many of the staff enthusiastically joined in to help as well. I am most grateful to Dr Christoph Heinz whose problem-solving tactics made a room available for the photography. Perhaps without his realising it, his kindness and his belief in my work have been a constant source of encouragement while writing the book. My thanks extend also to Dr Peter Zangger, who so readily agreed to his patients taking part.

A big thank-you goes to all the patients whose action pictures appear in the book and make it alive and real instead of a theoretical dissertation. I am most grateful to the relatives of those patients who were still not able to sign for themselves for granting me permission to use the photographs. A special word of thanks is due to three patients, Rien Buren, Dr Andreas Kasiske and Dr Fritz-Martin Mueller, who with such determination continued to work with me for some years and thus stimulated new ideas on how to adapt the treatment successfully during each stage of progression. The illustrations of patients in the primary acute phase were possible thanks to Professor Joachim Eckhart, who kindly allowed patients in his very modern and efficient intensive care unit to be photographed while being treated. I am also grateful for the time and trouble taken by his assistant Dr Neeser to ensure the success of the whole undertaking.

I thank Hans Sonderegger for all that I have been privileged to learn from him during our long association, especially during the many courses we taught together, for staying on to be photographed in action, and finally for agreeing to translate the book into German. I am particularly grateful to Dr Jürg Kesselring for contributing to my theoretical knowledge in the field, for stimulating new thoughts and searching out up-to-date literature for me. He has indeed been my "source of all knowledge", and I thank him for his enthusiastic support of my approach to the treatment of patients with brain damage and for agreeing to check the manuscript.

It has been a joy for me to work with my photographer, Rainer, who was a pillar of strength and patience during the long and often stressful hours. I thank him not only for his excellent professional achievements on my behalf but also for the great kindness and concern he showed towards the patients. I am also most grateful to his parents, Clara and Manfred Gierig, for the swift and efficient development of the photographs and for all their personal efforts to ensure the quality of the illustrations.

I very much appreciate the help of Inge Schnell, who gave up many hours of her limited and precious free time to assist with the photographing of patients. I thank her and the other Bobath instructors, Nora Kern, Lone Jorgensen, Karen Nielsen and Violette Meili, who agreed to demonstrate the treatment of patients for the illustrations.

Thank you, Jonathan and Jane Miall of the Arcade Bookshop in Chandler's Ford, England, for tracing and sending the many books I needed so promptly and efficiently. Their speedy arrival was a great help.

I feel a deep sense of gratitude to my publishers, Springer-Verlag, for the immense support and encouragement I have received with the production of this book and those preceding it. I thank Bernhard Lewerich for the many stimulating ideas, for sharing his wealth of experience with me and above all for agreeing to the many illustrations which I know will be a great help. I am most grateful to Marga Botsch for her personal and professional efforts on my behalf and for keeping in touch always, despite the long distances involved. I thank my copy editor, Alison Hepper, for her many excellent suggestions and for making the correction of the manuscript a pleasure instead of a burden. In addition, I should like to express my appreciation to Jaroslav Sydor, for producing the book with its numerous figures and to all other members of staff who have contributed towards its final appearance.

I am deeply indebted to the late Bertie and Karel Bobath who first opened my eyes to the possibility of changing muscle tone and facilitating normal movement instead of accepting and compensating for lost functions. Perhaps the greatest message that these two wonderful pioneers passed on to me was the need to keep searching for answers in order to develop their concept still further and not to stay complacently static. As Bertie explained in her last known publication, sent to me by Jos Halfens, the senior Bobath instructor in Holland, their concept was in a constant state of development and change throughout its history. In a survey of changes which the neurodevelopmental treatment underwent from the beginning in 1943, she describes how she and Karel, although never changing their basic concept, learned from and were influenced by the originators of many other methods as well as by observing their own mistakes. I will always be grateful to the Bobaths for their positive reaction to my earlier works and for their encouragement to continue teaching and developing their concept, which I have faithfully tried to do.

Thank you, David Butler, for teaching me how to mobilize the nervous system which has made such an amazing difference to the patients' movement possibilities, and for writing the Foreword for my book despite your many commitments.

Contents

1 Getting in Touch Again

Touch has been defined in *The Shorter Oxford English Dictionary* as being "That sense by which a material object is perceived by means of the contact with it of some part of the body, the most general of the bodily senses, diffused through all parts of the skin, but, (in man) specially developed in the tips of the fingers and the lips". Below the meanings, an illustrative quotation, dated 1599, includes poetic words of wisdom which emphasize the importance of the sense: "By touch the first pure qualities we learn Which quicken all things..."

Touch is indeed the most trustworthy of all the senses, unlike the others whose information can be deceptive at times, through illusory effects such as in the case of an optical illusion. For the nervous system to learn, mature and remain viable, the reception of tactile information is indispensable. The other sensory modalities are not essential for development but facilitate task performance and learning and certainly contribute greatly to life quality. The ability of the blind and deaf to lead independent lives, follow successful careers, participate in sport as well as achieve success as musicians and artists is clear evidence that visual and auditory information cannot be prerequisites for learning in general nor for acquiring motor skills, as is sometimes thought.

In the treatment of the brain-damaged patient the term "getting in touch" is, therefore, particularly significant and has a two-fold meaning. Firstly, the staff caring for the patient must make contact with him, whether in the isolation of his coma to establish a dialogue or later when he regains consciousness, to communicate with him more appropriately. Secondly, the patient will need to get in touch with his environment again so that an interaction can take place to make learning and adaptive behaviour possible once more.

Because the sense of touch is so diffuse and so intimately involved with function, it is invariably disturbed or distorted in some way by a brain lesion, with far-reaching effects. By the same token, however, its widespread distribution and relationship to activity can be utilized effectively in the treatment situation to ensure a meaningful input through appropriate stimulation.

Disturbances of Tactile Input

Perhaps because of the great number of sensory receptors in the skin, and underlying tissue, which provide such a variety of information, several different terms are used in clinical practice to describe the sense of "touch" with its wide range of sensations and all that it makes possible to differentiate between. The *tactile/kinaesthetic system* refers to touch and movement, respectively, information about the latter being supplied by muscles and their changing tension, joint positions and the stretching of underlying tissues. *Superficial sensation* usually refers to light touch, pin prick or two-point discrimination, while *deep sensation* describes the appreciation of pressure, with recognition and localization of vibration requiring a combination of the two. *Proprioception* is another term used for the appreciation of joint positions and movements. Regardless of the descriptive words, basically sensation has to do with the organism knowing where its body and limbs are in relation to one another and in space, that is, information provided through sources within the organism itself or information provided through direct contact with the environment, i.e. from sources outside the organism.

Assessing Sensation

Every patient who has suffered a brain lesion will "feel" differently from the way he did prior to the lesion, but in some cases the difference will be more marked than in others and the consequent problems more obvious. Slight changes in sensation will not be noticed in any of the standard tests presently in use, as Brodal (1973) points out with reference to personal observations made following his own stroke. In fact, because of the incredible complexity of human sensation, any attempt to test its complete integrity is virtually impossible or at best will only provide very limited information about specific qualities in a given situation and at a certain time. A patient who responds correctly as to where and when he is being touched, reacts to a painful stimulus and knows whether his great toe or his limb is being moved up or down cannot be judged as having intact sensation and the same applies to more refined forms of testing. All too often, a patient who has scored well in a test — for example, he may even have differentiated between a paperclip and a safety pin of the same size placed in his hand with visual feedback excluded — can then be observed leaving the room with the same hand caught in the spokes of his wheelchair without his noticing it. Nevertheless, while realising the limitations, it is advisable that one form of testing sensation be selected and repeated at intervals with the results recorded accurately, so that comparison becomes possible and improvement can be verified for statistical purposes.

For treatment purposes, the only way in which the therapist can gain insight into how the patient searches for and deals with tactile information is by observing him in many different real-life situations. Video recordings of his performances enable the members of the rehabilitation team to analyze his motor behaviour and coping strategies in more detail afterwards by replaying short sequences for closer observation. Listening to the patient describing what he experiences, his relatives relating things that have happened or the nurse reporting incidents on the ward can all add considerably to the therapist's knowledge and understanding of his sensory difficulties. Moore (1980) stresses the importance of listening to the patient and warns how vital information can be lost forever "if the reports offered by the patient concerning aberrant feelings or lack of functional abilities fail to correlate with the rehabilitationists' or researchers' perceptions of how things should be". Clinical interpretations of remaining functional capabilities may be "biased by what can be observed, palpated, or interpreted from multiple clinical tests coupled with the examiner's knowledge of the nervous system". As Moore explains, if the examiner has been trained to look at and mainly test the motor side of the nervous system, for example, then his mind will be preset to hear, feel and understand only that which he knows and he will have "a predilection for ignoring or dismissing that which is conflicting, strange or different".

Other Perceptual Disturbances

Many and varied disturbances of perception related to specific modalities have been recognized, described and given individual names, such as the apraxias, the agnosias, and visual and spatial neglect as well as a number of attention and memory-specific disorders. Distortion of body image and difficulties with spatial orientation have also received considerable attention. Concrete tests have been devised to evaluate the functions in normal as well as brain-damaged subjects, but a great deal still remains unresolved with regard to the organization of actual goal-directed movements. Referring to the contents of his comprehensive book on the subject, Jeannerod (1990) admits openly in the preface that "Many questions have been raised (very few are answered) concerning the motor mechanisms and their implementation in goal-directed actions".

Perhaps because it lends itself to testing in a laboratory situation more easily, considerable research has been undertaken to gain more knowledge about visual perception in particular. As a result, visual perception has been given a disproportionate emphasis, particularly with regard to motor learning, despite the obvious evidence that vision is not in fact essential for motor learning, namely, the normal motor development of nonsighted children and the ability of blind adults to acquire new motor skills. Dennet (1991) in his inimitable way, sums up the problem in a nutshell: "Vision is the sense modality that we human thinkers almost always single out as our major source of perceptual knowledge, though we readily resort to touch and hearing to confirm what our eyes have told us. This habit of ours of seeing everything in the mind through the metaphor of vision (a habit succumbed to twice in this very sentence) is a major source of distortion and confusion, as we shall see. Sight so dominates our intellectual practices that we have great difficulty in conceiving of an alternative".

In fact, the ability to use vision, to recognize things and their form, to judge distances and aim at targets is only possible because of the previous tactile/kinaesthetic experiences during development. "There is, to use an old phrase, a great deal more to vision than meets the eye", as Zekir (1992) so rightly says, after explaining that, in order to obtain its knowledge of what is visible, the brain cannot merely analyse the images presented to the retina but that "Interpretation is an inextricable part of sensation".

It can in fact be said that the sense of touch and movement is involved in some way and to a certain degree in all forms of perceptual processing regardless of the prime modality, whether in the development of the processes or to allow their optimal functioning. Even for the performance of relatively simple visual tasks such as target tracking, head movement and position are important and references from the position of the neck and trunk required (Jeannerod 1990). So important is the information provided by the cervical area, that a change in muscle tone and sensation on one side of the neck can seriously impede visual fixation. Vibration applied to the posterior neck muscles of normal subjects unilaterally caused an illusory displacement of a luminous target in a dark room. The subjects reported an apparent displacement of the fixation light usually in the horizontal dimension and to the opposite side to that of the vibratory stimulation, but by altering the location of the vibrator, illusions of vertical and diagonal movement could be produced (Biquer et al. 1986, 1988).

For the brain-damaged patient, disturbances of sensation, whether superficial, deep or proprioceptive, will therefore have profound consequences, and successful rehabilitation will require the implementation of specific treatment measures to enhance and improve tactile/kinaesthetic input. "He who would grasp must be able to feel" (Von Randow 1991) and functional use of the hand is indispensable for independence. Without feeling, not only grasping but many other skilled activities are impossible as well, such as those which entail letting something slip through the fingers in a controlled way. Von Randow quotes the example of a robot, so highly developed that it can play the organ and even sightread music with its video eyes, but which cannot turn the pages of the notes because that task is too difficult for its feelingless hands.

Problems Related to Disturbed Tactile/Kinaesthetic Input

Incongruous Behaviour and Movement

Clinical experience and observations have indicated that *any behaviour or movement which is bizarre* or is not in accordance with what is expected of a patient is the result of some perceptual disorder, and either directly or indirectly related to the tactile/kinaesthetic system.

It is not the degree of motor paralysis and his dependence upon others which makes the patient unpopular with members of staff and causes a disinclination to accept the burden of caring for him. A patient with a high cervical cord lesion who is artificially respirated and able only to move his face will have many willing helpers to feed, wash, lift or turn him in his total helplessness and the patient will be admired for his bravery and uncomplaining behaviour. In the case of the brain-damaged patient it is the presence of perceptual disorders that causes difficulties and the feeling of irritation, which leads to others being loath to treat or help him (F. Kraus, personal communication).

In fact, if staff are heard complaining that a patient is "difficult", is "lazy", "won't do anything for himself", "could do better if he tried" or that he expects his wife to do everything for him, that patient will invariably be found to have profound perceptual problems. The same applies to patients who appear to be unmotivated or who constantly need to use the toilet as if to escape their therapy sessions or who even become abusive or physically violent.

Once it is accepted that all these are nothing more than symptoms of the patient's lesion, as are the other more obvious signs of paralysis and spasticity, it is far easier for the therapist and other members of the team to cope. All that the patient is really saying is, "I can't, I can't", "I don't know how" or ultimately "I am so afraid". Although such an interpretation of aberrant behaviour may be accepted and understood in theory, it is frequently more difficult to apply in practice because of very normal reactions on the part of members of staff when they feel personally slighted or if it seems as if their professional ability is being questioned. In such a situation it is wise to remember the patient's lesion consciously and think out how the same task could be done differently in the future to avoid the patient's desperate reactions.

Spasticity

Spasticity, one of the commonest and most troublesome symptoms, can cause problems at all stages of the patient's rehabilitation. It makes active movement difficult and may precipitate the development of secondary complications such as contractures, pressure sores and heterotopic ossification if adequate therapeutic measures are not taken to minimize or inhibit hypertonus. Spasticity, with such variations in its development, degree and clinical manifestations is still not fully understood, but disturbance of both feedback and feedforward mechanisms are generally accepted as playing an important role. Abnormal sensation is frequently the underlying cause of the hypertonicity.

People with an intact nervous system will also exhibit hypertonus when for some reason they are unable to feel some part of their body and will often increase tension deliberately in their attempts to regain feeling or move the part into extreme positions. A common example is that of someonewho awakes from a deep sleep with an arm and hand completely devoid of sensation and makes strenuous efforts to revive the "dead" limb. Typically, the person makes a fist, tenses the whole arm and moves it vigorously up and down in the air through large ranges of movement. People whose leg has gone to sleep after sitting for a long time with crossed legs will stamp their foot on the floor, tense the leg muscles and bend and straighten their knee until sensation has returned. Even the localized loss of feeling in the lip following an injection at the dentist worries the victim, who will spend the next hour or so tensing his lips, pressing them against his teeth and moving them forcefully in all directions. If the patient cannot perceive his limbs or they feel strange, he will likewise press them hard against firm surfaces in the vicinity, move them restlessly or have markedly increased tone in the muscles.

People will also have increased tone in situations where sensory input is confusing and unfamiliar and the ground beneath their feet is no longer stable. Apart from the tension experienced during different "rides" at a local fairground and when learning to windsurf or ski, being a nervous passenger in an aircraft which encounters bad weather provides a clear example of such hypertonus. As the plane tilts, sways and drops down from time to time, clouds swirl past the windows and the engine changes pitch, the passenger presses his feet against the floor tensely, clutches the armrests and pushes back desperately against the backrest of the chair in the search for reliable information. The patient, too, will become more spastic in any situation where no absolute information is available to him or when the information he receives through the various sensory channels is conflicting and unfamiliar.

Preventing excessive increases in tone or reducing hypertonus can however, only be successful if additional contributory factors are taken into consideration as well and eliminated as far as possible. Human beings also demonstrate hypertonus under certain other circumstances and in similar situations, so too will the patient but in his case, because of his central nervous system lesion with loss of inhibition, the increase in tone will be more exaggerated and appear as spasticity in stereotyped patterns.

Additional Factors Contributing to Increased Tone

Acquiring a New Motor Skill

Normal Subject. When someone is learning a new motor activity which is difficult for him, he performs the required movements with far too much effort and his whole body tenses. For example, when learning to drive a car, everyone holds the steering wheel with a vice-like grip at first, and the actions of the foot on the accelerator, clutch or brake pedals are forceful and uncoordinated. In fact the learner's whole body is held rigidly, with even the neck muscles in a hypertonic state.

Patient. If the patient tries to perform an activity which is too difficult for him, tone will increase markedly. Gradual progression after preparation of the motor components together with the correct type and amount of support will avoid the problem. The occurrence of associated spastic reactions, therefore, inform the therapist or helper that either the activity needs to be changed or additional assistance given.

Loss of Balance or Fear of Falling

Normal Subject. When people lose their balance or are in danger of falling, muscle tone increases rapidly. Their body stiffens in extension, and their arms fly upwards and outwards as a result of the primitive "startle reaction" which has been described by K. Bobath (1974), although in adults the elbows tend to remain partially flexed. The reaction can be observed when someone slips on the ice and falls, for example, and, even if a person feels afraid while walking on a narrow board high above the ground, the same position is adopted.

Patient. Because humans have an innate fear of falling, the patient who is unable to maintain his balance will demonstrate increased spasticity in any upright position if he is not adequately supported. His trunk may extend but as a result of the fear, flexor hypertonus may be dominant and cause a flexed position of the arms and trunk. If the patient unfortunately falls at some stage, the fear and resulting hypertonus increase still further. With more appropriate support provided by the close proximity of pieces of furniture or the helper, tone is immediately reduced. As the patient learns to balance again through the retraining of balance reactions in physiotherapy, the spasticity becomes proportionately less. Until he is able to maintain his balance safely, the patient should never be left sitting or standing alone even briefly so that any danger of his falling is eliminated.

Pain or the Expectation of Pain

Normal Subject. When people hurt themselves, the immediate reaction is to clutch the painful part in their hand or against their body with an increase in flexor tone, for instance if a finger has been slammed in a car door or an elbow hits against a hard object. Flexion is also seen if someone has a headache or a stomach cramp. If a sharp pain is anticipated, tone rises quite dramatically, a common experience for many while the dentist is probing to locate a cavity in a sensitive tooth.

Patient. If pain is elicited by the therapist, doctor or nurse during assessment or treatment procedures, tone rises in the form of a protective spasm or a reflex withdrawal, which may well be the only avoiding behaviour possible for the patient. Once he has experienced a painful procedure, his tone will increase in expectation of the pain prior to each and every repetition of that procedure.

Recent research on the treatment of babies and young children in intensive care has revealed that a great number of painful procedures are carried out routinely without any form of pain relief being administered, and about 50% of patients showing an adverse response according to the nurses' notes (*The Independent*, 1993). The procedures which cause pain include puncturing the skin to put in and take out drains, inserting catheters etc. One baby alone underwent 159 interventions likely to have caused pain while in hospital for nearly a year. The professor of paediatrics who led the research explains the problem of babies and children under five not being able to express pain as adults or older children do by saying, "I want you to stop".

The comatose or barely conscious patient in intensive care is in the same dilemma as he too is unable able to protest verbally nor move actively to avoid the pain and following head trauma will be subjected to many other painful stimuli in addition, such as those routinely applied to test his level of consciousness in the widely used Glasgow Coma Scale (Teasdale and Jennet 1974). To check eye opening in response to pain, painful stimuli are applied to either the chest or limbs, while the patient's motor responses are judged almost exclusively by his reactions to painful stimuli generally applied to the nail bed, or movements which he makes in an attempt to escape them. Some responses are differentiated by noting whether the withdrawals from the painful stimulus take place in a stereotyped mass pattern of flexion rather than in one of total extension. Not only is tone therefore liable to be increased at regular intervals by pain or the expectation of pain but, in more severe cases, spasticity is repeatedly being elicited and thus reinforced. The same can be said of the "generalized responses" to painful stimuli included in part of the Rancho Los Amigos Scale (Hagen et al. 1972).

If a progressive increase in hypertonus is to be prevented, it is obvious that noxious or unpleasant stimuli must be avoided as far as is feasibly possible within the framework of medical care, and certainly not included in the assessments carried out by therapists in the way recommended by Giles and Clark-Wilson (1993), which would surely be counterproductive: "When the patient is not responsive to auditory and non-noxious tactile stimulation, the therapist could then elicit motor responses via more intense tactile stimulation. Each extremity may be tested to determine the patient's ability to localize noxious stimuli. Noxious stimuli could include supraorbital pressure, pressure to the nailbed (administered with the eraser end of a pencil), sternal rub or pin prick". Such testing will provide no useful, new information, since it will have already been carried out and recorded by medical staff, but instead it will tend to increase spasticity and be yet another unpleasant experience for the patient. Furthermore, should he be in a condition to recognize the therapist administering the tests, he may understandably be less willing to cooperate with her in future therapy sessions. Because pain causes increased tone, great care must be taken during passive mobilization and positioning to avoid hurting the patient and any use of force or stretching techniques are contraindicated.

Adverse Mechanical Tension in the Nervous System

Normal Subject. The nervous system as a whole has the property of adaptive lengthening to allow the unimpeded conduction of impulses in all postures and during every possible movement or combination of movements (Butler 1991). Following any injury to neural structures, adverse tension within the system develops which limits full mobility and interferes with adaptive lengthening in various parts of the body, not only at the injury site but anywhere within the continuum of closely linked nerves and surrounding tissue. A predisposing factor appears to make some people more prone to increased adverse tension. The patterns of limitation of movement closely resemble those caused by increased tension or hypertonus in muscles.

Patient. The patient with brain damage is particularly susceptible to a marked increase of adverse tension in the nervous system, such tension being further aggravated by the immobility or reduced mobility which usually follows the accident or illness. With the neural structures under tension the patient's limbs and trunk are pulled into and held in postures closely resembling those attributable to spasticity, and active movements against the resistance of unyielding nerves are performed in patterns similar to those of the total mass synergies generally associated with hypertonus. The adverse tension not only causes loss of range of motion but appears to increase tone in the musculature as well. Mobilization of the nervous system is therefore an integral part of the treatment to prevent or reduce hypertonus and should be included from the start in the ways described in Chaps. 3 and 4.

A Sudden Loud Noise or a Loud, Imperative Voice

Normal Subject. The sudden slamming of a door will make anybody in the vicinity jump with a quick surge of extensor tone and the same occurs with any unexpected crash or bang, whether from a firecracker going off, a gun being fired or a porcelain vase crashing to the floor. A person, suddenly addressed in a loud imperative voice will start, with increased tone causing his body to stiffen involuntarily. A loud command is also followed by a tense reaction, such as when the sergeant-major calls the troops to attention. Knott and Voss (1968) actually used the effect of strong, sharp commands in treatment to simulate a stress situation as a way of stimulating the patient maximally and increasing the demand for effort.

Patient. Care must be taken that the patient is not startled by sudden noises or people banging against his bed as both are likely to elicit a spastic reaction. The staff, for the same reason should never shout in order to attract his attention should he fail to acknowledge other stimuli, nor should they speak loudly when encouraging him to try harder to perform some activity. A normal speaking voice should be used when addressing him, and in fact lowering the voice in a soothing manner can even help to reduce tone.

Long Verbal Instructions or Explanations

Normal Subject. If a traveller asks the way in a strange city he becomes confused and agitated with a resultant increase in tone if the person giving directions uses long sentences without pausing to draw breath before describing the next landmark. The new owner of a complicated video recorder also suffers from raised tone if the technician gives long explanations as to how different programmes can be preset to record at various times without allowing time for notes to be taken.

Patient. Therapists and nurses tend to give the patient a long verbal explanation before some procedure or activity is carried out, and he is often unable to follow what may seem to be simple instructions. Instead tone rises in anticipation of effort or because he is not sure what is expected of him or what is about to happen. The verbal explanations are frequently not required at all and can be omitted in favour of performing the action manually with the patient or should be broken down into separate short instructions which apply only to the very next step of the movement or procedure.

Trying To Do Something in a Hurry

Normal Subject. Under pressure of time, trying to perform a task in haste, the performer becomes tense and his movements less skilful, particularly when another person is urging him to hurry for fear of being late for an appointment or missing the train. Searching desperately for the car or house keys his arms may be seen to flex as tone increases.

Patient. The patient is often expected to hurry to fit in with the hospital routine or to be on time for his various therapy appointments. He must be dressed and shaved for the doctor's round, he must eat his breakfast quickly to be in time for physiotherapy and the toilet visit is often a disaster because the nurse is looking at her watch and repeatedly enquiring as to whether he has finished yet.All of these things serve to increase tone in a rehabilitation setting which is designed to improve active movement and independence. Careful organization of the patient's programme and cooperation between the various members of staff can eliminate the need for rushing and thus reduce spasticity considerably.

Emotional States

Normal Subject. Strong emotions whether pleasant or unpleasant, tend to increase tone, as implied by commonly used phrases such as "jumping for joy", "in fits of laughter" "worried stiff", "convulsed with sobs" or "cringing with fear" and many others. Rage and frustration are very much associated with raised tone so that someone may be seen shaking his fist tensely, hitting the table far harder than intended or kicking at a machine that refuses to work with such force that he injures his foot.

Patient. With both motor and sensory difficulties to contend with, the patient can easily become frustrated when even the simplest of tasks requires so much time and energy and can easily go wrong. He should, therefore, not be left on his own to struggle unsuccessfully with activities of daily living in the hopes that he may learn by his mistakes. He will only become increasingly spastic, and all that he will learn from the experience is that he is doing something wrong, but not how to correct his performance. Fear of falling should be reduced by sufficient support at all times and falling out of bed avoided by the continued use of cot sides until all danger is past, bearing in mind that many patients will still be disorientated at night although seemingly safe during the day.

Unfortunately, if the patient laughs heartily, particularly if he does so on an intake of breath as many do at first, marked hypertonus throughout his body is often the result. The staff and his relatives may be so happy to hear him laughing that they repeat the same joke over and over or re-enact the funny event to make him laugh again. Great care must be taken to keep the patient's laughter within bounds as an appropriate response to genuine humour and spontaneous happenings and not by those around him creating artificial situations, tickling him or making fun of his mistakes.

Constant worry about constipation or possible incontinence can be an unrecognized cause of increased tone and the two problems must be dealt with through appropriate therapeutic management to alleviate the patient's concern (see "*Faecal incontinence and/or constipation*", this chapter).

Meeting People and Establishing Contact

Normal Subject. When meeting someone for the first time many people feel rather stiff when approaching and shaking hands, particularly if the occasion involves consequences which could be significant. A visit to a new doctor, an interview for an important job, the first music lesson with a famous teacher will all be accompanied by increased tone. Just as the first day at a new school during childhood evoked hypertonus so a therapist attending a postgraduate course will feel tense as she enters the room, is introduced to the instructor, sums up the other participants and searches for a vacant seat. With time, the feeling of belonging to the group allows the newcomer to relax, a process which in both cases occurs far more quickly during shared or concerted activity, the child playing with the others during break and the therapist practising manual techniques with the other students.

Patient. In the early stages, the patient is in the hands of a constant stream of professionals, each of whom is a stranger to him, from the changing nursing staff, the various medical specialists, the laboratory and respiratory technicians to the therapists and on-call therapists, each of whom has duties to perform which require touching him in some way. It is easy to understand how the summation leads to an ever-increasing degree of hypertonus. Whenever possible without affecting optimal total care, the patient should have a nurse, doctor and therapist who remain constant, and the number of other staff who handle him should be reduced. As has already been stated with regard to repeated testing for level of consciousness by different professionals using painful stimuli there is considerable overlap and redundancy in other routine procedures as well, many of which are liable to elicit spasticity. A typical example is the number of times each and every doctor who examines the patient tests for a positive Babinski sign. although the result of thus scratching the sole of his foot has already been clearly recorded. Flexor spasticity in the lower limb is continually reinforced because, "if hypertonicity of a spastic nature is present there will be dorsi-flexion of the whole foot accompanied by flexion of the knee and hip" (Atkinson 1986).

Once the patient no longer requires intensive care, it is advisable for him to be treated daily by the same therapists for a period to avoid the frequent meetings and adaptations to new people and the necessity for repeated assessments. Hypertonicity will be less of a problem and the therapist will be in the position to know which activities best normalize tone and facilitate movement for that particular patient. It is, however, most important for therapists to change at intervals to avoid the danger of possessiveness and routinization of treatment procedures as well as for the beneficial effects of another therapist taking a fresh look at the patient's difficulties and introducing other treatment strategies.

Unfamiliar Situations and Strange Apparatus

Normal Subject. It may be remembered that the nervous passenger became hypertonic in the aircraft when stormy weather was encountered, but the flight steward will almost certainly have remained calm and relaxed because it was a familiar situation for him. Anything which is strange and unaccountable will tend to cause a feeling of uneasiness accompanied by an increase in tone. For instance, having been invited to spend the evening with new friends, a person arrives at the strange house and finds all in darkness and no-one there although the door is ajar. Pressing the light switches fails to turn on any lights. When paying an educational visit to a coal mine, someone descends a mine-shaft in a fast lift which rattles and shakes and the sense of unease heightens while traversing the dank tunnels and listening to the earth rumbling.

Strange or unfamiliar apparatus will also have the effect of increasing tone, not only in situations where it will be used on a person's own body, such as during cobalt therapy, but also when a person is attempting to use a complicated newly acquired gadget or machine. Attempting to cook a conventional dinner in an unfamiliar modern electronic oven can be a nerve-wracking experience.

Patient. Hospitals in general and the intensive care unit in particular are not only an unfamiliar experience for most patients but both contain a great variety of strange and rather daunting apparatus. To be totally helpless, lie naked in front of strangers and be submitted to procedures, both uncomfortable and bewildering, would be sufficient to increase tone without the strange sight, noise and magnitude of the machinery of modern medical technology in addition. The therapist introduces something more familiar in the form of movement, and the more she incorporates real-life tasks in her treatment, the better she will be able to reduce hypertonus and encourage the return of active movement. Even in the restricted setting of intensive care, goal-orientated activities involving well-known objects will stimulate awareness without increasing tone and help the patient to understand what is expected of him. For the same reason, the therapist should move the patient in the way he would previously have moved on his own to allow him to experience and relearn the normal movement patterns which are so familiar to him. Special methods of moving may lighten the load on the staff, but can be confusing for the patient who may resist the imposed change or restriction strongly or exhibit increased hypertonus. If a tilt table is used to bring the patient into a standing position, for example, his feet will often plantarflex so strongly that it is impossible to bring his heels down on the supporting surface. It is a very strange feeling to come directly from supine lying to upright standing without any forward inclination of the trunk, as therapists who tried it out for themselves reported, and all of them observed how their toes flexed strongly when the table was brought rapidly up to a vertical position.

Ataxia or Tremor

Ataxia is closely associated with inadequate afferent feedback and also with hypotonia. "Hypotonia and ataxia are so closely allied that they may be considered together", according to Atkinson (1986) who in addition to the abnormal postural tone emphasizes the problem of inadequate feedback. "Even less appreciated is the importance of afferent information. If there is no appreciation of the position in space the necessary steps to alter it cannot be undertaken. Moreover, if inadequate information is forthcoming during the performance it can be nothing but crude and wide of the mark since no corrective measures can be taken". Although it has been suggested that vision can be used to compensate for the loss of feeling, it can only be for gross or single joint movements which do not require fine control. With regard to hand function, Jeannerod (1990) found position sense to be an "essential aspect of visually goal-directed actions" and that "the visual signals relating to the shape of the object to be grasped could not be used to correct motor commands for the fingers". It has wisely been pointed out that, although normally visual and kinaesthetic sensations collaborate for movement control, visual cues cannot substitute for kinaesthetic cues, "simply because we never have looked at the movements of our fingers....but always at the result we are accomplishing. Consequently we have no association between the visual sensation of the moving fingers and the proper impulse to set the muscles into coordinated action" (Woodworth 1899).

Molcho (1983) explains how normally when someone reaches for an object, such as a glass, an electronic camera recording each phase of the movement reveals that the hand continually corrects its course by making small, adjusting movements along the way until the glass is actually grasped. The author describes the adjustments as being due to visual information which tells the subject that his hand must move more to the left or right to reach the goal, indicating that visual correction only takes place after the incorrect movement has been observed. Another interpretation of the deviating movements along the way is that they provide information by changing the amount of tension or stretch placed on the structures. The patient with impaired tactile/kinaesthetic sensation will make the far larger and more obvious corrections described by the term ataxia or tremor, because with hypotonia and decreased sensation the signals provided by smaller movements would not be appreciated. When a patient attempts to use visual information to guide a movement, the delay in correction can be observed because he will have difficulty in changing direction quickly and so will overshoot the target and then return towards it, maybe even requiring several motions back and forth of gradually decreasing range. For example when trying to place his foot on a step or on to the footrest of his wheelchair, he will lift it far too high in the air, see the error and then lower it again until eventually attaining the correct height. Tensing the whole body is another way in which patients will attempt to increase tone, or by fixing different parts such as elevating their shoulder girdle strongly. Others may press down hard against a surface or grasp a nearby fixture tightly while trying to move in a more controlled manner.

With some forms of tactile disturbance, it can be observed that the patient lifts his fingers off a hard surface and they are held in extremely extended positions to the extent of being bent backwards. The same patient may also lift his feet off the floor when sitting or away from the bed when lying on his back. It is as if he were trying to avoid a contact which is unpleasant or most disturbing and using the end position of his phalangeal joints for increased information. He will usually exhibit ataxic or athetoid type movements as well because the limbs in motion can be more clearly perceived than when they are held still in the air.

Activities Performed Slowly and with Undue Effort

Whereas normally tasks are performed with the minimum of effort required and at the most economic speed possible, the patient who cannot feel adequately will often move slowly and deliberately, with far too much effort for the task involved.. He will lift any object, for instance a gymnastic ball, as if it weighed a ton and can frequently be observed pressing his hands or feet down hard against any available surface even when a task is comparatively simple. Putting on his clothes may take an hour and cause him to perspire with effort, while meal times become a concentrated, marathon event. The effects are clearly noticeable when the patient speaks, as his speech is slow and associated tension can be observed in many other parts of his body. Disturbances in sensation are particularly significant during eating and speaking because of the quick, coordinated movements inherent in both, the necessity for tactile feedback and the impossibility of any form of sensory substitution.

Dizziness and Nausea

The capability of controlling posture and motion in relation to the surroundings is achieved by reflex and voluntary control systems, the responses of which are based on sensory information received from the vestibular end organs, visual afferents and somatosensory perception, the three sensory systems being the basis of the balance system (Pfaltz 1987). Conflicting sensory information resulting from damage to these systems due to injury or disease can cause symptoms of dizziness, nausea, vomiting and perspiration, similar to those of motion sickness, which is also believed to be the result of a "neural mismatch" (Reason 1978). "However, it has to be emphasized that the conflict is not just between signals from the vestibular apparatus, the eyes, and other receptors stimulated by forces acting on the body, but that these signals are also at variance with those which the central nervous system *expects* to receive" (Benson 1984). Such symptoms are usually far less marked when a patient is performing a task in a confined space than when he is standing or walking in free space.

Persistent Incontinence

To be continent is a learned ability of such complexity that it takes the normal child about 5 years of constant instruction and encouragement to master completely. It is not surprising, therefore, that the patient with perceptual problems will likewise have considerable difficulty in managing independently all that continence implies both physically and cognitively. Not only must he plan in advance, wait for a suitable time, find the right place, manage his clothing, contract and inhibit muscles in perfect sequences, but will often have an additional problem to solve because he requires the help of another person. Getting dressed is a task of approximately the same degree of complexity, so that from a perceptual point of view it would be unusual to find a patient able to dress himself without any help at all from start to finish but still incontinent.

Memory Disorders

Loss of memory or an inability to retain newly learned information is common and can pose great difficulties for the patient in rehabilitation where he is required to learn or relearn how to perform tasks in a certain way to enable him to function optimally during and after treatment in hospital or rehabilitation centres. Not being able to remember is very demoralizing for the patient who will often become frustrated and even aggressive if confronted with having forgotten, while others will cover up the fact by constantly telling jokes, making witty remarks or inventing unlikely reasons for their failure. Because memory problems are so diverse and often related only to specific subject matter, they are difficult to understand, and it is still not certain how storage of information takes place or how the stored information can be recalled for utilization at a later stage. It has long been known that memory and learning are not localized to specific regions of the brain but that the properties responsible for both are widely dispersed throughout many areas (Franz 1902). As even Giles and Clark-Wilson (1993) concede, "Given the frequently diffuse nature of traumatic brain injury following trauma, it is not surprising that a particular individual's memory deficits are not perfectly predictable from the type of injury or location of brain damage".

What is frequently baffling and incomprehensible for the staff and relatives is the patient's ability to remember certain facts well, such as names, telephone numbers and seemingly unimportant incidents, while not recalling that he made a pizza or rode a horse for the first time the previous day. The diversity is easier to understand and influence by treatment when the findings of Damasio (1992) are taken into consideration, namely that "What counts is how the brain acquires the knowledge. The brain lays down knowledge in the very same systems that are engaged with the interactions". As an example, the memory of a kitchen spatula is cited where the memory resides in that part of the cortex that originally processed how the spatula felt and how the hands moved it, thus activating the areas governing movement and touch.

The patient who is unable to move, manipulate objects and/or feel them adequately will have difficulty in recalling events which required tactile/kinaesthetic experience, while those which were perceived visually or auditively can be remembered. Improvement in memory will, therefore, not be achieved through practice in remembering visually presented facts or things that he hears but by being helped to search for and receive more tactile/kinaesthetic information. "Together with the internal representation of the goal and the motor program that initiates the neural commands to the muscles, position sense will be shown to be part of a complex proactive rather than retroactive mechanism, which acts not only in the short term for steering movements, but also in the longer term in processes like motor learning and motor memory" (Jeannerod 1990).

Behavioural Problems

Of all the problems resulting from brain damage, those affecting the patient's social behaviour would appear from the literature to be the most disturbing and upsetting for his family and for the rehabilitation team as a whole. Despite their efforts to help him, the patient refuses to cooperate, screams or hurls abuse at them, attacks them physically by biting, hitting or pulling their hair or throwing things in their direction. Inappropriate sexual advances are an embarrassment as are any vulgar or obscene remarks coming from someone who would never have uttered them previously. The patient's refusal to carry out activities of daily living which he would be capable of doing physically is hard to accept if the underlying perceptual disorders are not understood. In dealing with such problems, all too often, despite affirmation to the contrary, human behaviour is seen as a "thing on its own" and the environment as an abstract geometrical zone with the behaviour of both in a sort of juxtaposition but with no direct influence on one another (Kesselring 1993). The author goes on to explain that man and his environment are, however, an integrated, stereodynamic system of information exchange so that behaviour can really only be understood if considered as an interaction between organism and environment. Unfortunately, the important role played by the environment is often forgotten when behaviour modification programmes are used to improve the patient's compliance and behaviour, with the result that he learns only what pleases or displeases the staff with a resultant reward or punishment, but without the actual cause for his undesirable behaviour being discovered and remedied. The circumstances which caused the outbreak of unwanted behaviour should always be considered and changed rather than an attempt being made to modify the patient's behaviour after the event. The patient's "good" behaviour may make life easier for those responsible for his treatment in an in-patient setting, but unless the underlying problems are recognized and dealt with, he will not be able to cope with the ever-changing and complex demands inherent in life outside the sheltered confines of the hospital or rehabilitation centre. Jacobs (1988) offers profound advice which should be carefully and honestly considered before any system involving punishment and reward is introduced: "Programmes and procedures must always be for the benefit of the client and not the convenience of the programme. It is always necessary to consider whether it is the client's behaviour or the programme's procedures that need modification. In many cases ambiguities or problems in the overall rehabilitation programme may be responsible for the noted aberrations on the part of the client. In such situations intervention must focus on programme modification rather than modification of the client's behaviour to conform to a substandard programme".

The patient's inappropriate behaviour is almost invariably the result of his perceptual disturbances which make him afraid, anxious and confused. Bannister (1974) describes such a state as being "perhaps the most disturbing and disorganizing experience that man can undergo" because to live in an inexplicable world is frightening enough, but to be inexplicable to oneself is even more frightening. Understandably, therefore, the patient will often react violently, much as a drowning man in his panic may attack his rescuer. In the expressive words of Grosswasser and Stern (1989), "The patient is physically, emotionally and cognitively dislocated. The only response to this situation could be that of extreme overt aggression brought on by anxiety".

The reactions of the staff to the failures caused by his perceptual difficulties will also influence his behaviour adversely. He may for example hear the word "no" countless times a day in response to everything he does or be aware of nonverbal signals such as sighs, eyes being rolled heavenwards or surreptitious glances exchanged between members of staff. When the treatment is appropriate and the patient experiences success instead of repeated failure his behaviour will improve alongside of his other abilities. (See Chap. 7 "A case in point").

Inattention or Shortened Attention Span

Two important facts need to be taken into account before the patient's apparent loss of the ability to attend can be realistically evaluated. The first is that there is no single "centre" in the brain responsible for attention nor, in the words of Wall (1987) referring to pain and its mechanisms, should it be "considered as a separate special system bolted onto the outside of the real brain" but should rather "be integrated into sensation and perception in general". Secondly, normal attention is dependent upon several factors, an important one being the activity or material which is supposed to be attended to and the conducive state of the environment at the time. People gathered at a political meeting will soon begin to talk and laugh amongst themselves if the speaker continues to utter meaningless platitudes which they have heard repeated innumerable times before. Likewise a group of housewives will not attend for long during a scientific lecture on the construction of a new type of double-sided, high-density microdisk for business computers, but will start to scribble down notes about what still has to be done that day.

In the first case, the audience was bored because the subject matter was already too familiar and nothing new was being learned, and in the second instance, the group was overloaded by information way above their level of knowledge. The same applies to motor activities where a child or adult will soon "give up" if the task is way beyond their capabilities and success out of reach. The ability to attend is seriously compromised if the surroundings are not conducive to attending. For instance, someone continuously talking to her neighbour during the microdisk lecture would shorten the attention span of the person in front of her still further, and loud extraneous noises make concentrating on a complicated task very difficult. Most people have suffered the effects of hot weather or pain when trying to attend, or experienced the frustration of being interrupted while writing an important letter by a friend asking what they would like for supper.

It is interesting to note that normal subjects are frequently unable to remember their own telephone numbers or other familiar information when striving to maintain balance in extremely unstable conditions in experimental situations. A patient will attend for longer periods if the task is meaningful for him and success is a possibility. It should be remembered that he will usually have many additional matters to contend with at the same time, such as maintaining the upright position, not falling over and using an impaired limb with sensory loss.

Luria (1978) makes the distinction between "elementary, involuntary forms of attention" and the "higher, voluntary forms of attention" and the distinction makes it easier to understand some of the deficits commonly exhibited by patients. Involuntary attention stimulated by a sight or sound can be observed at a very early stage of normal development such as a baby within the first months turning its eyes and head towards a visual or auditory stimulus with a cessation of other irrelevant forms of activity. It is not until about 5 years of age, however, that the child is easily able to eliminate the influence of all irrelevant, distracting factors, although signs of instability of higher forms of attention evoked by a spoken instruction may still continue to appear for a considerably longer time. Luria found that higher, voluntary attention, as demonstrated by physiological changes which formed gradually, only appeared in a precise and stable form at the age of 12–15 years. He postulates that in fact, "unlike the elementary orienting reactions, voluntary attention is not biological in its origin, but a social act, and that it can be interpreted as the introduction of factors which are the product, not of the biological maturing of the organism, but of forms of activity created in the child during his relations with adults, into the organization of this complex regulation of selective mental activity".

A learned ability or behaviour so complex that it requires years to become stable, will surely be one that is markedly affected by disorders of sensation as are many other social or adaptive behaviours. Whereas normally a student will continue to attend despite the shortcomings of the teacher and the unsuitability of the tasks required of him, suppressing both his irritation and frustration to remain socially acceptable within the group, the patient will not have the same inhibition and will be easily distracted by other stimuli and no longer attend to the task in hand.

Attention does not, as has been suggested, require effort if the subject is fascinating for the student and he is learning at the correct level for his individual ability which means that what is presented or that which he is required to do is neither too easy or already known to him nor so difficult that comprehension and execution are impossible.

Lack of Motivation

As is the case with attention, lack of motivation is not caused by damage to some hypothetical centre in the brain as is sometimes supposed. Motivation is very much a by-product of the patient's environment and the way in which he is helped to achieve realistic goals. Motivation is directly related to that amount of effort required to achieve an aim, being in proportion to the reward or satisfaction which achieving the aim would bring. A few examples may help to illustrate the point. On a very hot day someone longs for an ice cream but the nearest supply is 5 km away and no form of transport is available. Because it would not seem worth walking all that way in the hot sun just for the ice cream the person lies down in the shade and does without it. Another person dearly wishes to learn windsurfing, but after falling into the water countless times, having to climb back on to the board and pull the heavy sail up again each time, the would-be surfer becomes less and less motivated until finally deciding after a week of such frustrating attempts to lie on the beach and read instead.

For the same reasons a patient with severely disturbed tactile/kinaesthetic perception may be unwilling to dress himself if it takes him an hour to do so instead of the normal five minutes and will either stay in his pyjamas or demand that a nurse or relative put on his clothes for him. Likewise, a patient with sensory problems who can only walk very slowly with great effort will continue to use a wheelchair for moving around and could be accused of not being motivated to walk.

People basically have an intrinsic desire to learn and to cooperate with others in their group, a characteristic that does not suddenly disappear as the result of a disabling condition but which can be suppressed by continued lack of success with eventual resignation. By changing the environment, in this case the treatment approach, to enable the patient to learn through successful accomplishment, any apparent lack of motivation will soon disappear.

Enhancing Learning in the Treatment Programme

The main aim of any treatment programme is to enable the patient to learn optimally, which automatically includes his physical well-being. Providing adequate nourishment, maintenance of full range of movement, the avoidance and alleviation of pain as well as the stimulation of motor activity are, therefore, most important areas in the overall management of the patient. Treatment measures to ensure the achievement of these goals are described in the chapters which follow, but specific therapy to facilitate learning will need to be incorporated if the outcome of rehabilitation is to be truly successful.

In order to provide the patient with enhanced learning opportunities, it is important to understand how people normally learn both during the course of development and later in adult life, not only because the patient will have to regain lost functions previously acquired during his early development but also because a close link appears to exist between the two types of learning. It has been found that "recovery following brain injury can be a long tedious process somewhat resembling our own growth, development and maturation" (Moore 1980), and more recently still, that one of the reasons for a new interest in learning and memory is "the evidence accumulating to suggest that mechanisms involved in the structural change in the nervous system that accompanies *learning* may strongly resemble certain steps in the nervous system's *development*. In other words, the sort of adjustments among synapses that account for learning may be the same as the 'fine-tuning' that occurs while the maturing system is assuming its unique elaborate form" (Ackerman 1992). Explaining how the human being, known to be the most helpless of living creatures at birth, is capable of such complex performances as an adult, Affolter and Stricker (1980) state that "acquisition, learning, development — these processes appear to evolve as a result of continuous interaction between environment and the individual", and emphasizes that such interaction requires contact, a word which means literally "to be in touch with", and which can be realized only through the tactile/kinaesthetic system.

Many complex factors and influences are involved in learning but primarily "the nervous system learns by doing", as Moore explains, adding that although learning by observation is possible "this has never been as effective as learning actively. The organism needs to 'get into the act' so to speak, and go through the process of an activity before permanent memory engrams are laid down:" It would be impossible for example, to learn to swim, to drive a car or to play tennis merely by looking at others, or for that matter by listening to verbal instructions. Vision does not seem to be an essential modality for learning, as has often been supposed. Damasio and Damasio (1992) believe that "there are no permanently held 'pictorial' representations of objects or persons as was traditionally thought. Instead the brain holds, in effect, a record of the neural activity that takes place in the sensory and motor cortices during interaction with a given object. The records are patterns of synaptic connections that can recreate the separate sets of activities that define an object or event; each record can also stimulate related ones", and that "the brain does not merely represent aspects of external reality; it also records how the body explores the world and reacts to it". As can be observed during the course of development, a child learns by touching, clasping and moving objects and later, "by changing relationships involving objects in their surroundings, their own bodies, and the mutual support, children begin to gain insight into the causes and effects which occur while they are interacting with the surrounding world" (Affolter 1991). Motor learning in both children and adults could well be seen as the result of an increase in knowledge about the environment or the conditions in which movement takes place, with motor representation being conceived as consisting of "units of knowledge" of interactions between the subject and the environment in "perceptual and motor schemas" (Arbib 1981).

Learning also requires repetition, and to learn a skill the process needs to be repeated over and over again but, as in the case of the child during its development, not repeated in exactly the same way, but always differently and in a variety of situations. Endless repetition would not only be too boring but the acquired skill would merely be a habit and not have the necessary adaptability required for functional use. "The nervous system adapts and habituates to that which is too repetitive or consistent. It begins to ignore or inhibit stimuli, especially when it is constant, aberrant or meaningless" (Moore 1980). Kesselring (1993), referring to the treatment of brain-damaged patients, describes the phenomenon as "input habituation whereby the stereotyped repetition of perceptual patterns with little variation suppresses and extinguishes attention".

In addition Moore presents two important considerations for treatment: "In order for learning to occur in the nervous system, that which is learned must have some meaning or degree of importance to the organism that is doing the learning" and "it is of little value to have a patient flex and extend or rotate an isolated part of an extremity over and over again in an attempt to regain function, because the nervous system is not organized in this manner". For learning to be facilitated, tasks must include a goal or an aim which can be clearly identified by the patient in his present condition which is equally important even in the early treatment because "apparently even the most elementary motor processes can be influenced (or penetrated) by specific cognitive states such as expectation, goal, or knowledge of the result" (Jeannerod 1990). The type of goal-orientated task selected at any stage of treatment is also important with regard to preventing spasticity and facilitating movement. Electromyographic (EMG) studies have shown bursts of antagonist activity with changes in amplitude and timing related to different voluntary movements, the task itself and the way in which the task is presented leading to the conclusion that the occurrence of the burst of antagonist activity is not part of an invariable motor subroutine, but depends on the task to be achieved (Meinck et al. 1984).

Lastly, real-life tasks must be chosen which by definition involve problem-solving to a greater or lesser degree of complexity. Normally, a person's day from the time of waking until going to sleep again at night is a constant stream of decision-making and problem-solving so that it would not be equitable with rehabilitation to try to eliminate problems from the patient's life because they are an indisputable part of living in reality.

Choice of Therapeutic Intervention

If all the above factors related to learning are taken into consideration and regarded as criteria, it is clear that no therapy based on reflex responses can help the brain-damaged patient to learn or relearn to function adequately and independently, because none of the criteria for learning are fulfilled. During normal development, even the reflexes of very young babies show accommodation and hence learning as they become increasingly organized and goal-directed, for example in the development of sucking from reflex to a direct action (Piaget 1969). Use of concepts such as that developed by Vojta and Peters (1992) or the sensorimotor patterning of the Doman-Delacato Treatment (American Academy of Pediatrics 1983; Maisel

1964) which do not include voluntary action or actual task performance are, therefore, not recommended because although some improvement in the movements elicited as reflex responses may occur in certain cases, without actual learning the patient's functional ability will remain unchanged. Normally, as Searle (1984) explains, motor actions are the result of intentionality so that a movement takes place because of someone's intention to do something.

Neuromuscular electrical stimulation (NEMS) and functional electrical stimulation (FES) have both become popular in the treatment of brain-damaged patients (Baker et al. 1983), but while electrical stimulation has been shown to change fast muscle fibres into slow ones or even strengthen muscles if tension is adequate (Lieber 1992), it cannot teach the patient to use those muscles for a particular functional activity. Lack of muscle strength is in any event rarely the reason why a patient is unable to perform an actual task.

Music therapy may be enjoyable for the patient, provide auditory stimulation and encourage him to participate actively but it cannot teach him to solve problems in the realm of daily life. In a similar way coma stimulation methods, whereby various isolated stimuli are applied to the different sensory modalities without being incorporated in an actual task or event, will not have a learning effect because normally, "we perceive events, not a successively analysed trickle of perceptual elements or attributes" (Dennet 1991).

In combination with the treatment of the patient's physical symptoms, specific therapeutic intervention is required for learning to be enhanced. If the criteria for optimal learning are to be fulfilled such intervention must provide the following:

- Interaction with the environment through contact
- Help with searching for, obtaining and organising tactile/kinaesthetic information in real life situations
- Successful performance of problem-solving tasks
- Repetition with variation
- Meaningful, goal-orientated activity

In the treatment of brain-damaged children and adults, guiding the patient's hands and body during the performance of actual tasks has proved to be amazingly successful. The unique method, discovered, developed and described by Affolter over many years is appropriate at any stage of treatment and enables the patient to improve both his physical and mental abilities (Affolter 1981, 1991; Affolter and Bischofberger 1993; Affolter and Stricker 1980). Used in conjunction with the treatment described in the subsequent chapters, the Affolter "concept" of **therapeutic guiding** will make a big difference to the course of the patient's rehabilitation from the intensive care stage through to the time of his discharge from a rehabilitation centre and will help him to achieve a more positive outcome.

Therapeutic Guiding

It is not possible to treat an apraxia or an agnosia as such, because each is a symptom arising as a result of a problem and not the cause. Just as massaging the painful area in someone's leg cannot cure his sciatica of spinal origin, so the patient's memory will not be improved by practice in memorizing or sensation restored by applying repeated isolated stimuli to the distal extremities. Treatment must be aimed at the root of the difficulty if any lasting functional improvement is to be achieved, and considered in a way similar to that which Maitland (1986) expresses in relation to his own concept, namely that "as the whole treatment is based on 'cause and effect' the importance and influences of the integrant parts must be thoroughly understood".

For the patient who is unable to learn through interaction with his environment because he cannot move or feel normally the therapist strives to make the necessary interaction possible. By guiding the patient's hands and body during the performance of an actual task, she ensures tactile/kinaesthetic input. The following example of a guiding sequence illustrates the underlying principles and practical application.

Pressing Juice from an Orange

- The patient sits at a table on which everything that is required for the task has been placed. The therapist stands close behind him so that she can move from one side to the other with her body in contact with his.
- On the table are an orange, a knife, an orange press, a glass and a damp dishcloth, the objects themselves making the task clear without verbal instructions being necessary.
- The therapist helps the patient to search for stable information before guiding any movement of his hands. With her body she eases his trunk forwards until his chest is against the table in front of him. She places one of her hands over his hand and, starting from his fingertips, moulds her hand to his as if she were trying to feel the surface of the table through his whole hand and test the stability of the surface. Her wrist and forearm do the same along the top of his forearm right up to his elbow, not pressing down hard, but ensuring a firm, even contact with the table. The therapist's upper arm is against the patient's, and with the front of her body and her shoulder she moves his trunk over towards the securely supported arm while maintaining the contact between his chest and the edge of the table. The therapist moves her foot round to the side of the stool on which the patient is sitting so that she is in close contact with the whole side of his body right down to his hip.
- It is then possible for the patient's other hand to be moved easily and the therapist guides it forwards with her free hand to reach for the orange (Fig. 1.1a). His fingers encircle the orange which is then drawn towards him without being lifted into the air.

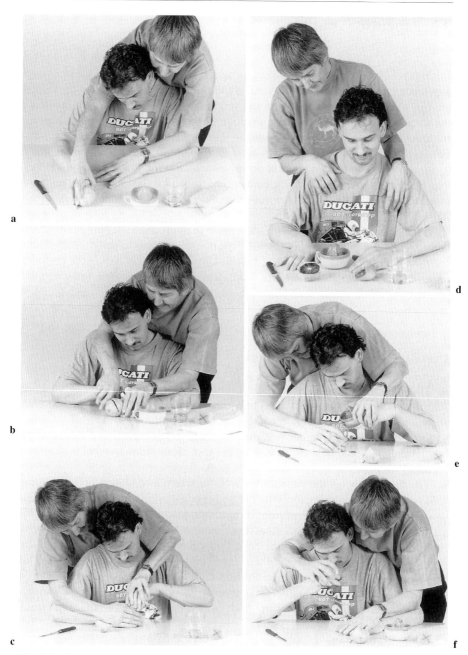

Fig. 1.1a–f. A patient with marked ataxia is guided while pressing an orange. **a** Adequate tactile information on his left side allows his right hand to move freely. **b** Only the patient's fingers are in contact with the orange and knife. **c** The press held firmly against his chest. **d** Pausing to take breath. **e** The press in contact with the glass. **f** Having a sip

- With the orange still in the same hand, the therapist moves round to that side of the patient so that she can assist him to search for stable information with that arm in the same way as she previously did with his other arm, starting distally and progressing upwards to his trunk.
- The therapist guides the patient's other hand to the orange and clasps it with all his fingers in contact with its surface. Her fingers do not touch the orange directly but are over the dorsal aspect of his hand and fingers to ensure a firm contact through them.
- Once again she moves round to start the search on the opposite side so that the patient's hand can be guided to take the knife and bring it to cut the orange in half (Fig. 1.1b). The knife is not moved through the air on to the top of the orange but instead its blade is pressed against the lower side and moved up into the correct position for cutting without losing contact.
- The same step by step procedure is repeated to seek information with each arm alternately while the other is moved as the knife is put down and the press drawn towards the patient to be held against his chest for stability.
- With the information provided through the side on which the press is being held, the therapist guides the patient's other hand to take the first orange half and press out the juice (Fig. 1.1c) and then changes sides so that the second half of the orange can be pressed with the patient's other hand.
- Because the movements have been carried out slowly with a renewed search for information before each step, the therapist should introduce a short pause after a sequence has been completed, that is, after a subsidiary goal has been achieved. She takes her hands from the patient's and stands upright to relieve the strain on her back, and can make a comment like "That was a juicy orange!" (Fig. 1.1d). Both she and the patient have been concentrating intensely and will need a moment to draw breath before continuing.
- Following the same principles, the glass is held in the patient's hand and the juice poured from the orange press (Fig. 1.1e).
- If the patient does not have swallowing difficulties, the therapist guides the glass to his mouth so that he can have a drink (Fig. 1.1f).
- If the patient is still not able to drink safely the therapist can guide him as he offers the glass of juice to someone else (Fig. 1.2). The act of drinking the juice himself or another person doing so rounds off the whole task satisfactorily and makes it more meaningful.

Tidying up After Completion of a Task

Whatever task has been performed, the patient can be guided to tidy up afterwards, not only because of the beneficial movements and problem-solving activities involved, but also because the relationship to real life is intensified.

- The therapist guides the patient as he places the used objects together, and wipes the table clean (Fig. 1.3a,b).

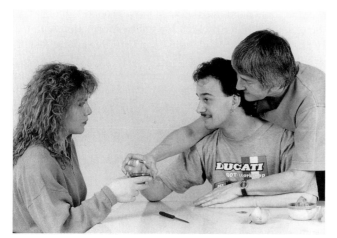

Fig. 1.2. Offering the orange juice to a friend

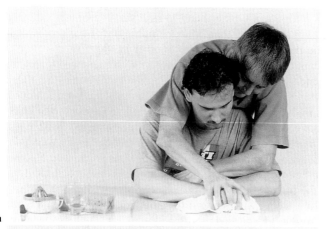

a

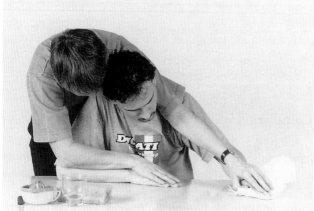

b

Fig. 1.3a,b. Searching for information on alternate sides while cleaning the table

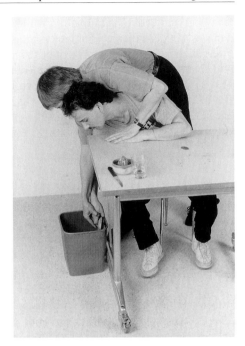

Fig. 1.4. Maintaining firm contact while bending down to put the peels in the wastebin

- The orange peels are put into a wastebin, which must be placed so that it is within reach before the commencement of the whole task and not need to be fetched by the therapist after the event. The therapist guides the patient's hand down towards the bin, without moving it through free space on the way. His hand travels down the leg of the table or chair until it encounters the side of the bin while his other hand is helped to remain in firm contact with the table top. The information thus provided from the surfaces of the receptacle and the table will facilitate the release of the patient's grasp and enable him to let go of the orange peel and drop the pieces into the container (Fig. 1.4).

If the patient is able to walk with assistance, the tidying-up process can be done by his being guided as he places all the utensils on a tray, stands up and walks with the tray to an appropriate place such as to a trolley for used plates or to a nearby sink.

Important Considerations for Guiding

Guiding is not only invaluable as a treatment intervention but also provides important information for the continuous assessment of the patient's level of performance. The therapist can feel sensitive changes in muscle tone, anticipatory behaviour and active participation, while close observation will reveal improvements as well as indicate what factors are still causing difficulty. For such detailed observations it is of inestimable value to have a video recording of the whole of the guided task which allows the therapist to analyse afterwards why certain sequences went well and others led to a breakdown in the performance. Studying the video film will enable the therapist to review the way in which she guided the patient so that she can alter or improve her handling as well as change the task and the way in which it is presented. The following are important considerations for successful guiding:

The Position of the Therapist and the Patient

Tasks can be guided in many different situations, with the patient lying, sitting up or standing, and much will depend upon the physical possibilities for ensuring the best tactile/kinaesthetic input and the nature of the task itself.

A solid table placed in front of the patient when he is sitting provides a stable surface and can be a realistic starting position for a great variety of tasks. The therapist can move freely from one side to the other and can use her hands and body to guide optimally without the patient being in danger of losing his balance.

If the patient is seated in a wheelchair, the person guiding him will have difficulty in reaching far enough forwards to guide his hands or establish contact between his trunk and the table and will be unable to use her own body against his side (Fig. 1.5a)

A wheelchair with an easily removable backrest can be a help, particularly during spontaneous guiding when the patient needs assistance with routine activities in his daily life (Fig. 1.5b). However, even without the back of the chair the helper's movements to either side are still restricted although she can guide the patient's hands on the table in front (Fig. 1.5c).

Transferring the patient from his wheelchair on to a normal upright chair allows more contact between the therapist's body and the patient's trunk but with the backrest in the way she cannot move him forwards and her flexed posture imposes an additional strain on her back (Fig. 1.6).

Ideally, the patient sits on a firm wooden stool which allows the therapist to move freely but still maintain close contact with the patient. When helping him to search for information on one side she can move right round to that side so that her leg is against his hip, her trunk against his and her hand and whole arm can cover his appropriately (Fig. 1.7a). When the role of the two hands changes, the therapist moves her feet round to the opposite side of the patient, so that she is in a balanced position to guide the next step (Fig. 1.7b).

When using other starting positions the same principles apply but the therapist will experience far more difficulty in establishing sufficient contact between the patient and his surroundings. For example, if the patient is standing, even with a table in front of him there will be an empty space in front of his legs which will need to be filled in some way with a board or other firm surface. Standing in a

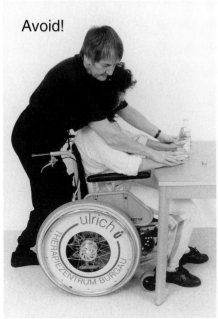

Avoid!

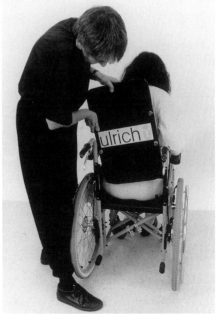

a

b

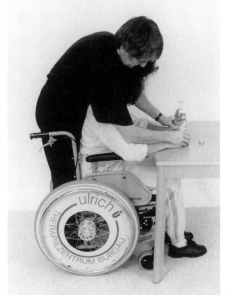

Fig. 1.5a–c. Guiding the patient in a wheelchair. **a** The backrest causes difficulties. **b** A removable backrest. **c** Contact with trunk possible

c

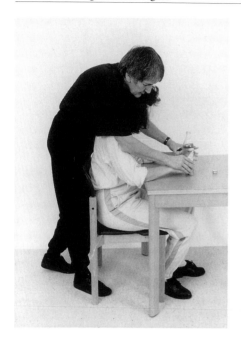

Fig. 1.6. Guiding with the patient sitting on a normal chair

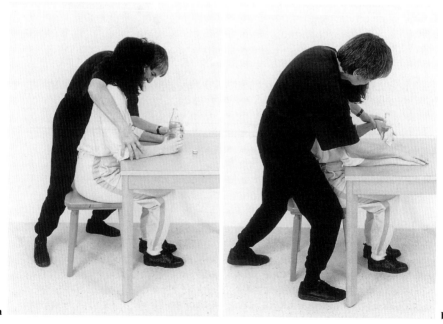

a   b

Fig. 1.7a,b. For therapeutic guiding a wooden stool is the ideal seat for the patient. **a** The therapist can move easily to either side. **b** Contact with the patient's whole side possible

kitchen area solves the problem as there are usually built-in cupboards against which the therapist can guide his thighs and knees with hers from behind, but only the patient's hands can easily be guided to seek information and not his whole arm and trunk. For therapeutic guiding, the therapist may therefore prefer to work with the patient in a sitting position even if he is able to stand well. The effect from a perceptual point of view will still be an increased input, and as a result influence standing and walking positively. In addition, when working in upright positions, such as required by the task, the walls and the corners of the room can be used to provide stable surfaces for the patient's trunk and arms as can door frames and tall cupboards.

Comprehension of the Ultimate Goal of the Task

The patient must understand what goal is to be attained by completing the task which will require a form of presentation of the problem appropriate to his individual level at the time. In the case of the previous example of making orange juice, the objects on the table made the goal clear. A verbal presentation, such as "Let's have a drink of orange juice" could be used at a more advanced level where the task involved finding all the necessary requirements and bringing them to the table or even meant going out to purchase the oranges. Between these two extremes are many other ways in which the problem-solving task can be presented to the patient with varying degrees of complexity.

Whatever the patient's level of ability it is important that the goal is clear. In the beginning it is usually necessary to have all the objects required within his visual field from the start. Practising grasping and moving different objects which have no connection to one another merely to exercise the motor components will not have the same learning effect (Fig. 1.8a).

When the patient has sat down or been transferred onto the stool at the table, adjusting the position of the table offers an excellent opportunity for a guided activity. The therapist guides first one of his hands and then the other across the surface of the table until the edge can be grasped to pull it nearer towards him, before repeating the procedure to grasp the opposite side. However, if there is nothing on the table to indicate the task to be performed, the patient is unlikely to pay much attention to the manoeuvre (Fig. 1.8b). As soon as the necessary objects are on the table, the situation changes because the reason for drawing the table closer becomes obvious (Fig. 1.8c).

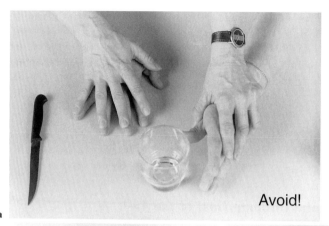

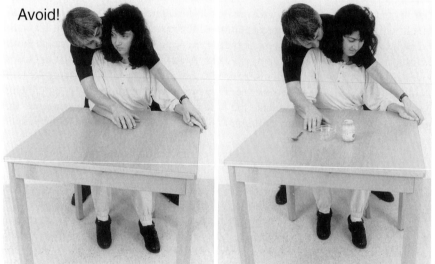

Fig. 1.8a–c. The goal of the task must be clear from the start. **a** Two unrelated objects fail to indicate a goal. **b** Without a meaningful task the patient is inattentive while drawing the table into position. **c** Immediate attention when the task is clear

One Hand Always Provides Information About the Stability of the Support

Whether the patient's problem is one of spasticity or ataxia the therapist should never move both his hands off the supporting surface simultaneously and manipulate the objects in the air, as both symptoms would be intensified due to inadequate information from the surroundings. She first guides the patient to seek a stable supporting surface before his other hand moves to perform the next step towards attaining the goal. For example, if the patient is required to pour a yogurt drink from its container into a glass, the therapist does not help him to do so by taking the yogurt in one hand and the glass in the other and transferring the liquid while both are being held in the air (Fig. 1.9a). Instead she takes time to guide the

Fig. 1.9a–c. One arm must always provide information about the stability of the supporting surface while the other is moving. **a** Both hands lifted simultaneously will increase ataxia or spasticity. **b** The patient's trunk and left arm guided to make contact with the table. **c** The right side providing information while the yogurt is poured into the glass

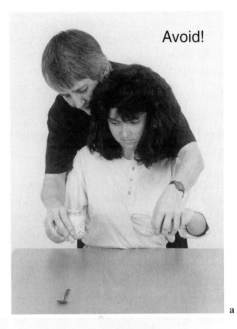

a

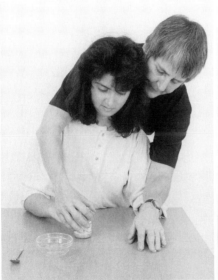

b

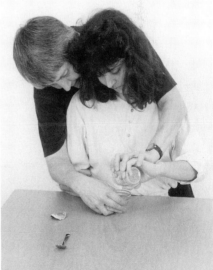

c

patient's trunk to approximate with the table and one of his arms so that the hand and forearm are in direct contact with the supporting surface before his other hand reaches for the yogurt drink (Fig. 1.9b). Only when both objects have been drawn close to him in this way is the liquid poured into the glass, while the hand holding it in position and the arm on that side are both in contact with the table (Fig. 1.9c). Sonderegger (1993) likens the movement sequences to a mountain climber scaling a cliff face, who never moves a hand or foot until he is very sure that his other three holds are absolutely secure. It should be remembered that the hand searching for and acquiring the information from the environment is more important for the patient's tactile perception than the hand which moves without a change in resistance through the air to fetch or carry an object. The therapist is frequently so intent on completing the task that she tends to focus her attention on the hand which is actively moving at the time, instead of on that which is feeling more.

An Instrument Is Only Necessary After A Problem Has Been Identified

The order in which the therapist guides the patient to reach for objects is relevant and not solely due to the fact that one is perhaps nearer at hand. During the pressing of the orange, for example, the knife would not be grasped as the first step before there was a reason for using it (Fig. 1.10). Prior to reaching out for the knife, the therapist guides the patient's hands to grasp the orange, examine it, try to open it up unsuccessfully and only then is a sharp instrument required to solve the problem of how to cut the orange in half. In other words any problem-solving strategy always follows an encounter with the problem, so that guiding a patient to open a door would not be a repetitive exercise in door opening and closing but must be necessary in order to let him pass through to fetch something or go somewhere for a reason.

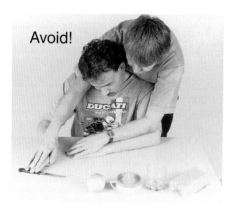

Fig. 1.10. The knife should only be included after the orange has been examined and the need for an instrument established

Right to the Fingertips of Both Hands

Because the tips of the fingers are exquisitely sensitive with a rich supply of receptors, they play an important role in touching, and therefore care must be taken that they are incorporated in any guided activity to ensure maximal tactile input. Through lack of emphasis or perhaps mechanical factors caused by the size of the patient and the relevant length of the therapist's arms, it can often be observed that his fingers are not in contact with surfaces or objects during a guided sequence (Fig. 1.11a). In fact in many cases his fingers will be seen to extend or move in the air instead of being moulded to the form of the object. It is imperative that the therapist cover the patient's fingertips with hers and guide them on to the underlying surface or to the contours of the object which is being held. She must avoid holding the patient's wrist and allowing him to grasp inappropriately and find a way to overcome any mechanical obstacles, usually made possible by her changing her own position. A short intensive period of input is far more effective in the treatment than guiding a whole sequence incorrectly.

Both hands are equally important during guiding because input takes place through both, and the difficulty is not specific to one side as is the case with muscle action. Information received through one side influences and is beneficial to both sides and will have a positive effect on the patient's sense of touch as a whole.

The Patient's Hand Should Feel Light and Be Easy to Move

When the guided search for information on one side is adequate and reveals that the support is stable, it will be easy for the therapist to move the patient's hand (or foot) on the opposite side. If at any stage his hand and arm feel tense, spasticity increases or the movements are ataxic, she must concentrate her attention on the source of

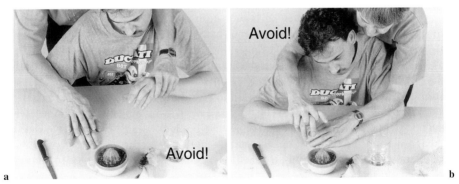

Fig. 1.11a. The therapist must guide both the patient's hands right down to the fingertips, whether searching for information or grasping an object. **b** The therapist should not hook her fingers through those of the patient to move his hand

information and not struggle to control or guide the movement with great effort. She should never be tempted, for instance, to interlace her fingers with those of the patient to enable her to lift his hand against a resistance (Fig 1.11b) because his hand and fingers would be prevented from making direct contact with the objects or the surface of the table. The therapist should not, in fact, touch the objects directly at all during a guided sequence but only feel them through the patient's fingers. Once a renewed and intensified search for information has been undertaken successfully, the patient's hand will feel light and ready for action, and the therapist will be able to move it without difficulty. It should be remembered that after a short time, perception of any surface begins to fade out so that the therapist cannot continue a movement with one hand for long but will need to change sides and alter the position, even if only slightly, before continuing.

The Patient, Guided by the Therapist, Performs Every Step of the Task

While performing a problem-solving task, it is important that no help be given by a third person or surreptitiously by the therapist when the going becomes difficult or if some extra implement is required. When mini-problems arise along the way then they too must be solved with the patient and not "for" him in order for the whole task to be meaningfully completed. It is hard for a helpful onlooker not to step in and push a necessary implement a little closer within reach, pick up an object which has fallen to the floor or hold a wobbly object steady. The solutions to such subsidiary problems form part of the whole task, so that the therapist guides the patient to solve any that might arise. In the orange-pressing task, for example, if the orange half should fall off the table, the therapist guides the patient to search for it and then finds a way for him to retrieve it in some way. Should the press be out of reach, either the patient must lie across the table to grasp it, the table must be pulled closer or turned or he must rise to his feet to be able to stretch further.

The therapist must resist the temptation to help by manipulating the objects surreptitiously while the patient is moving them, because by so doing she will change the input of their weight, how to turn or tilt them and what is required to use them. A common example is that when pouring a drink from a full bottle, the therapist hooks her little finger underneath it to take some of its weight as she feels unsure as to whether she can lift it with the patient's hand beneath hers. Another would be her holding the orange with her index finger placed in front of the patient's because she is afraid of cutting his.

Whether an outsider places a cup or glass nearer, something that has fallen down suddenly appears on the table again or a heavy bottle becomes strangely light, such "magical happenings" will impede the patient's learning by creating gaps in the problem-solving task with missing tactile links in his stored experience (memory) of the performance.

Verbal Input Is Avoided During A Guided Activity

As is the case in normal daily life, many tasks presented to the patient will be self-explanatory because of the situation and the combination of objects. Should the task to be performed by its nature require a verbal explanation, the therapist tells the patient clearly and concisely what has to be done. During the actual guiding, however, she should not talk to him because either he will not hear her as he is so absorbed by what he is doing or he will need to stop attending to the task in order to listen to what she is saying. It is most distracting, as most people will have experienced, to have someone talking to them while they are performing an extremely demanding task which requires absolute concentration. In the short intervals following completion of a stage of the task the therapist may make a spontaneous comment and then as the work proceeds she is silent once again.

The therapist must talk if the task performance breaks down completely, particularly if the patient becomes agitated or panics, in order to reassure him. Even in a less extreme situation where for some reason the guided performance cannot be completed and has to be left unfinished, she will need to say something appropriate to explain to the patient why the task is being discontinued. For example she might say "this cream isn't fresh and won't thicken. We'll have to get a new pint" or "we'll try with an electric beater, I'll bring mine from home tomorrow".

The Therapist or Helper Must Feel Relaxed and Confident

The therapist's own emotional state can make an enormous difference to the guiding and she must therefore try to be relaxed and calm. If she is worried that the task she has selected will not work out well, that it is taking too long and she will be late for the ward round, or if she is simply tired and irritated that day, the patient may react adversely. He could show signs of distress, become tense or be unable to perform as well as he had on a previous occasion. These factors should be taken into consideration if the patient's performance is being used for assessment purposes or when the therapist is selecting a task. Tension is frequently the result of both the therapist and the patient striving too hard to complete the whole task in one go and both must understand that it is perfectly acceptable to achieve only a part and continue the next day. For example, reaching for the orange and examining the possibility of opening it may for some patients be sufficient for one therapy session, with the knife and press used the following day because on no account should the process be rushed.

Feeling Through an Intermediary Tool, Object or Substance

At a certain stage in its development, a baby discovers that the manipulation of one object can affect other objects whereby cause and effect relationships are expanded (Affolter and Stricker 1980). The ability to "feel" clearly when using instruments allows the performance of countless skilled tasks ranging from eating with a knife and fork to performing intricate brain surgery. Gibson (1966) comments on the remarkable fact that, "when a man touches something with a stick he feels it at the end of the stick, not in the hand". By the same process it is possible for a driver to note via the steering wheel when the wheel of his car is against the curb, or for a pedestrian to recognize what is underfoot through the thick sole of his shoes. The ability which Dennet (1991) calls the "wand" phenomenon and Affolter the "stick phenomenon" is made possible through the unique qualities of the tactile/kinaesthetic system. The sense of touch with a "wand" is so sensitive that when starting to cut a banana for example, exactly the right amount of pressure is exerted to dissect the peel (Fig. 1.12a), and an automatic adaptation takes place when the soft flesh is being sliced, ending with a cessation of pressure at the moment when the knife touches the plate which provides the information that the action has been completed (Fig. 1.12b).

The "wand" phenomenon is important with regard to guiding for several reasons. As in normal development, using an intermediary tool constitutes a more advanced stage than direct contact with the objects themselves so that in the early stages the therapist selects tasks for the patient which can be performed with his hands and body and do not involve manipulating one object with another. Using a knife, fork or spoon is dependent upon the "wand" phenomenon as is working with a hammer or pair of pliers, but so is the simpler act of adjusting the position of a saucer with a cup or drawing a cross with a pencil. Because of the "wand" or "stick" phenomenon it is also possible to guide a patient who has a plaster cast either to stabilize a fracture or to overcome a contracture as the changing resistances and consistencies can still be perceived through the hard material resulting in meaningful tactile/kinaesthetic input.

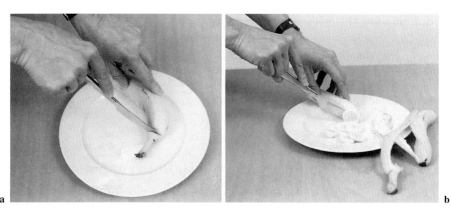

a   b

Fig. 1.12a,b. The "wand" phenomenon. **a** Even through the knife the consistency of a banana is appreciated. **b** The total resistance of the plate is registered indicating completion of the slice

Choosing a Suitable Task

Because of the infinite number and variety of tasks and their wide range of complexity, selecting one which is appropriate for the individual patient in his present condition will need careful thought.

Mechanical Factors

On a basic level, such factors as the size and compressibility of the objects must be taken into consideration. If the patient is very spastic and unable to participate, it would be far easier to work with a cucumber than a banana and guiding his hands to take yogurt from a firm glass jar would be more successful than if the yogurt were in a soft, plastic container.

For a patient who is unable to swallow at all, tasks which do not involve his eating or drinking would be more meaningful unless he had reached the stage of being able to enjoy offering what he has made to another person (See Fig. 1.2).

Standing can be included in the guided sequence with positive results, but if the patient requires leg-splints in order to stand then it is usually better to have him in the upright position with the splints already bandaged in place before guiding commences (See Fig. 4.12). For other patients, standing up from sitting is actually facilitated by the task necessitating the action.

Degree of Complexity

A problem-solving task becomes more complex according to how many objects and steps are involved, whether the necessary objects are all within the patient's immediate field of vision or only some of them, and even more complex when the task requires finding what will be needed in some other location. For example, the simplest level would be a glass and a bottle of water standing on the table directly in front of the patient and at the other end of the scale would be inviting friends for lunch, planning the menu, purchasing the ingredients and then cooking and serving the meal. Learning and attention are optimal when the learner is working at the limit of his ability or ceiling performance level with the task providing a challenge and a novelty factor (Affolter and Stricker 1980).

It should also be remembered that a person's level of ability will not always be identical, so that even a Wimbledon tennis champion has "good" days and "bad" days. The complexity of a task may be increased by extrinsic factors such as loud noise from a building site nearby or a wobbly chair or by intrinsic factors such as lack of sleep, constipation or pain. In the case of the brain-damaged patient, simply the enormous amount of effort and concentration which he requires just to get through a routine day will affect his level of performance at times.

Judging the Suitability of a Task

The suitability of a task can only really be judged by observing the patient while he is performing it, just as in any learning situation the behaviour of the students will reveal whether the subject matter and the teaching method are ideal. The learner's attention is a prerequisite for effective learning which implies his understanding because that which is not understood cannot be stored and learned, as Affolter (1991) formulates. Judgement of the patient's attention while he is being guided is based on the following observations:

- He is quiet and does not talk.
- His eyes are directed towards the task and not looking at other people or objects in his vicinity. His eyes may move away from the working area but appear not to be seeing, as if he were thinking or even be closed as if to shut out visual input.
- Irrelevant motor activity ceases or is reduced to a minimum including involuntary movements.
- Tone normalizes so that hypertonus decreases and if hypotonicity was a feature before the start, a certain alert tenseness is felt.
- The therapist may feel anticipatory movements in the appropriate direction or notice a slight turning of the patient's head towards the object required for the following stage of the task.

If the task or its presentation is *too complex* for the patient, one of the following behaviours will usually be observed or some of them occur in combination:

- The patient talks about something quite irrelevant or gives some reason as to why he cannot perform the task. For example, if the task has to do with the preparation of food, he may explain that his wife takes care of all culinary matters and that he never even enters the kitchen.
- He often complains of feeling too tired to continue.
- He may express a sudden urge to visit the toilet
- He may try to push his chair away from the table and refuse to participate altogether.
- He becomes violent and hurls the objects off the table.
- He is aggressive and hits out at the therapist or shouts and swears.
- He may scream or cry and become very spastic.

Should the task be *too easy* and familiar the following behaviour is more likely:

- The patient chats and jokes with the therapist or anyone else in his vicinity.
- He looks around continuously and greets or makes comments to other patients.
- He moves restlessly or fiddles with his clothes or face.

The therapist, when preparing to guide the patient for the first time will have to estimate what she thinks will be suitable for him and then alter the subsequent tasks according to what happens. To discover where the patient's difficulties lie, it will be necessary to attempt a task which places him at the limits of his performance ceiling because it is easy to overestimate his ability if he appears to cope well with a relatively simple task and his real problems are not revealed.

Interpretation of Behaviour Signals

A conclusive interpretation cannot be made on the basis of an observation made in only one situation. The patient's behaviour can only be interpreted and his actual difficulties evaluated after numerous observations have been made in a variety of different situations. A typical misinterpretation made on the basis of one observation is that of the patient being lazy and not liking to work. A good example is the case of a young patient who refused to dress herself and always waited for someone to come and help her, which soon led to her being called lazy. However the patient had been a gold-medal athlete before her lesion, so it seems highly unlikely that she was someone who was lazy by nature. A more logical explanation for her refusal, as verified later, was that she was unable to perform the complex task of dressing although her motor function appeared to be adequate. Another error commonly resulting from a single observation, or observations made in identical situations is an interpretation based on the assumption that the patient does not like doing some activity. His lack of compliance will invariably have a very real basis which will be discovered by further assessment.

For accurate assessment and hence appropriate treatment, care must be taken to differentiate between an interpretation and an observation. "The patient looks unhappy" is an interpretation. "The patient is sitting in a wheelchair in a flexed position with his head down and his face immobile" is the actual observation. Many an aphasic patient is interpreted as being able to read the newspaper merely because he has been observed holding the paper in front of him every morning, with his eyes directed towards it and turning the pages from time to time.

Ways in Which Guiding Can Be Implemented

Therapeutic Guiding

A specific task can be selected for the patient, carefully prepared and then guided therapeutically during any therapy session. Depending on the patient's condition he can be guided while still in the intensive care unit, on the ward or in the occupational therapy or physiotherapy department. To help make the situation as realistic as possible, the task should be performed in the right place and at the right time whenever feasible. Preparing a salad would therefore be undertaken in the ward kitchen or the one attached to occupational therapy and not with the patient seated at a plinth in the middle of the gymnasium. Should he have been helped into his clothes a few moments before, it would be unrealistic for him to be guided while undressing and dressing again with the occupational therapist. Her session should rather be arranged to coincide with his being brought out of bed, or before he lies down again. In the same way, if he has just finished his lunch guiding him while he makes a ham sandwich would not be ideal.

Spontaneous Guiding as a Way of Assisting

In the patient's daily life in the hospital or rehabilitation centre there will be many moments when he requires assistance with some activity and whoever is with him at the time can guide him instead of taking over and completing the task for him. The patient will most frequently require some help with activities centred round transferring to or from his wheelchair, personal hygiene, dressing and eating and moving about in the hospital, all of which can provide ideal opportunities for guiding. Such an extension of therapy in real-life situations when problem-solving tasks confront the patient quite naturally will be of great benefit and establish a carryover from therapy sessions into daily living. All members of the team including the patient's relatives should be on the lookout for such opportunities and be prepared to step in and guide him spontaneously. For example, a patient may be trying unsuccessfully to summon the lift and someone in the vicinity automatically takes his hands, uses the surrounding walls and door frame as information sources and guides the activity to a successful conclusion; or, for example, at lunch, the patient's table napkin falls on to the floor and the person assisting guides the necessary action to retrieve it; or while brushing his teeth, the patient requires some more toothpaste and instead of putting it on the brush for him the helper guides the sequence with him, the basin, neighbouring wall and the cupboard above lending themselves well to providing stable surfaces for information.

Teaching Relatives How to Guide

Members of staff should all be familiar with the concept of guiding and after both theoretical and practical instruction be able to incorporate the principles when working with the patient. It is equally important that his family and friends who spend considerable time with him should be taught to guide the patient as well, so that they too can help him and communicate with him in a more meaningful and therapeutic way. Through guiding they will also gain a deeper understanding of his difficulties and the nature of the unseen problems which cause them. Careful instruction which includes actual handling is essential because it is not possible to learn how to guide optimally simply by watching someone else at work or being told what to do:

- The therapist guides the relative exactly as she would the patient himself, so that the person concerned feels for him- or herself the speed of the movements, the amount of contact with the various surfaces and the constant proximity of the therapist (Fig. 1.13a). Several tasks should be performed in this way so that the person concerned experiences how the input changes when different objects are manipulated in different ways.
- The patient's relative guides him while he performs the same task which he or she has just experienced. The therapist can place her hand over that of the relative during the guiding to adjust the amount of contact, pressure and move-

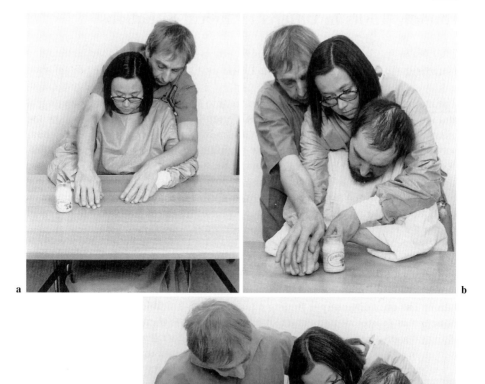

Fig. 1.13a–c. Teaching a member of the family to guide. **a** The therapist guiding a patient's wife to enable her to understand the principles. **b** The unconscious patient is guided by his wife while the therapist gives tactile help. **c** The patient's wife continues on her own with stand-by assistance

ment without any distracting verbal interruptions and to make learning through feeling possible (Fig. 1.13b).

- The relative continues the guiding on his or her own, with the therapist giving stand-by assistance and only stepping in again if required (Fig. 1.13c).

Guiding Tasks in Different Clinical Situations

Guiding in the Intensive Care Unit

The therapist will need to use her imagination to select tasks which are meaningful and suitable within the rather unreal and certainly unfamiliar surroundings of the intensive care unit. Spontaneous activities such as brushing the patient's hair, washing, applying cream, wiping away perspiration with a towel can provide opportunities for guiding or some specific task can be chosen which offers more change in resistance and hence tactile information which can be more easily appreciated. However simple the task, it must still fulfil the criteria of being goal-orientated, requiring problem-solving and providing tactile/kinaesthetic input, all within the framework of a real or actual event.

Whether the patient is unconscious or demonstrates only slight signs of starting to regain consciousness, he can still be guided during the performance of tasks even while lying in bed or when sitting in a wheelchair for very short periods at first and thus helped to be in touch with the world again through meaningful, tactile stimulation. The only difficulty is finding a task which is suitable for the situation. The presence of plaster of Paris casts should not deter the therapist from guiding the patient because tactile input is possible despite the cast through the "wand" phenomenon as has already been explained. Indications are that patients regain consciousness sooner and are certainly less spastic if meaningful tasks are guided in the early stages. The following guided tasks illustrate the possibilities.

With the Patient Still in Bed

Example 1. The patient switches on the radio.

- A portable radio is put on the bed in front of the patient who is lying on his side.
- The therapist places her arm through beneath the patient's neck to guide his search for information on the underneath side with her other hand free to move his other hand.
- The patient's hand is guided to grasp the radio and move it until it is right against his body (Fig. 1.14a).
- After interchanging the moving and information sides appropriately during the course of the activity, the therapist guides the patient's hand along the top of the radio to find the on/off switch (Fig. 1.14b).
- Once the correct switch has been located by the patient's fingers, it is pushed down as required into the "on" position while his other arm continues to keep the radio firmly in contact with his body (Fig. 1.14c).
- The music starts, and the task has been successfully completed. At that stage it is not unusual for the patient to show some sign which could be interpreted as recognition or satisfaction, either by opening his eyes or a change in his facial expression or perhaps only by an alteration of pulse rate or respiration (Fig. 1.14d).

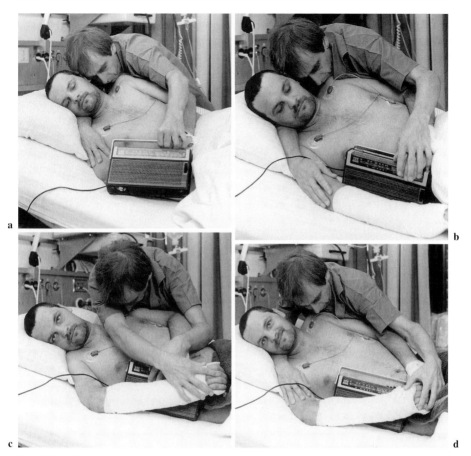

Fig. 1.14a–d. Guiding an unconscious patient in the intensive care unit. **a** Information search on the right side while the radio is drawn towards his body. **b** Feeling along the top of the radio to find the switch. **c** The patient's eyes open as the switch is located and pressed down. **d** The sound of music indicates the successful completion of the task and the patient reacts with a smile

Example 2. The patient applies eau de toilette before his girlfriend's visit.

- While the patient is lying on his side, the bottle of men's eau de toilette is placed on his bed within reach. The therapist guides his uppermost arm to seek information, pressing it against his body with his hand in contact with the surface of the bed (Fig. 1.15a).
- The therapist guides the patient's other hand to grasp the bottle and move it up towards his neck ((Fig. 1.15b).
- She eases the patient's index finger in to place on top of the bottle to press the spray mechanism and helps him to bring his hand into the correct position before spraying the eau de toilette on to his neck and behind his ear (Fig. 1.15c).

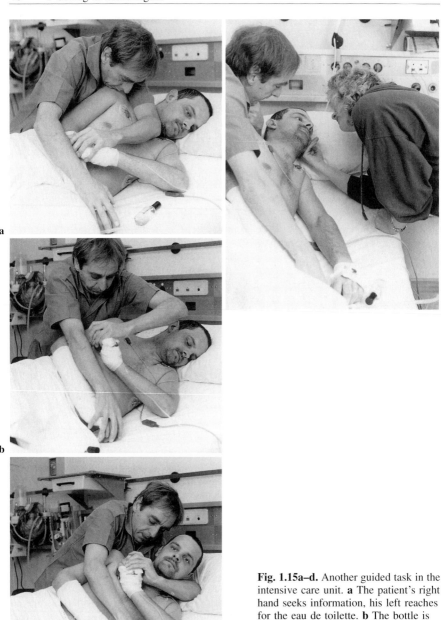

Fig. 1.15a–d. Another guided task in the intensive care unit. **a** The patient's right hand seeks information, his left reaches for the eau de toilette. **b** The bottle is moved into place and the index finger finds the spray button. **c** Spraying on the toilet water. **d** His girlfriend greets him and the event is a successfully concluded

- When the patient's hands are lying on the bed once again and the bottle has been released, as arranged in advance his girlfriend walks up to the bedside to greet him, thus bringing the task performance to a satisfactory conclusion (Fig. 1.15d).

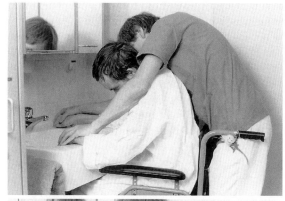

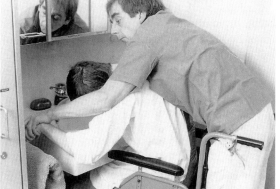

Fig. 1.16a,b. Guiding the unconscious patient in a wheelchair. **a** Using the basin as a source of tactile information while moving to reach the tap. **b** Reaching for the towel after washing hands and face

When the Patient Is Sitting Out of Bed for a Short Period

Example. The patient washes his face and hands at the washbasin.
- The patient, seated in a wheelchair, is brought as close as possible to a basin in the vicinity of his bed and the therapist guides one of his hands to test the stability of the edge of the basin nearest to him. She guides his other hand along the surface of the basin to the tap which he then turns on (Fig. 1.16a).
- After filling the basin, testing the temperature of the water and washing, with the therapist guiding each movement, the patient is helped to reach for his towel (Fig. 1.16b) and then dry himself.

Guiding to Overcome Difficulties with Sitting Posture

Many patients will have difficulty in sitting upright in a wheelchair at first and will tend to be either too flexed or too extended. Ways in which the wheelchair can be adapted or the patient supported to achieve an improved posture are described in

Chap. 2. It is of no avail to try to fix the patient forcibly in a corrected position in some way, as any mechanical fixation will usually worsen the situation. In the case of his head and trunk being too flexed, a strap around his head to hold it up will only serve to provide a resistance against which he will press his head even more strongly, and if he pushes into extension when sitting he will push his head relentlessly back against any form of headrest attached to the chair. Both postures indicate that he is trying desperately to gain more information as to where exactly he is in relation to his surroundings through the extreme positions of his neck and trunk. Guiding the patient while he performs tasks that require him to lean forward, should he be always pressing back in extension, or to look up and extend his trunk, should he be constantly in flexion, will help to solve the underlying problems. Preventing the development of incorrect postures is a priority in treatment and their prevention is far easier and less distressing for all concerned than is the arduous work required to overcome the problems later. It should, therefore, be borne in mind that such problems are seldom seen in patients who have been moved correctly, sat out of bed and stood with support during the early stages following the traumatic or other type of lesion, in ways which will be described in the subsequent chapters.

The following example illustrates how an existing problem of extreme extension can be helped:

- A patient who lay supine in bed for many months is unable to flex either his neck or his trunk actively or allow them to be flexed passively. He has so little cervical flexion that the nurse cannot lift his head to put a pillow under it in bed. Therapeutic and functional activities are not possible because he is unable to lean forwards to use his hands on a surface in front of him (Fig. 1.17a). The

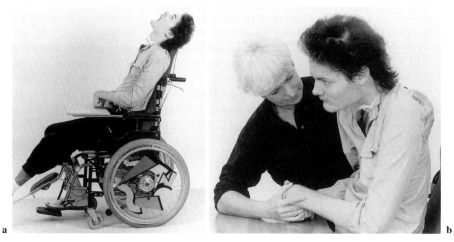

a   b

Fig. 1.17a,b. Hyperextension of the trunk and neck. **a** Abnormal posture in sitting. **b** Therapist unable to correct the patient's posture manually

patient's mouth is wide open all the time in combination with the extreme cervical extension, and he is unable to take food by mouth.

- Despite his cooperation, the patient's trunk cannot be brought forwards to a table placed in front of him and he pushes back even more strongly when the therapist tries to overcome the enormous resistance physically (Fig. 1.17b).
- The patient's great height presents an additional problem without neck and trunk flexion, as he is over 2 m tall.

The Effect of a Guided Task on the Patient's Sitting Posture

Example:The patient brushes his hair:

- The patient is transferred from his wheelchair to sit on a stool with a table in front of him, and the therapist stands close behind him to keep him in position.
- A man's handbag, which contains a hairbrush amongst other articles, is already lying on the table and no verbal instructions are given to the patient so that he does not know what the goal of the task is.
- Without saying anything, the therapist immediately starts to guide the patient, one arm to make contact with the table top and the other moving to explore the handbag (Fig. 1.18a).
- Following the previously described principles of guiding, the patient's hands move or seek information alternately until the bag can be opened. Already the extension of his neck and trunk becomes less extreme, and his mouth is closed (Fig. 1.18b).
- Moving slowly and carefully while maintaining close contact with the patient's body and between his body and the table, the therapist guides the necessary movements to take the brush out of the bag (Fig. 1.18c).
- The patient brushes his hair with the therapist guiding and the extensor hypertonus diminishes even further (Fig. 1.18d).
- After being transferred back into his wheelchair, the patient's sitting posture is remarkably improved with both trunk and neck being far more relaxed. (Fig. 1.19).

Guiding in Conjunction with Walking

Ways in which guiding can be used when the patient is standing in the early stages are explained in Chap. 4. The aim is to enable the patient to stand in a more upright position and for longer periods than when practising standing as an activity in itself. For many patients, walking can be a very frightening experience as very little information or stable support is provided through contact with the surroundings, and there may be conflicting information through different sensory channels. With only one foot in contact with the ground, the patient is otherwise totally dependent on the sources of information provided from within his own body and these are frequently disturbed or not working in unison with one another. What the patient perceives visually as he moves may contradict what he feels

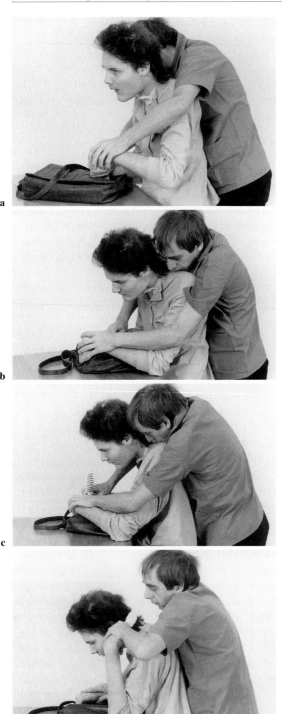

Fig. 1.18a–d. A guided task to correct sitting posture. **a** Guiding a 2-m tall patient to explore a man's handbag. **b** Discovering how to open the handbag. **c** Finding the hairbrush and taking it out. **d** Trunk and neck flexion achieved as the patient brushes his hair

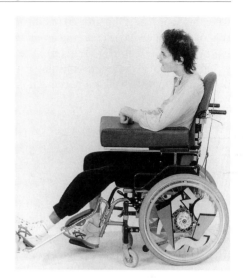

Fig. 1.19. Immediately following the guided task the patient's posture in the wheelchair is markedly improved. (compare with Fig. 1.17a)

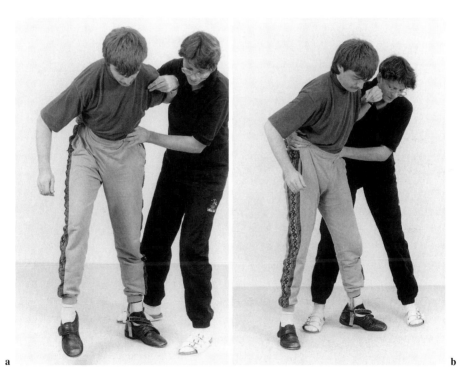

a   b

Fig. 1.20a,b. Patient MC, with marked disturbance of tactile perception is terrified of walking. **a** Taking a step with his right foot, the therapist scarcely able to support him. **b** Trying to move his left foot (see "A case in point, in Chap. 7)

when his foot meets the ground and he gives an impression of insecurity reminiscent of someone who is teetering along on very thin ice, terribly afraid of its breaking beneath his feet (Fig. 1.20a,b). The fact that the therapist is supporting him efficiently and giving him constant verbal reassurances does nothing to lessen his fear. Once he is walking because it is a part of an actual task with the therapist

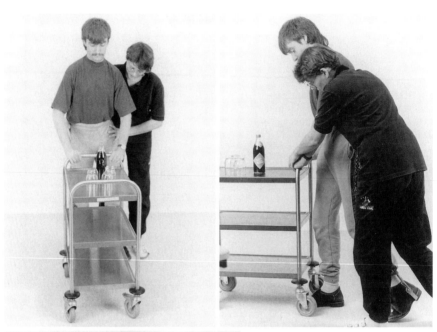

a

b

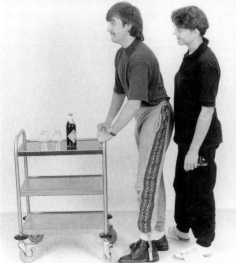

c

Fig. 1.21a–c. Patient M.C. walking while performing an actual task.
a Pushing a trolley to serve drinks.
b The therapist, with her body close to his facilitates walking. **c** Patient continues to walk without the help of the therapist and shows no signs of fear

guiding his movements he is far less likely to feel afraid or panic and the walking pattern itself becomes more normal and relaxed.

One example of a task which necessitates walking would be to load a tea trolley with cool drinks and glasses and then walk to serve drinks to others. In order to bring the drinks to the people, it is necessary for the patient to stand up and take the trolley to them (Fig. 1.21a). Because the patient has a goal to reach and because he is holding the trolley which he pushes in front of him he is able to walk confidently with very little assistance from the therapist who perhaps need only to hold his hand in place (Fig. 1.21b). The patient who, moments before, was terrified to take a step with either foot with the therapist barely able to support him may be able to walk confidently without her help in the course of completing the task (Fig. 1.21c).

While Regaining Independence in the Activities of Daily Living

How the patient is helped to dress, have a shower, shave or wash can make a difference as to how soon he achieves independence in the activities of daily living (ADL). From the start the activities should be performed in such a way that he will gradually be able to take over more and more sequences himself as he starts to participate actively and will not have to learn a completely new procedure.

Before the patient shows signs of regaining consciousness, the therapist or whoever is with him will have to complete the tasks for him from start to finish, but even then there will be opportunities to guide him, as was shown in Fig. 1.16. When the patient can help in some way by moving actively then he should be encouraged to do so even though the therapist or nurse still has to carry out the task itself for him.

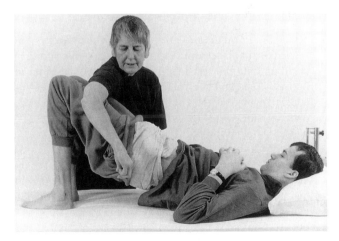

Fig. 1.22. A patient with marked ataxia lifts his hips off the bed for his trousers to be pulled up over his buttocks

For example, when someone is putting on the patient's trousers for him in bed he can be asked to hold his leg in the air so that she can slip the trouser-leg over his foot. In order to pull the trousers up, the therapist places the patient's feet on the bed with his knees well flexed and asks him to raise his seat in the air. Holding his legs in place against her body she can then draw the trousers over his buttocks (Fig. 1.22). If he can use his hands on his own, he can help by grasping the waistband and pulling with her.

Guiding While the Patient Is Getting Dressed

In the very early stages, although she still has to dress the patient, the therapist can guide those parts of the activity which are feasible from a physical point of view and are possible without rushing in the time available.

- *Example 1. Putting on shoes and socks.* If the patient is still not able to sit upright even with the support offered by his wheelchair then the therapist brings him into a sitting position on the bed. Supporting his trunk with her body in close contact with his, she guides his hand to put on his sock after helping him to find a stable supporting surface on the other side (Fig. 1.23a).
- *Example 2. Putting on a tracksuit top.* Having transferred the patient into his wheelchair, the therapist places the top of his tracksuit on a table in front of him. With the armrests of the wheelchair and the table providing firm supporting surfaces the therapist guides the patient while assisting him to put on the jacket (Fig. 1.23b).

As balance improves and the patient is able to sit confidently in his wheelchair, he can progress to dressing in sitting and standing positions with more movement involved. He should also be guided to select his clothes from the cupboard and take them to a nearby table before starting to dress.

- *Example 1. Standing to pull up a pair of trousers.* After the patient has been helped to put his feet into the trouser legs while sitting in his wheelchair, he can stand up with the assistance of the therapist in order to pull them up over his buttocks. The table in front of him will facilitate his standing up from the chair and will provide a point of reference while he is balancing in standing in order to complete the task (Fig. 1.24). The therapist adjusts his position to ensure that weight is taken through both legs.
- *Example 2. Putting on shoes and socks in sitting.* In order to put on his socks or shoes, the patient will at first need to cross one leg over the other as he will usually not be able to hold his foot actively in the air. The therapist guides his hand down to pick up his sock, keeping it in contact with his leg or the wheel of his chair all the way down to the floor to avoid moving through the air. She helps the patient to lift one of his legs and place it in the other and then, standing close beside him, draws his weight over towards her and guides his hand to pull on the sock (Fig. 1.25a).

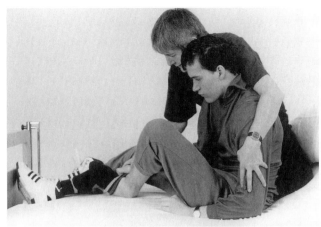

a

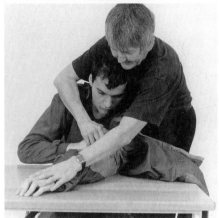

b

Fig. 1.23a. The therapist guides the patient when helping him to put on in his socks. **b** He sits in his wheelchair to put on his tracksuit top while she guides the task therapeutically

- *Example 3. Fastening shoes.* Tying shoe laces is a very complex task, and one which the normal child can only perform correctly at the age of about six years. Making the knot and the bow are almost impossible for the therapist to guide and the patient's repeated, unsuccessful attempts to tie the laces on his own can be very frustrating. Velcro straps to fasten the shoes or a strap with a buckle are far simpler to manage, and the therapist can guide the movements of his hands if necessary. Velcro straps can easily be sewn on to a normal lace-up shoe to avoid the expense of purchasing an additional pair which already has a Velcro-type fastener as a standard fitting.

Standing close to the wheelchair, the therapist slides the patient's hands down his legs one step after another until he reaches his foot. Holding one of his hands against his leg she guides the other hand to grasp the strap and press it firmly into place (Fig. 1.25 b).

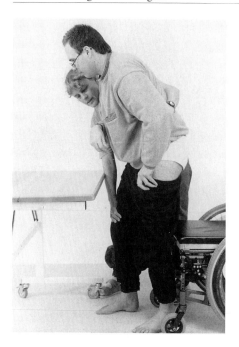

Fig. 1.24. A patient with right hemiplegia stands to pull up his trousers with the help of the therapist. A table in front of him makes balancing easier

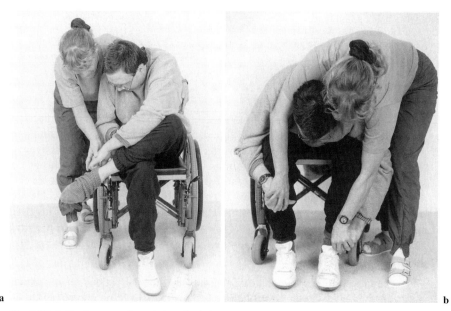

a   b

Fig. 1.25a,b. Putting on socks and shoes in sitting. **a** Pulling up a sock with one leg crossed over the other. **b** When bending down to fasten a shoe, the patient's hands slide down his legs

Increased Tactile Information to Maintain Lying Positions

Patients who have very disturbed sensory input will often be extremely restless in bed as they search desperately for stable surfaces to provide some orientation in the inexplicable world in which they find themselves, the strange and frightening world of distorted or absent sensation (Fig. 1.26a). Many people who walk in their

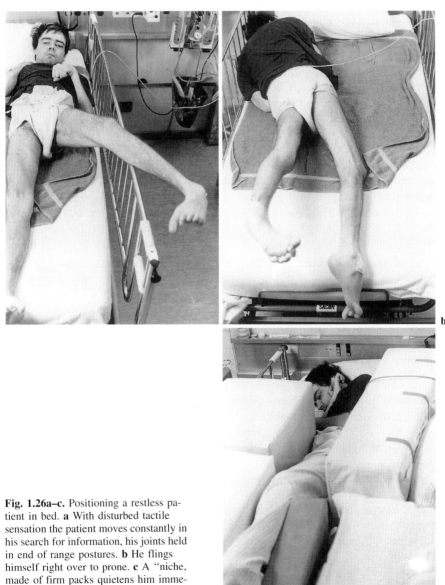

Fig. 1.26a–c. Positioning a restless patient in bed. **a** With disturbed tactile sensation the patient moves constantly in his search for information, his joints held in end of range postures. **b** He flings himself right over to prone. **c** A "niche, made of firm packs quietens him immediately after his leg briefly explores the opening

sleep and wake up in the dark somewhere other than in their beds show a similar reaction to the disturbing situation in which they find themselves, one of not knowing where they are and why. Instinctively they too will move their arms and legs about rather wildly in an attempt to make contact with objects in their vicinity which if familiar could provide information as to their exact whereabouts or the location of the nearest light switch.

The patient "exists in a state of chaos in which everything is mixed up with no order or logic. The patient feels totally exposed to his environment, unprotected against an unsympathetic world" (Grosswasser and Stern 1989). It is easy to understand why some patients, when lying on a soft mattress in the seemingly vast expanse of the bed, will not always stay quietly in the same position in which the nurses have carefully placed them, but will be in constant motion (Fig. 1.26b). It can be difficult for the staff to cope with such a patient who will be in danger of falling out of bed or could injure himself during his uncontrolled movement excursions. He should not be tied down to the bed, because the bindings will only make him more restless and he will tend to fight against the restraining ties. By surrounding him with firm packs so that he lies in what Affolter refers to as a "niche", immediate contact is established between him and his environment and because he no longer needs to search for information, will usually quieten down at once and go to sleep (Fig. 1.26c). Replacing the guardrails on the sides of the bed with wooden boards will tend to have the same effect. Care will need to be taken, however, that the patient is not left lying in bed with too little stimulation because it could be such a relief for all concerned to have him staying quietly in one position at last that they prefer not to disturb him.

The Problem of Incontinence

The voluntary control of the bladder and bowel is an extremely complex mechanism which is still not fully understood. The spinal cord segments as well as the peripheral nerves responsible for micturition have been located and described in many textbooks, but uncertainty remains as to which areas of the brain govern continence as a whole. Diagrammatic representations merely indicate afferent and efferent signals to and from unspecified "higher centres". In actual fact, it would seem that almost the entire brain is involved when considering that, according to one author, these higher centres are found in the cerebral cortex, basal ganglia, hypothalamus, mid-brain, pons and cerebellum in either an inhibitory or facilitatory manner. Ruch and Patton (1970) give an idea of the complexity, stating that "the micturition reflex is tonically influenced from at least 3 levels of the brain stem, and successive levels are alternately inhibitory and facilitatory. The reflex is also influenced by 2 suprasegmental structures — the cerebellar and the cerebral hemispheres". On a physical level, to be continent involves inhibiting the detrusor muscle contraction and activating the sphincters to prevent excretion until both time and place are appropriate and then, in a highly coordinated manner, relaxing the sphincter(s) and allowing contraction of the relevant muscles to empty the bladder or the bowel. However, in addition to the motor act many cognitive task performances of a highly complex nature are required. For people to be continent of urine they must be able to carry out the following:

- Think in advance that they will soon need to empty their bladder.
- Choose and wait for a suitable moment.
- Go to a toilet, which, if they are not in familiar surroundings, will require finding one.
- Open the door, enter the bathroom, close the door and secure the lock.
- Remove such clothing as is necessary.
- Adjust their position to pass water in the correct receptacle and maintain their balance.
- Perform the synchronized motor activity.
- Clean themselves with toilet paper.
- Adjust their clothing again.
- Flush the toilet.
- Wash their hands.
- Unlock and open the door and close it behind them after leaving.

It is important to remember that continence is a learned ability, one which takes the normal child about five years to achieve with absolute certainty and that it is influenced by many psychosocial factors. "The humiliation of involuntary or untimely excretion has been so pounded into us by years of zealous toilet training that to avoid it we have learned absolute control, iron control, control so rigid that neither our bladder nor sphincter dare to let go even while we are asleep" (Friday 1981). Because continence is such a complex task performance it is easy to understand that the patient with severe brain damage will frequently be incontinent, particularly in the early stages of rehabilitation. Independent dressing is a task of approximately the same level of complexity so that a patient who can choose and put on his clothes without any help is likely to have voluntary control over urine and faeces as well.

Persistent incontinence can be demoralizing for the patient and most distressing for his relatives. The passing of urine and faeces at inappropriate times can also be a contributory cause of skin breakdown or infection, and much treatment time is lost if the patient requires frequent cleaning and changing. Adequate management of the problem is, therefore, essential from the beginning.

Urinary Incontinence

Because urination occurs more frequently during 24 hthan does defaecation, loss of bladder control is a far greater problem. The urinary problems are aggravated by the fact that the patient is required to have a catheter for urinary drainage during the period of coma to enable fluid intake and output to be accurately measured. Having regained consciousness he is therefore liable to have already existing tissue irritation and minor infections, both of which will precipitate micturition.

Considerations for Management

1. The patient does not have a neurogenic bladder such as that resulting from a spinal cord injury but rather one which can be likened to that of a developing child who has not yet learned to control or inhibit spontaneous emptying of its bladder. Just as the baby will pass water at any moment due to some stimulus, even though his bladder is not necessarily full, so the patient will urinate at irregular intervals in response to a variety of stimuli such as pressure and movement, tension or relaxation. Because his incontinence is the result of perceptual disturbance and disorganization, treatment aimed at overcoming the patient's disordered perception as a whole will automatically improve his ability to control his bladder. The concept of guiding should be incorporated in many different situations for optimal results and not concentrate solely on using the toilet as such if frustration is to be avoided. On no account should the patient be reprimanded should "accidents" occur, just as the very young child is never punished for wetting its nappy, nor should he be accused of being "naughty" or inconsiderate. His incontinence is neither a form of carelessness or disobedience, nor a voluntary reprisal, but is a symptom of his brain lesion in the same way as is the spasticity or paralysis of his arm. He has not yet regained the high level of cognitive performance required for continence and careful analysis will reveal that he also fails in other tasks of equal complexity.

2. As soon as the patient regains consciousness or no longer requires intensive care the catheter should be removed and not left in situ merely as a means of keeping him dry. The only reasons for continuous catheter drainage are measuring the fluid balance in the acute stage and draining the bladder in the case of acute retention, a problem which very rarely arises after head injury (Schlaegel 1993). While lying in bed a bottle can be placed to catch the urine and during the day a disposable napkin of absorbent material should be used and changed regularly whenever wet. A condom urinal with a leg-bag attachment, such as recommended for paraplegics (Bromley 1976), may be worn only if the patient is at such a stage that he does not constantly attempt to pull it off, but he should still be encouraged to pass water at regular intervals and not be lulled into a sense of security by the appliance.. Female patients have no alternative but to use the absorbent padding material until they have regained the necessary degree of control.

3. The complexity of the task is reduced if the patient is offered a bottle or taken to the toilet at regular intervals, for example every 2–3 h, and helped to undress and transfer. It is interesting to note that patients at home will often be kept continent because their close relatives are able to notice any signs indicating that they need to pass water and react immediately, whereas one of the same patients may become incontinent again during a subsequent period in hospital. Nursing staff taking care of a number of dependent patients would not be able to give him the same degree of attention on a one-to-one basis as he received at home.

4. With regard to psychological factors, if the patient is dressed in his own clothes and not left to sit in a hospital nightgown he is also less likely to be incontinent. The way in which he is helped has also been shown to make a significant difference, so that all who work with him should be prepared to assist him at once in a friendly and encouraging manner, despite their workload and the pressure of time.

5. To avoid embarrassing accidents, the patient should visit the toilet or use a bottle before attending a therapy session. Should he indicate that he needs to pass water during therapy, the opportunity should be taken to guide him therapeutically in the situation and should not be regarded as an irritating interruption. A supply of clean diapers should be kept in the therapy department so that in the event of an accident, the patient can be changed without having to return to the ward or his room and thus less time will be lost. If the patient is liable to become wet when in one of the various departments it is advisable for him to carry a clean pair of trousers with him in the wheelchair.

6. Bladder training such as that used for patients with spinal cord injury, whereby the bladder is emptied at regular intervals by applying compression or stimuli to elicit a reflex emptying, is not applicable for the patient with brain damage. Unlike the patient with a spinal cord lesion, the brain-damaged patient has an intact spinal cord and his difficulties arise from a loss of cognition and not from alterations in the activity and tone of the muscles of the bladder and its sphincters or a loss of peripheral sensation. In order to facilitate bladder emptying, the patient will therefore need to be relaxed and calm and not be in a hurry, and soothing sounds such as that of running water will help him to initiate urination rather than direct manipulation of his bladder through the abdominal wall or stimulation over surrounding areas.

7. Any urinary tract infection must be treated accordingly to eliminate the frequency associated with infected urine. Subsequent infections can easily occur if the patient has neurogenic dysphagia and has difficulty in drinking enough. Intensive treatment for the sensory/motor problems of his face and mouth, with particular reference to the selective movements of his tongue should be commenced at an early stage and continued until he is able to swallow fluids easily (see Chap. 5). Ideally he should drink approximately 2 l per day and if he has no form of substitute feeding it will be encumbent upon all members of the team to encourage and help him to drink small amounts at frequent intervals during the day to ensure an adequate fluid intake. Unfortunately, it is sometimes erroneously thought that the patient should drink less so that he need not pass water so often, but the dangers inherent in such a strategy must be carefully explained to all who work with him. Not only will the risk of repeated urinary infections be increased, but his kidneys could be damaged as a result.

Faecal Incontinence and/or Constipation

Untimely bowel actions can be most unpleasant for both the patient and those working with him, but fortunately it is possible to establish a routine such that his bowels are emptied at a set time once a day or every second day and the danger of accidents thus eliminated. Almost all patients will become constipated due to their immobility, the lack of roughage in their diet and the difficulty in swallowing fluids. Psychological factors also play a significant role in the development of constipation and, as a result, many people without neurological impairment experience the same difficulty. Examples of such psychological factors are:

- An unfamiliar toilet particularly if the door cannot be locked.
- A change in the time of rising and having breakfast.
- A different type of breakfast, without enough tea or coffee or perhaps without the usual fruit juice.
- The presence of another person.
- Trying to use a bedpan in a lying position following surgery.

The patient will have to contend with all or some of these factors until he has recovered sufficiently to manage on his own because of the hospital routine, his swallowing difficulties and inadequate balance. He will not be able to be left alone on the toilet or lock the door for fear of his falling and injuring himself.

As well as delaying the return of continence, constipation must be stringently avoided because of its adverse side effects, which include the following:

- Particularly in the early stages, but also during later rehabilitation the patient may feel nauseous, vomit and even suffer an obstruction with serious consequences.
- The discomfort and pressure of an overloaded bowel increases spasticity.
- Bad breath as a result of constipation can be most off-putting for the patient's family in an already sensitive situation.
- Bladder drainage via a urinary catheter may be impeded.
- The patient without a catheter may need to pass water more frequently, with his bladder capacity reduced by the loaded bowel. He may have difficulty in initiating urination.
- Because he is worried about the constipation, the patient will be less able to concentrate during therapy sessions. He may continually ask to be taken to the toilet and remain there for long periods without success which can be very depressing for him.
- Apparent diarrhoea can be the result of too fluid faeces by-passing the hard stool within the bowel, leading to frequent soiling. Treatment time is wasted by the patient having to be cleaned and changed repeatedly. If the cause of the diarrhoea is misunderstood, the situation can be worsened by the administration of medication to harden the stool.
- If laxatives in various dosages are given at irregular intervals to relieve severe constipation, the patient may have to remain in his room for the whole day because the result was so vigorous that he is constantly passing liquid

faeces. On the other hand, should the dose have been insufficient to move his bowels, he will be unable to give his full attention to the therapist, as he is so afraid that he might soil himself at any moment.

Considerations for Management

1. Preventing constipation:
   - While the patient is still unconscious the problem of constipation must be anticipated and measures taken accordingly. A nonchemical laxative is administered after it has been noted that no stool has been passed, and abdominal compression, assisted expiration and passive movement of the trunk are instituted after 12 h to facilitate a bowel motion. Should no motion be passed, a manual evacuation is performed and the dose of the laxative increased for the next attempt. The laxative should be given in the evening and the bowel action achieved in the early morning to establish a routine in preparation for the future, when the patient has regained consciousness and is participating in an active rehabilitation programme.
   - As soon as the patient can be sat up out of bed, he should be transferred on to a commode and helped to have a bowel motion each morning, after either his oral or tube feed. The nurse or therapist flexes his trunk forwards and assists deep expiration by compressing his thorax. The patient is encouraged to bear down actively if he is able to participate.
   - Should the attempt be unsuccessful, a glycerine suppository is inserted and will often provide the necessary stimulation for defaecation to commence. In the event of nothing being passed, either a manual evacuation or an enema should be used to empty the bowels. The amount of laxative should not be increased day after day without the bowels having been evacuated. For the next attempt however, it should be noted that an increased dose is required and after some trial and error the amount necessary to produce a soft, formed stool at one sitting can be established and used repeatedly.
   - The physiotherapist should practice transferring the patient from his bed to the wheelchair in the easiest possible way and show the nursing staff how to help him in the same way. Once the patient can be transferred onto the actual toilet he will be better able to have a spontaneous bowel action although someone will have to remain with him for safety reasons. The assistant must have enough time so that she does not need to hurry the patient, keep looking at her watch and ask him repeatedly if he has finished yet, all of which would have a very inhibitory effect.
   - Learning to balance in sitting during therapy sessions will enable the patient to have some privacy while on the toilet, even though the door is not locked because he will no longer need to have someone standing beside him all the time.
   - As before, treatment of the face and mouth are most important because once the patient can chew and manage solid foods as well as swallow fluids easily he has less tendency to become constipated.

- The more the patient moves and stands, the less he will suffer from constipation as a result of immobility.
- When the patient is eating and drinking, standing and moving with support and able to press actively to move his bowels. the dose of laxative medication is gradually reduced and eventually stopped altogether. Close watch must, however, be kept because with any change of the patient's routine, such as cessation of tube feeding, moving to another ward or to a rehabilitation centre, the problem could arise again and pass unnoticed.

2. Overcoming existing constipation. A patient may be admitted for rehabilitation at a later stage and have an already existing problem of persistent constipation through lack of adequate treatment. In addition, to avoid the possibility of repeated soiling, some patients themselves, their relatives or nursing staff have ill-advisedly adopted a regime of having a bowel motion only once a week, usually with the aid of an enema or manual evacuation each Saturday, the patient remaining constipated for the rest of the time. A normal routine should be re-established as soon as possible to avoid the unwanted side effects. Before starting a regime to retrain regular, timed bowel actions, it is important that the patient's bowels be emptied completely, by means of an enema or manual evacuation if necessary.

- In the evening of the assisted evacuation on the usual day, the patient takes an estimated dose of a plant laxative, judged on the basis of how long he has been constipated, how hard the stool generally is and what medication he has taken previously.
- The following morning after a hot drink or a tube feed, if he is still not able to swallow, he is transferred on to a normal toilet and supported to ensure his safety.
- He is encouraged to breathe deeply, with assistance if required, and asked to bear down. A suppository may be needed to initiate the act of defaecation at first.
- Because of the time which could be involved due to the uncertainty as to the correct dose, the patient's therapy must be cancelled in advance for that day or he should be treated on the ward.
- If he does not succeed in having a bowel motion, manual evacuation or an enema is required. An increased dose of the laxative is administered and the same procedure followed on the next day until he is able to pass a formed but softish stool without the additional measures being necessary.
- If the dose has been too high, then the patient will need to remain on the ward that day and the nursing staff deal with the repeated bowel actions.
- The unpleasantness of the diarrhoea and its consequences will be most frustrating for the patient and he will need plenty of encouragement and sympathetic understanding from the staff if he is expected to continue and not give up before the correct dose has been established. The patient, his family and the staff must all be convinced of the importance of changing the previous routine and understand the reasons for its being changed.

- The patient's diet plays a significant role in maintaining regularity. Once again the treatment of his mouth should be intensified if dysphagia is a problem and one of the reasons for the constipation. In the same way, if frequent diarrhoea is a problem then advice on diet is essential. The patient who is being tube fed will frequently suffer from diarrhoea and may require medication if continence is to be achieved. With intensive orofacial treatment he should be helped to take food by mouth as soon as possible so that his diet can be normalized and the problem overcome.

Avoiding the Negatives Associated with Post-traumatic Epilepsy

Some patients will unfortunately have to contend with the added complication of epilepsy following traumatic brain injury or other forms of brain lesion. The attacks are most likely to develop within the first 12 months after brain damage, frequently commencing during the first week. Such epileptic attacks, known as post-traumatic epilepsy (PTE), are most distressing for the patient, causing problems above and beyond those already confronting him. For successful rehabilitation and later, reintegration in life outside the sheltered confines of a hospital setting, it is of the utmost importance that PTE be managed in the best way possible.

The number of patients who will suffer from PTE is disputable and the reasons for the selectivity remain unclear. Some studies have shown that early epilepsy occurs in about 5% of patients admitted to hospital with head injury, and about one quarter of these cases will continue to have seizures, with epilepsy more likely to occur after open rather than closed head injuries (Shorvon 1988), a likelihood previously noted by Jennet (1979). Armstrong et al. (1990), on the other hand, in a study involving a large number of patients with blunt head injury who were admitted for rehabilitation in an "adult head trauma unit", found that 37% of the patients developed PTE. The higher percentage was almost certainly due to the fact that "the study population was comprised of patients with more severe head injuries and, thus, a higher proportion of risk factors for PTE".

Certain factors have been found to increase the risk of PTE, and the type of lesion and its localization appear to play a significant role (Karbowski 1985). For example, "brain abscess may result in epilepsy in about three-quarters of survivors" (Shorvon 1988). Other risk factors include post-traumatic amnesia lasting more than 24 h, skull fractures and intracranial haemorrhage as well as penetrating injuries and bilateral involvement.

Prophylactic medication is sometimes administered to patients routinely during the first years following brain damage, but the preventative value has not been verified. Despite medication, the incidence of PTE appears to remain unchanged.

Problems Related to PTE

Because it is not yet possible to prevent the development of PTE, it becomes even more important that the associated problems are avoided or minimized in the most effective way. Unless management of the condition is optimal the patient who already has difficulties as a result of the initial brain damage will be ill-equipped to cope with the problems related to the seizures themselves, the anticonvulsant drugs and the attitudes of others towards him.

The Seizures Per Se

The epilepsy in itself with isolated seizures does not seem to cause a deterioration in the majority of patients' cognitive ability. Bourgeois et al. (1983) found no deterioration in intelligence quotient (IQ) in a large group of children with epilepsy, except for those with poorly controlled seizures, and control of seizures was noted to be associated with a stable or increased IQ for patients in remission, but with a decreased IQ in patients whose epilepsy was inadequately controlled (Rodin et al. 1986). It is likely that the frequency of seizures play a role in memory disorders as well, both directly and indirectly. "Directly because seizures with loss of consciousness distort mental functioning, not only during the seizure but also afterwards, sometimes for several days. When a test is carried out after a seizure, the score is lower than when obtained far from it: and when seizures are frequent, far away is never far" (Loiseau et al. 1988).

Indirectly, frequent repeated epileptic attacks may cause cerebral damage which could lead to impaired performances, for example Mouritzen Dam (1980) describes the cell loss in the hippocampus, a structure closely associated with memory processes. Epileptic attacks can also be very demoralizing for the patient as he gradually regains independence. The suddenness of an attack which leaves him lying helpless on the ground at unexpected moments can result in his being unwilling to venture out in unfamiliar or exposed surroundings, particularly if he has been incontinent during an attack. Later, if PTE is not adequately controlled, his potential for independence is limited by his not being able to drive a car, while the dangers inherent in taking a bath or living on his own impose still further limitations.

Anticonvulsant Drug Therapy

To avoid the complications arising from repeated epileptic attacks, drug therapy becomes a necessity, the difficulty being that most of the commonly used prescriptions have been shown to have neurobehavioural sequelae, and a deleterious effect on cognitive functioning including memory. Sedative antiepileptic drugs have been reported as having detrimental effects on memory by Loiseau (1988) who explains that the main antiepileptic drugs are in fact sedative. Normal, healthy volunteers taking certain of the prescriptions demonstrated prolonged reaction times (Iderström et al. 1972; MacPhee et al. 1986), and rated themselves as more sleepy and less able to concentrate. In other studies, subjects rated themselves as being more tired, anxious and depressed, significantly so with regard to the tiredness (Trimble 1988).

Mueller, a neurologist himself, took anticonvulsants prophylactically for 1 year after sustaining a head injury with resultant hemiplegia and makes an interesting observation about the tiredness he experienced. He reports that despite his knowledge of the possible side effects, he was not consciously aware of being tired until the medication was stopped, and only then realized by comparison how very tired he had in fact been (F.-M. Mueller, personal communication). The observation reveals that even if a patient denies being tired, his response does not necessarily provide evidence that he is not suffering from the side effect which can adversely influence his rehabilitation.

Some patients may be taking a combination of drugs and, as Trimble (1988) points out, "although individual drugs may have a different effect with regards to cognitive function, polytherapy itself may be an important variable". An improvement in the mental state of chronic epileptic patients whose polytherapy was reduced to monotherapy was noted by Shorvon and Reynolds (1979) with particular reference to alertness, concentration, drive, mood and sociability. Such symptoms as nystagmus, ataxia and speech which is not clearly articulated may well be the expression of a drug intoxication with the need for a reduction or change in medication (Karbowski 1985).

Because of the different effects of the various medications as well as the different reactions of individual patients to a specific anticonvulsant, the choice of drug can play an important role in rehabilitation. Repeated assessment and reports of observations from all members of the team will provide valuable information for the doctor responsible. As three-quarters of the patients will cease to have seizures after a time (Shorvon 1988), a slow reduction of medication should be attempted but should only be considered after 6 months at the earliest (Schlaegel 1993)

The Attitude of Others Towards the Patient with PTE

Certain studies have indicated that patients with PTE will have less successful rehabilitation outcomes than those without PTE (Armstrong et al. 1990; Dikmen and Reitan 1978). Unfortunately the results tend to be self-fulfilling in that the rehabilitation team may have a less positive attitude towards patients who develop seizures in the early stages. Long and Moore (1979), for example, found that parents of epileptic children have diminished expectations for their child's academic performance, so that "the IQ deterioration might not therefore be linked causally to epilepsy but to the psychosocial consequences of the disease" (Ossetin 1988)

It is most important that all who are involved in the care of the patient should concentrate on the patient's possibilities for improvement and not on the difficulties which might arise as a result of PTE. Firstly, it should be remembered that test batteries relating to cognitive function frequently are not related to actual functional activities in real life and secondly that statistics do not refer to individuals, so that many patients with PTE will do extremely well. Despite the somewhat negative statistical results of the Armstrong study, the authors point out that the patients in both groups, those with and without PTE, demonstrated "significant treatment gains on measures of PT [physiotherapy], OT [occupational therapy], speech, psychology, therapeutic recreation and nursing", and emphasize that; "both groups were able to participate in the rehabilitation program and to make significant functional gains which resulted in greater independence at discharge" (Armstrong et al. 1990).

The patient with PTE should be treated in the same way as his non-PTE counterpart and thus be given an equal chance of a successful outcome. The way in which the patient is treated during and after an epileptic attack can help to make the experience less traumatic for him and the after effects less discouraging.

During an Attack

The therapist, the nurse and the patient's relatives should be carefully instructed as to how to behave in the event of a seizure occurring while they are with the patient. It can be very distressing or even frightening for someone, for example the therapist, to be faced with the situation of a patient having a severe seizure while she is treating him if she has not had adequate preparation and does not know exactly what to do and how to react. She should lie the patient down on the floor, as he might otherwise fall off the plinth and injure himself. After placing pillows strategically to prevent his hurting himself against nearby furniture or the floor, she must call the doctor responsible for the patient or ask another person to do so for her.

If there are other patients in the vicinity a screen should be placed to shield him from view in order to avoid their being upset and behaving differently towards him after the event. The therapists who are with the other patients should explain to them calmly that nothing serious has happened and that all will be well in a short while, that the patient concerned has just had a slight attack.

The therapist remains close to the patient, in contact if possible, and, as he starts to come round, talks to him calmly and confidently in a normal tone of voice, explaining what has happened and telling him that he is quite all right again.

Should the patient not regain consciousness immediately after the seizure has subsided, he must be positioned on his side to avoid the danger of aspiration. Once the attack has passed, and the doctor has checked the patient, it is advisable not to have an emergency trolley rushed in to transport him back to the ward. It is important that the patient does not become alarmed and think that something serious has occurred, because he will otherwise be terrified of having another seizure.

After the Attack

The patient will often feel tired and rather disorientated after a major attack, and it should be remembered that certain cognitive performances such as memory and attention may be reduced for some time thereafter. The therapist should adjust the tasks she sets the patient appropriately so that he will not be disappointed in his achievement or become frustrated when he is unable to complete a task which he had been able to complete successfully only the day before.

Conclusion

Disorders of perception are closely linked to the many and varied problems which arise as a result of brain damage, whatever its cause may be. It could in fact be said that perceptual disturbances are at the root of all the patient's difficulties including the loss of motor abilities. Although teaching the patient to walk again has always been a major goal in rehabilitation, it should never be forgotten that the ability would be of little use to him if he were unable to communicate his wishes when he arrived at his destination or perform the task which was the reason for his walking somewhere in the first place. Certainly, the disturbed perception and its symptomatic manifestations are the most difficult for those who care for him to deal with or accept because it is for them as if his mind and hence his personality has changed. The patient is however the same person with the same stored experiences and character traits, only he is now desperately trying to cope with an "inexplicable world" and his place in it without all the necessary processes required for exploration, adaptation and organization.

Because the brain functions as a whole and not as a mosaic made up of separate parts which function in complete isolation, damage to one area will affect the smooth, efficient working of the others to a greater or lesser degree. The patient will, therefore, never have difficulty with only one task but will reveal similar difficulties with other tasks of equal complexity. In the same way, treatment aimed to improve any function will effect other functions as well, so that, for example, input through the patient's hand while he is sitting down may result in better balance in a standing position or his being able to articulate more clearly when speaking.

The possibilities for treatment are therefore endless and although it can be said that any input or stimulation is better than none at all, the more direct the input the more successful the treatment will be. No other sensory modality is as direct as that of touch, and it is the only modality that can be manipulated directly. The therapist cannot move the patient's eyes in such a way that a visual input is ensured, nor can she be certain that he is receiving an auditive stimulus merely because she has directed his ears towards a sound. If, however, the patient's hands and body are guided in contact with his surroundings and actual objects, then some tactile input is assured.

Above all, whether the patient is still in coma, or has already recovered sufficiently to carry out simple everyday tasks, perhaps even complex ones, he remains a human being no matter how helpless or different he may be at that time. Great care must be taken to treat him with kindness and respect at all times, because the words of Bentham (1789) are equally applicable to all patients who have suffered brain damage: "The question is not, Can they reason? nor, Can they talk, but Can they suffer?"

2 Early Positioning in Bed and in the Wheelchair

It is essential for the patient who is unconscious or still unable to move himself actively to be positioned correctly at all times, and to have his position changed at regular intervals. A routine should be established so that he is turned every 2–3 h in the early stages as Bromley (1976) describes for the treatment of paraplegia and tetraplegia of spinal origin. The routine turning must be continued until the patient regains consciousness and is able to turn over on his own.

Turning and Positioning in Bed

Supine Lying

The supine position should be avoided whenever possible because it is the position which has many incipient dangers for the patient. With the neck in extension, extensor tone throughout the body tends to be increased although the patient's arms will frequently pull into flexion. If the patient is nursed exclusively in a supine position, there is a very real danger that his neck will stiffen completely with no flexion possible at all and that his arms will develop marked flexion contractures (Fig. 2.1). Should the patient vomit while lying on his back, the risk of an aspiration pneumonia will be greater. Pressure sores can easily develop over the bony sacrum and on his heels. Sustained neck extension can cause severe headache and facial pain later, particularly if the patient has suffered a traumatic brain injury, because in such cases the cervical spine will invariably have sustained some damage as a result of the forceful injury to his head (Schultz and Semmes 1950). A neck which has become fixed in an extended position is associated with difficulties in mouth closure, eating, drinking, breathing, speaking and sitting in a wheelchair (Fig. 2.2), as well as with maintaining balance in all positions.

Through prolonged immobilization in bed, lying supine, the patient's thoracic spine becomes rigid in extension. In addition, there may be distortion of the ribcage, which is typically flattened from anterior to posterior, resulting in decreased respiratory function. The concomitant retraction of the scapulae and loss of upper trunk rotation are difficult to overcome later and can delay full functional use of the hands in front of the body (Fig. 2.3).

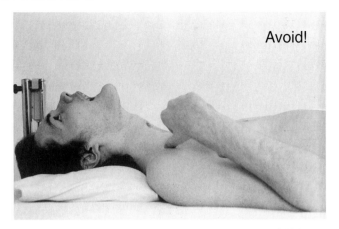

Fig. 2.1. A patient nursed exclusively in supine with only one small pillow exhibits rigid hyperextension of his neck and trunk with flexion contractures of his elbows

Nursing and medical procedures will necessitate the patient's lying on his back at certain times but the periods can be shortened as much as possible. As soon as the required procedures have been completed, the patient should be turned onto his side once again.

It is a common practice in some intensive care units for the patient to be nursed in supine with only a small flat cushion beneath his head (Fig. 2.4a). When he is obliged to lie on his back for certain periods, the position of his head and neck

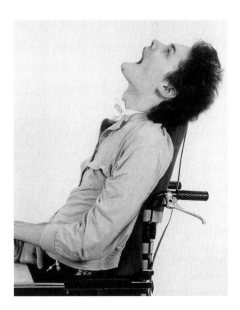

Fig. 2.2. The hyperextension of neck and trunk causes problems in sitting and impedes mouth closure, swallowing and speaking

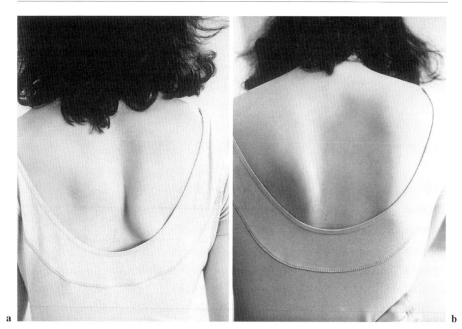

a   b

Fig. 2.3a,b. Thoracic spine fixed in extension with scapula retraction after prolonged immobilization in supine. **a** Scapulae crossed in upright positions. **b** Marked limitation of scapulae protraction is still a a problem 3 years after brain injury

should be optimized by supporting his head instead on a large pillow so that the neck no longer lies in extension and the resultant problems can be avoided (Fig. 2.4b).

Side Lying

When the patient lies on his side, spasticity is reduced and there is no pressure on the sacrum. Lying first on one side and then the other assists drainage of secretions from the lungs, which is particularly important for the tracheostomized patient or for the patient who is unable to cough adequately. Physiotherapy to assist removal of secretions should be performed before and immediately after the patient has been turned onto his side.

Turning the Patient onto His Side

At first, when the patient is deeply unconscious, he will need to be turned over passively by two assistants, either nursing staff or a therapist and nurse. As soon as he appears to be reacting to stimuli, no matter how slight his reaction may be, the

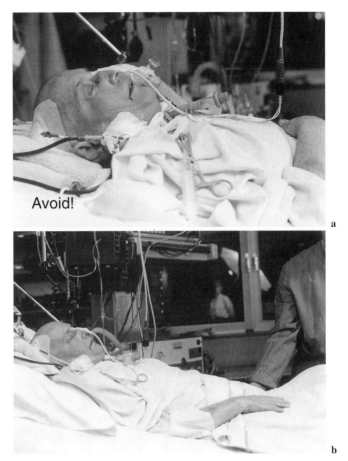

Avoid!

a

b

Fig. 2.4a. With only one small pillow beneath her head, the patient's neck is hyperextended.
b A large pillow corrects the position

therapist provides the opportunity for him to participate actively in some way. The amount of active participation is gradually increased until he is able to turn over on his own using a normal pattern of movement.

Rolling over onto his side and back again is an important activity for the patient in that it incorporates many of the active movements required for walking and balancing. Considered in relation to normal development, it is the young child's first independent form of locomotion as he moves to reach an object, and forms the basis for walking later. For the patient, rolling over is a relatively simple movement sequence which, if taught correctly from the start, will make other functional activities such as turning over in bed, sitting up from lying and walking, easier for him.

Turning the Unconscious Patient

The patient's head is turned to the side towards which he is being turned and supported on a pillow. His knees are flexed, and one of the assistants turns them to the side while the other assistant turns the patient's shoulders and upper trunk (Fig. 2.5). The patient is then moved back towards the edge of the bed and the necessary pillows placed in position.

If it is difficult to hold the patient's head because of skull fractures, open wounds, surgical incisions or operative removal of bone a towel can be placed beneath the head. The assistant can then hold both ends of the towel, one on either side of the patient's head and uses it like a sling when turning him to the side (Fig. 2.6).

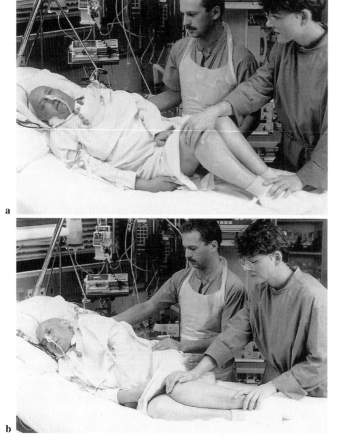

a

b

Fig. 2.5a,b. Turning an unconscious patient onto her side. **a** Both knees flexed, head turned in preparation. **b** Two helpers required, one for the lower limbs, one for the shoulders

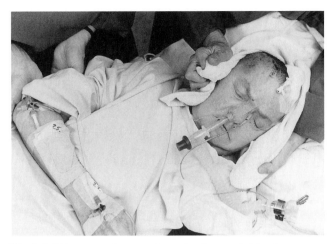

Fig. 2.6. Using a towel to turn the patient's wounded head

Stimulating Early Active Participation from the Patient

As soon as the patient shows signs of regaining consciousness, even if he can only open his eyes or move one of his limbs, for example, the therapist can try to stimulate some active movement when turning him onto his side. She places his limbs in an optimal position to facilitate the movement after reducing any overt hypertonus (Fig. 2.7a). She holds his legs in such a position that they will not impede the turning movement in any way, and then calls on the patient to turn towards her, guiding his uppermost arm forwards as she does so (Fig. 2.7b,c). The patient's head may not turn at once, but it is possible that if the therapist allows him a little time and waits for a reaction, then he will actively turn his head.

It should be remembered that carrying out a change of position swiftly may be easier for the assistants, but will give the patient no chance to take part actively in the procedure.

Turning with More Active Participation from the Patient

The therapist can encourage the patient to rotate his head and shoulders to one side actively as if to start turning over. She assists the movement by placing one of her arms behind his upper trunk and head to facilitate flexion with rotation. With her other hand she draws his uppermost arm and shoulder forwards (Fig. 2.8a). Once the rotatory movement is flowing easily, the therapist asks the patient to try and remain in the position with his head and shoulders turned to one side while she lessens the amount of support she is giving (Fig. 2.8b). The therapist moves the patient's leg forwards and, as she moves it, she calls on him to turn his head and shoulders actively (Fig. 2.8c).

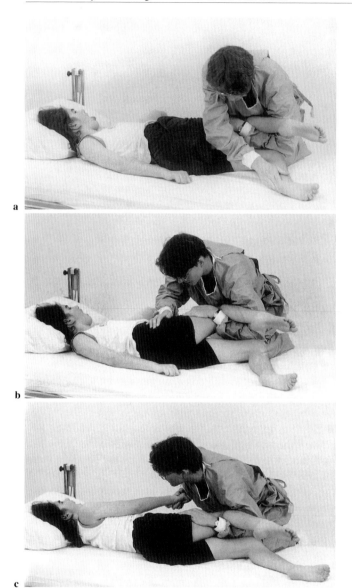

Fig. 2.7a–c. Facilitating early active participation when turning. **a** Legs in step position after inhibition of spasticity. **b** Drawing the pelvis forward with the weight of the leg supported. **c** Guiding the arm forwards to encourage the patient to turn her head

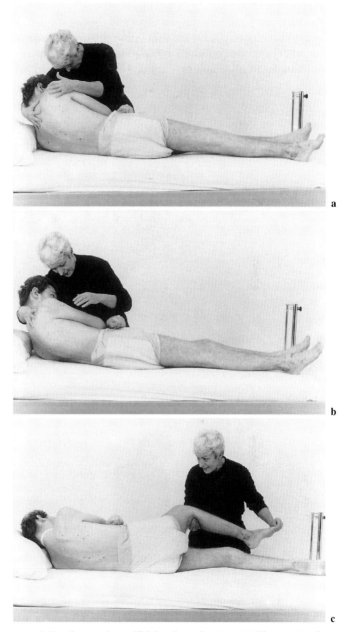

Fig. 2.8a–c. Stimulating more activity when turning. **a** Helping the patient to rotate his upper trunk.
b Instructing him to hold the position. **c** Assisting the forward movement of his uppermost leg

Turning Over Actively in a Normal Pattern

The therapist facilitates the movement by tipping the patient's head forwards lightly with her fingers and at the same time rotating it in the required direction. With
her other hand she helps him to leave his undermost arm lying relaxed on the bed at
right angles to his trunk (Fig. 2.9a). The patient should lift his moving leg off the

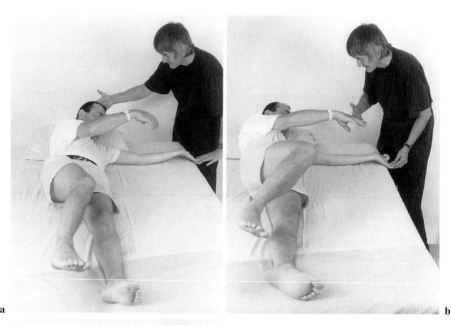

a   b

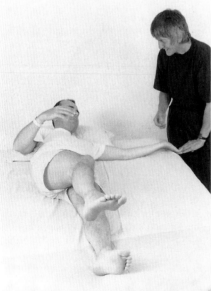

Fig. 2.9a–c. Facilitating active turning in
a normal pattern. **a** Guiding the head
movement. **b** Drawing the uppermost arm
forward **c** Returning to supine with the
c   arm remaining in abduction

bed, without pushing off with his foot as he does so. The therapist guides his upper-most arm forward as he brings his leg forwards with only slight flexion of the hip and knee, and lowers it onto the bed in front of him in a controlled way (Fig. 2.9b). When returning to a supine position, he once again lifts his leg into the air and rotates his trunk backwards at the same time, holding his head in flexion until his leg has been slowly lowered to lie extended on the bed before letting it relax down on the pillow (Fig. 2.9c). He then repeats the movement without the thera-pist's assistance.

Positioning the Patient on His Side

Position A
For the majority of patients the most satisfactory position is lying right on the side with both knees flexed and a large pillow placed between them (Fig. 2.10). With his knees and hips flexed the patient's legs are less likely to push repeatedly into ex-tension, which often causes him to roll back into the supine position.

The patient's head is supported on a large pillow so that it lies somewhat higher than his trunk. In this way lateral flexion of the neck to both sides is maintained, a movement which can easily become limited otherwise.

A pillow is tucked in firmly behind his back to hold his trunk in the correct position, i.e. lying at an angle of 90 to the surface of the bed, parallel to the edge of the bed and with the spine neither too flexed nor excessively extended.

One or two pillows are placed between the patient's knees to prevent any pres-sure over their bony medial aspects and also to maintain some degree of abduction of his hips, which will help to prevent increased extensor tone in his legs.

A pillow placed over the patient's trunk supports his uppermost arm and the other arm lies comfortably in some degree of flexion at his side.

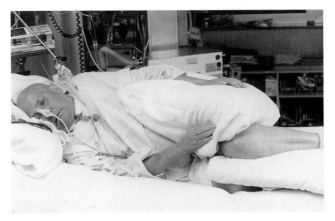

Fig. 2.10. Side lying position with both knees flexed and arms in slight flexion. The patient's head lies on a large pillow

Position B

If the patient's arm shows a tendency to pull into flexion, it can be supported in such a way that it remains in extension (Fig. 2.11a). The therapist or nurse first releases the flexor spasticity by pushing gently but firmly down on the patient's sternum with one of her hands, while at the same time she places her other hand under his scapula and draws it well forwards (Fig. 2.11b). The patient's own weight will keep the scapula in protraction and the elbow will no longer pull into flexion.

Many hospital beds have a removable footboard which can be used to support the extended arm. The nurse places one end of the board underneath the mattress, on a level with the patient's shoulder (Fig. 2.12a). The patient's arm can then lie at right angles to his trunk, supported on a rolled pillow which is placed upon the board to ensure the correct height (Fig. 2.12b,c).

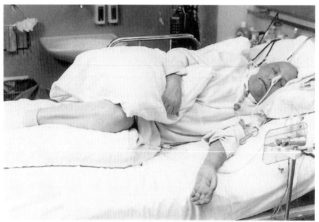

a

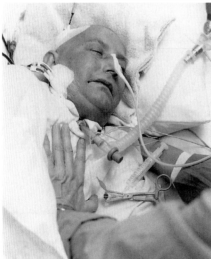

b

Fig. 2.11a,b. Side lying with one arm in extension. **a** Scapula protraction, the arm lies at right angles to the trunk with the wrist extended over the edge of the bed. **b** Pressure over the sternum to facilitate scapula protraction

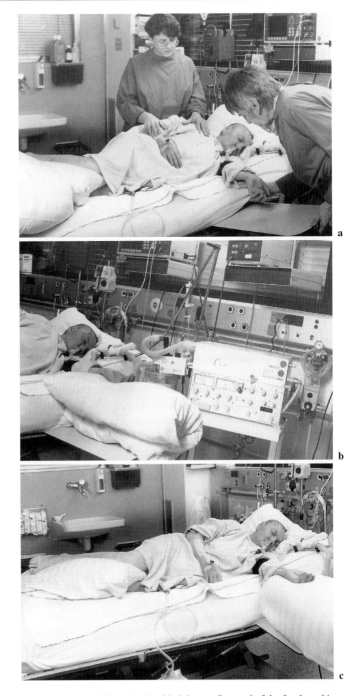

Fig. 2.12a–c. Supporting the extended arm with patient in side lying. **a** One end of the footboard is placed beneath the mattress. **b** A rolled pillow supports the extended arm. **c** The arm well supported in the corrected position

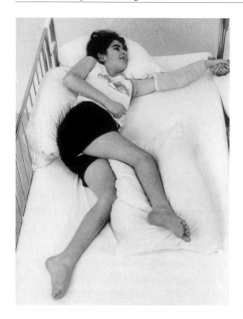

Fig. 2.13. Side lying with one leg in front of the other for the patient with less extensor spasticity

Position C

If extensor spasticity does not present a problem, either right from the beginning or later as the patient's condition improves, then it is desirable to place his legs in a step position, that is with the undermost leg in hip extension and his other leg lying on a pillow in some degree of flexion of the hip and knee. The pillow not only supports the uppermost limb but also prevents the lower one from pulling into flexion (Fig. 2.13).

Overcoming Difficulties in Maintaining the Position

Marked Extensor Spasticity

Increased tone in the extensor muscles of the trunk and legs will cause problems for the nursing staff and the therapist both when turning the patient onto his side and when trying to maintain the patient's position on his side. The patient's legs push so strongly into extension that he will often end up lying on his back in total extension (Fig. 2.14a). For such patients it is particularly important that they are not left to lie on their back and so a way must be sought in which the problem can be solved. A self-reinforcing situation will otherwise occur in that the patient who has strong extensor spasticity will lie continuously supine, the very position that increases extensor tone.

PROBLEM SOLVING

When lying on his side, the patient's head and neck are flexed and his arms are folded across his chest. Both hips and knees are flexed and two or three large pillows are placed between his legs. The wide abduction of the hips will decrease

Fig. 2.14a–c. Side lying when marked extensor spasticity is a problem. **a** The helper unable to flex the trunk or limbs. **b** Flexion of neck and arms inhibits mass extension with two large pillows between the legs for increased abduction. **c** The patient remains in the corrected position

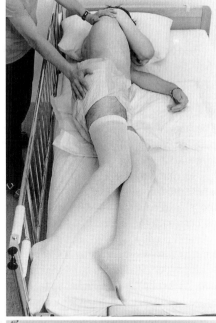

a

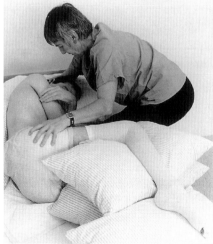

b

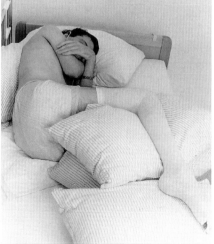

c

the extensor thrust in the lower limbs (Fig. 2.14b,c). It is easier to achieve the fully flexed position if the therapist first inhibits the spasticity by flexing the trunk and limbs with rotation (see Figs. 3.7 and 3.28). In some cases it may only be possible for the therapist to flex the neck, trunk and limbs if the patient is first turned onto his side.

When turning the patient on to his side and then correcting his position, the whole procedure is performed slowly and quietly, and once the patient is in the correct position the nurse or therapist stays next to him with her hands maintaining contact with his trunk. Only when she feels that he has relaxed again does she slowly and carefully move away.

The bedclothes should be in place before she takes her hands from his body. If they are suddenly pulled up over the patient, the stimulus may elicit a strong extensor reaction once again.

Restlessness and Hyperactivity
The patient who moves excessively in the bed, turning over constantly from one position to the other, presents a big problem for the staff (Fig. 2.15a–c). Such movements can be interpreted as being a desperate search for information from his surroundings. The behaviour of normal subjects who are in a strange room when the lights suddenly go out or if they are blindfolded is very similar. They too turn themselves in all directions and seek information by touching nearby objects with their hands and feet to establish where they are.

PROBLEM SOLVING
Firm padded blocks can be placed around the patient to reduce the open area of the bed, so that he lies in a niche, so to speak. In most cases, the patient will lie quietly as he has direct contact with many parts of his body. The packs cannot fix him mechanically in any position but quieten him by providing the information as to where he is in space, which the mattress and open area of the bed do not do. (Fig. 2.15d).

The patient should never be tied down as he will only fight against any such restraint and in so doing impede his circulation and injure his skin.

A point which is often overlooked in the acute care of the patient is that he will become restless and move about constantly if he is kept in bed without any form of exercise or distraction. The patient who is hyperactive in lying should not be sedated but should be sat out of bed, be helped to stand and be taken around in the wheelchair for a change of scene instead. Any one of us would become restless if kept in bed day and night with absolutely nothing to do! It is most rewarding to observe how a patient who has worked hard during appropriate therapy will fall asleep immediately when he is put back to bed, almost before his head touches the pillow!

Prone Lying

It is of great benefit to the patient to lie prone for some periods each day. He should be carefully positioned on his stomach as soon as he is not being artificially respirated and as soon as any additional fractures have been stabilized. A tracheostomy alone does not contraindicate lying in a prone position as the pillows can be so arranged that the patient can breathe freely (Fig. 2.16). In fact, drainage of secretions from the respiratory tract is facilitated by the position and a shallow receptacle or draw-sheet can be placed appropriately to collect them.

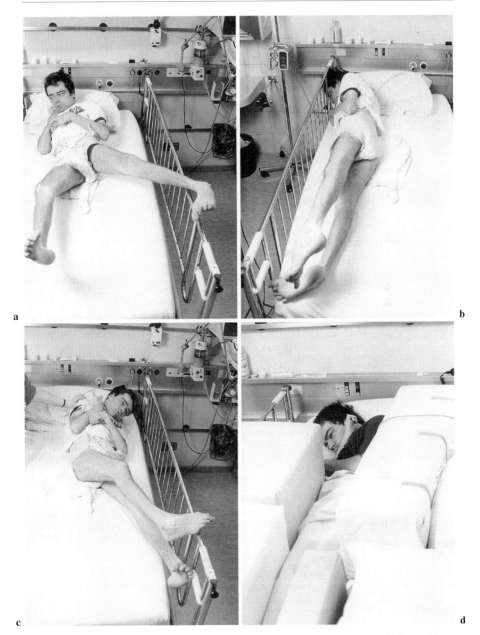

Fig. 2.15a–d. Positioning the very restless patient. **a** Patient's legs held in extreme joint positions. **b** Constantly turning over. **c** Feet always moving on and over the cot sides. **d** With firm packs surrounding him, the patient calms down and sleeps

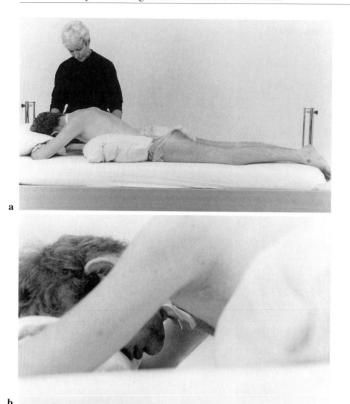

Fig. 2.16a,b. Patient with tracheostomy lying prone. **a** Pillows under his chest and forehead leave the airway clear. **b** Tracheostomy free and limitation of range in shoulders accommodated

Turning Over to Prone

When the patient is still unable to move actively at all, two assistants are required to turn him to ensure that his shoulders and hips are not traumatized. One assistant stands at the head of the bed, from which the headboard has been removed. When rolling the patient over his right side to prone, she turns his head to the right and places his right arm in elevation. The other assistant lifts the patient's left leg, supporting it adequately beneath the thigh as well as below the knee (Fig. 2.17a). As she moves the leg forwards, the first assistant moves the patient's left shoulder and arm forwards, and draws the whole limb into elevation as he turns over completely onto his stomach (Fig. 2.17b). The position of the hips and shoulders is then adjusted by the assistants to ensure that they are lying comfortably in a relaxed position (Fig. 2.17c).

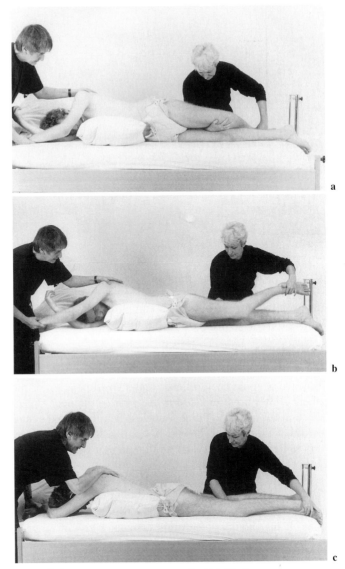

Fig. 2.17a–c. Turning the patient into a prone position **a** Standing at the head end of the bed a helper takes care of his shoulders **b** A second helper lifts his leg up and over the other. **c** Straightening out his thorax and legs with his feet over the end of the mattress

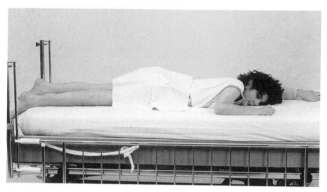

Fig. 2.18. Prone lying position with only a small pillow required beneath the abdomen to allow catheter drainage

Position in Prone

Ideally, if there are no secondary complications, the patient lies flat on his stomach with a pillow underneath his trunk to allow free drainage of the catheter if one is present (Fig. 2.18).

The patient's head can be turned either to the left or the right, but the side to which it is turned should be varied regularly in order to avoid the asymmetrical influence of tonic neck reflexes and a fixed position of the cervical spine. If the patient shows a preference for one side or the neck appears to be stiffer in one direction the head should nevertheless be placed to that side as well, but for short periods at first until it relaxes. A small pillow placed under his cheek allows the head to lie with less cervical rotation to that side, until it can remain easily in the correct position.

His arms are positioned with the shoulders in elevation and some abduction. They should not lie at the patient's sides because the position reinforces medial rotation of the shoulders and increases the kyphotic position of the thoracic spine. If his shoulders feel tight or have a loss of range of movement, a pillow or even two pillows placed beneath his trunk enable the arms to lie in a relaxed position with less elevation until full range of motion has been regained (see Fig. 2.16a).

The patient's legs are extended with the hips abducted and placed so that his feet lie over the end of the bed in some degree of dorsiflexion, the footboard having been removed for this purpose.

Problem solving

Even if a patient does not have full range of motion in his limbs, it is most important that he lie prone, particularly if hip and knee flexion contractures have already developed (Fig. 2.19). It will, however, be necessary to arrange pillows or packs in such a way as to make the position possible at first (Fig. 2.20). Accord-

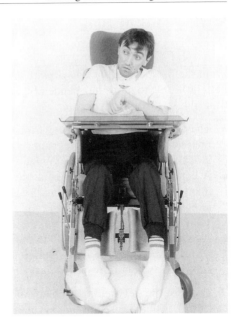

Fig. 2.19. It is important for a patient with severe contractures to sit out of bed and to lie prone

ing to the degree and location of the contractures, the therapist and nurse use their ingenuity to enable the patient to achieve the prone position, and then gradually remove the supports as his mobility increases until such time as he can lie completely flat on the bed. It is well worth the effort involved for the staff because many contractures can be overcome to an amazing degree simply by lying the patient in the prone position every day, slowly increasing the time he spends in the corrected position.

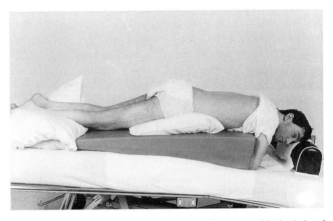

Fig. 2.20. Despite the severe contractures, the same patient is able to lie prone with the help of different supports

Sitting Out of Bed

From the intensive care stage onwards, the patient must sit out of bed every day until he is able to move independently. Transferring him directly into a wheelchair from the start has many advantages:

- The patient can be moved away from the bed, which enables the therapist or his relatives to guide him in a greater variety of situations. The change of scene alone will provide further stimulation.
- A better sitting posture can be achieved in a wheelchair because there are so many possibilities for adjusting the height and inclination of the backrest, the armrests and the footplates, and for using the numerous adaptations which are available, such as a fitted table.
- As soon as the patient is able to move actively in some way, the wheelchair allows him to start moving himself from one place to another, usually long before he is able to walk independently.

Many of the devastating problems which make the later rehabilitation of the patient so difficult arise through his being kept lying in bed for too long. He must be moved out of bed and positioned in the wheelchair, even if he is still apparently unconscious. All too frequently, the patient is nursed only in bed for weeks if not months following his accident. Increased hypertonus, contractures, decubitus formation and even the development of a bite reflex result from the immobilization and the lack of any meaningful stimulation.

Communication within the team is essential if the above-mentioned situation is to be avoided, and it should be carefully considered if there is really a reason why the patient cannot sit up out of bed. Just as patients with other severe injuries or those who have undergone extensive surgical procedures are brought out of bed at a very early stage, so too should the brain-injured patient be sat out of bed early with appropriate support. There are in fact very few contraindications to sitting. Alarming hypotension or an associated bilateral pelvic fracture would make a sitting position untenable, for instance, but the commonest reason given as to why the patient was left in bed for so long is that he was unconscious or attached to a respirator. With careful handling and positioning, these two reasons are not valid, and any associated difficulties can be overcome with a little effort and initiative. The patient's whole future may depend upon the engagement and willingness of the staff at this stage.

Transferring the Patient from Bed to Wheelchair

Moving from Lying to Sitting

When the patient is still unconscious or unable to move in any way, the therapist brings him to a sitting position passively.

The patient is turned onto his side with his hips and knees flexed. Standing beside the bed the therapist encircles his knees with one arm while her other arm is placed around behind his neck, with her hand on his thoracic spine (Fig. 2.21a).

The therapist moves the patient's legs over the side of the bed and by transferring her own body-weight laterally at the same time, she brings his trunk up to an upright position (Fig. 2.21b,c).

With her legs pressing against his knees, she can prevent the patient from sliding forward off the bed, and can support his head against her shoulder while her hands behind him maintain the position of his trunk (Fig. 2.21d).

Moving to the Edge of the Bed

Before she can transfer the patient into a wheelchair, the therapist must first move him forwards to the edge of the bed so that his feet can be placed flat on the floor. She does so by bringing first one of his buttocks forwards and then the other, shifting his weight well over to the opposite side each time she does so.

The therapist stands in front of the patient with his head resting on one of her shoulders and one arm placed over his shoulders with her hand on his thoracic spine. The patient's trunk is supported by her arm as she places her other hand under his trochanter to lift his buttock on the opposite side and draw it forwards (Fig. 2.22a). She then changes the position of her hands appropriately in order to move his other buttock forward in the same way, as though he were "walking" on his buttocks (Fig. 2.22b).

Recommended Transfers

The transfer into the wheelchair is performed quietly, calmly and slowly so as not to alarm the patient. Some assistants say that they prefer to carry out the transfer at speed to lessen the strain on their back, but the sudden movement in space can be very frightening for the patient. Reported incidents where a patient has bitten a helper may well have been caused by his literally "hanging on by the skin of his teeth" because he was terrified of falling while being moved suddenly through the air.

Fig. 2.21a–d

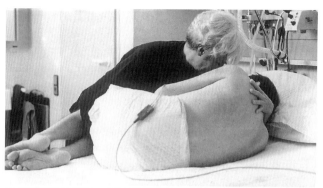

a

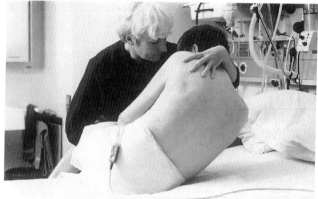

b

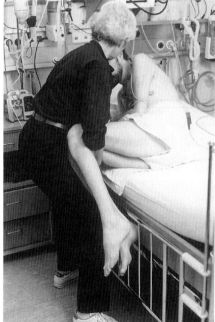

c

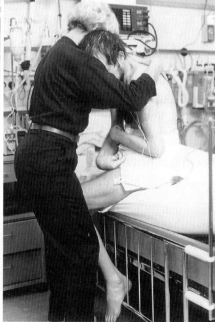

d

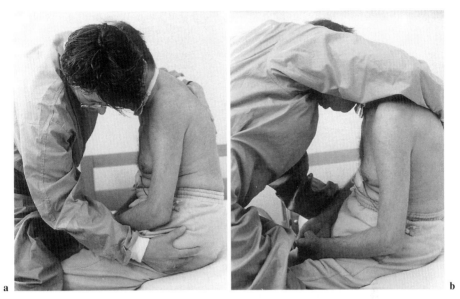

a   b

Fig. 2.22a,b. Moving the patient to the edge of the bed. **a** The therapist lifts one of his buttocks forwards. **b** Her arm around his shoulders prevents his overbalancing

Method 1. With the Patient's Arms Resting on the Therapist's Shoulders

The unconscious or severely disabled patient can usually be transferred from his bed by the therapist alone without too much difficulty. If, however, for any reason she feels uncertain that she can move the patient on her own, an assistant stands in the "V" formed by the chair and the edge of the bed, and places one hand under each of the patient's trochanters.

The wheelchair, with the nearside armrest removed, is placed in line with the bed and as near to the patient as possible. The footrests must always be turned right back or removed altogether to prevent either the patient or the helper from injuring their ankles against them (Fig. 2.23a).

With her knees pressed against the patient's knees and his arms resting on her shoulders, the therapist presses down over the patient's scapulae and uses her knees to extend his until his seat leaves the bed. His head rests on one of her shoulders. As the therapist leans the patient forwards, the assistant helps to lift his bottom off the bed and turn it towards the wheelchair (Fig. 2.23b).

The therapist turns the patient, pivoting him around until she can lower his bottom well back into the wheelchair (Fig. 2.23c).

◀ **Fig. 2.21a–d.** Bringing the patient from lying to sitting. **a** The therapist's arm around his flexed knees, her other beneath his neck. **b** His legs over the side of the bed. **c** lifting his trunk towards the vertical. **d** Preventing his knees from sliding forwards while supporting his head and trunk

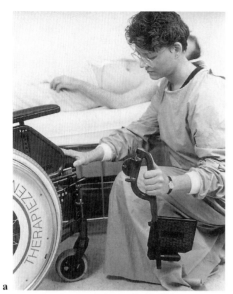

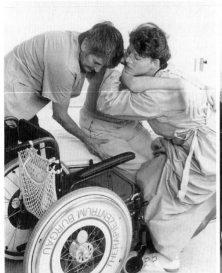

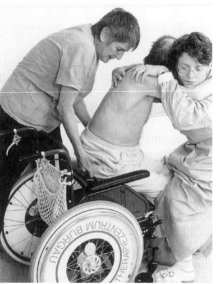

Fig. 2.23a–c. Transferring a severely disabled patient. **a** The wheelchair is placed close to the bed and the footplate removed. **b** An assistant helps to lift his bottom. **c** His seat is turned and lowered well back in the chair

Method 2. With the Patient's Arms Down in Front of Him

If the patients shoulders feel at all stiff or have marked limitation of movement, the therapist leaves his arms in front of his body when transferring him. As before, she moves him forwards by lifting first one trochanter and then the other until both his feet are flat on the floor (Fig. 2.24). Standing in front of him she presses her knees

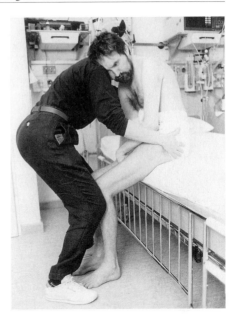

Fig. 2.24. Moving the patient so that his feet are flat on the floor

against the front and slightly to the side of his. One of her arms is placed round behind him so that her hand is over his thoracic spine (Fig. 2.25a). Her other hand pushes forwards and downwards over his scapula as she uses her knees to extend his knees so that his weight is taken through his legs (Fig. 2.25b). She pivots the patient round and lowers his seat well back into the wheelchair (Fig. 2.25c).

Method 3. With the Patient's Trunk Flexed

Another useful and safe way to transfer the patient is for the therapist to lean him well forward and use her hands over his trochanters to lift his seat as she presses her knees against his (Fig. 2.26a,b). The patient's head is supported against the side of the therapist's trunk and/or hip, as she turns him towards the chair or bed (Fig. 2.26c).

Method 4. Using A Sliding Board

When a patient is extremely heavy, the therapist and a helper can use a sliding board made of solid, polished wood to take the patient's weight when transferring him. The bed is lowered to the same height as the chair and the board is placed so as to span the distance between them. The patient's bottom is edged onto the board so that he can slide along it into the chair (Fig. 2.27a). The therapist stands in front of the patient and keeps his trunk flexed forwards as she uses her hands to slide him along the board (Fig. 2.27b). Her knees against his prevent his seat from slipping forwards off the board. If necessary, a helper stands behind the patient and can help to move his bottom along the board or prevent his trunk from extending suddenly.

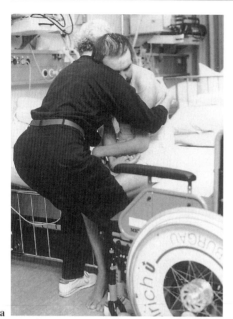

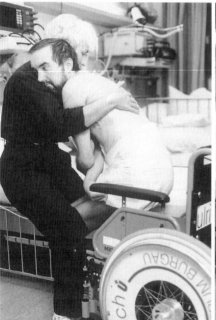

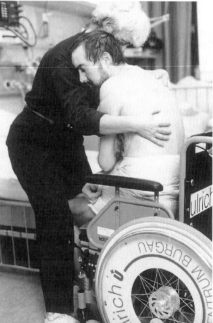

Fig. 2.25a–c. Transferring the unconscious patient whose shoulders feel stiff. **a** His trunk brought forwards, head supported and arms left down in front of him. **b** The therapist extends his knees with hers while her hands press his thorax forwards. **c** Placing his seat well back in the chair

Fig. 2.26a–c. Transferring the patient
with his trunk flexed forward. **a** The
therapist flexes his trunk and supports his
head against her side. **b** She puts one hand
under each trochanter. **c** Pressing her
knees against his she lifts and turns his
seat onto the bed

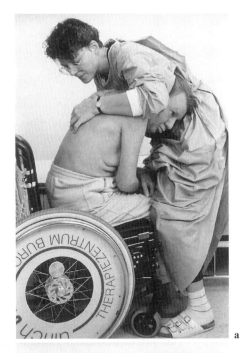

a

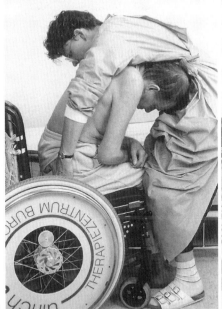

b

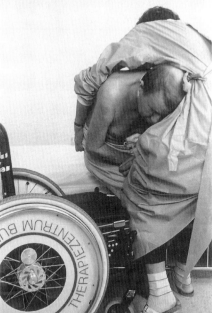

c

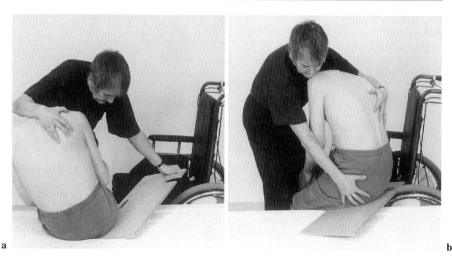

a   b

Fig. 2.27a,b. Using a sliding board. **a** One end of the board is placed beneath the patient's buttocks.
b Sliding along the board

When the patient is being put back to bed the same methods are used to transfer
him from the wheelchair and to move his seat back on the bed. Such transfers can
also be used when the patient is being moved onto the toilet, transferred to another
chair or even into a car.

Position in the Wheelchair

The patient should be seated well back in the chair in an upright position with his
arms supported on a table in front of him. The table provides constant information
for the patient and will also lessen the likelihood of his seat sliding forwards out of
the chair (Fig. 2.28a).

When the patient is being moved from one place to another in the wheelchair, a
table fitted to the arms of the chair can be used (Fig. 2.28b). With his arms supported on a table the posture of his trunk is improved. Ideally, his trunk should be as
upright as possible and his head free to move. The height of the wheelchair table
should be such that his arms can rest on it without his shoulder girdle being elevated yet sufficiently high to allow his trunk to remain upright.

The patient sits with his hips at an angle of approximately 90 with the whole
length of his thighs supported by the seat of the wheelchair. The thighs should be
parallel to one another, neither pulling in towards one another nor pressing outwards in abduction against the sides of the chair. The footrests are adjusted so that
his knees form an angle of 90 flexion or slightly more. The patient's feet are well
supported on the footrests with his ankles in dorsiflexion.

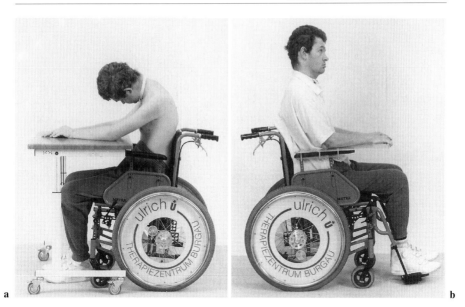

a   b

Fig. 2.28a,b. Sitting position in the wheelchair. **a** With a table placed in front of the patient. **b** With a table attached to the wheelchair arms

The ideal position in the wheelchair may be difficult to achieve when the patient is first brought out of bed, even more so if he has been left in bed for a long time and has developed secondary complications. It is essential that the nurses together with the therapist strive to sort out the problems with imagination and enthusiasm, guided by their observation of the patient when he is sitting, and by trial and error.

If the patient's posture is grossly abnormal, attempting to feed him or carry out oral hygiene will surely end in failure, as will any therapeutic procedures aimed at improving his ability to speak (Fig. 2.29). It is most detrimental to the patient if he is left sitting for long periods in an abnormal posture (Fig. 2.30). Increased spasticity with concomitant contracture development in the arms and legs are almost inevitable. Spinal deformities arising from prolonged sitting in asymmetrical or kyphotic postures can be difficult to correct later. The sustained head position with the neck in flexion, extension or lateral flexion can cause severe headache of cervical origin or intense pain in nerve root distribution, both of which are often erroneously thought to be symptoms arising from the brain lesion itself.

It should be clearly understood that the patient cannot be tied in place or wedged in with a pummel between his legs if he tends to slide out of the wheelchair. Such short-term solutions will only lead to skin damage or pressure areas and the patient will fight against painful restraints of this type. In the same way, if his head is strongly flexed a firm collar does not solve the problem but only causes pressure sores under his chin. Should the patient's head push backwards, fixing a headrest on the back of the chair will increase the neck extension tendency as he will push his head back even harder against the solid support.

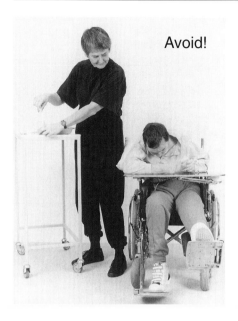

Fig. 2.29. An incorrect sitting posture makes oral hygiene or feeding impossible

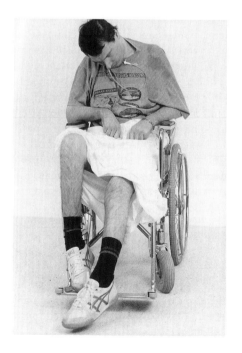

Fig. 2.30. An abnormal posture in the wheelchair increases spasticity and can lead to the development of contractures

Choosing a Suitable Wheelchair

The first line of approach when attempting to improve the patient's sitting posture is selecting the right wheelchair for him. There are numerous models available and the therapist must choose which of them is most suitable. It is important to try out several types of wheelchair before the final choice is made and the manufacturers and their representatives are most helpful in this respect.

Points to Consider

- The patient's motor abilities will tend to improve with time and treatment, so that the wheelchair chosen to suit his needs at one stage will need to be reviewed at regular intervals and adapted or changed for another model as required.
- Most patients will learn to walk again, so the wheelchair should be the right one for the present and need not be selected with an eye to the distant future. For example, the therapist may think that the patient sits well in a certain wheelchair but decides against it because it would be too cumbersome for his relatives to lift into the boot of the car. The patient, however, might not yet be at the level where an outing in a car would be feasible. An example would be a patient who has been lying in bed for months, and has severe contractures of his upper and lower limbs and pressure sores. While these problems are being overcome, the therapist may choose a special type of chair to enable him to start sitting out of bed for some periods (Fig. 2.31) and then, as his condition improves, select a lighter, more mobile chair so that he can be taken out and about.
- The wheelchair should be as light as possible without loss of stability, so that the patient or others helping him may push it more easily.

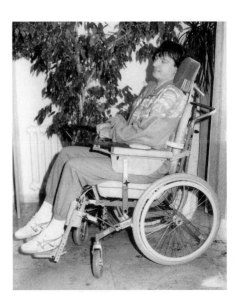

Fig. 2.31. In a more suitable wheelchair the same patient sits correctly (see Fig. 2.30)

- A backrest that can be reclined backwards is useful particularly if the patient has difficulty in holding his head up. An extension for the backrest should be available for a very tall patient.
- For guiding the patient when he is eating or washing himself, it is useful if the backrest can be removed easily (see Fig. 1.5b,c).
- The arms of the wheelchair must be removable so that the patient can be transferred to and from his bed or the toilet without difficulty. It is a great advantage if the height of the armrests is also adjustable for optimal support of the patient's upper limbs with or without a wheelchair table.
- The wheelchair table itself should be inherently stable and long enough to enable the patient's arms to be adequately supported when his trunk is inclined forwards. It is important that the fitting by which the table is attached to the chair is not only stable but also allows easy removal and replacement.
- The seat of the wheelchair must be firm enough so that it does not sag down in the middle causing the patient's legs to adduct mechanically. A thin wooden board can be cut to the correct size, covered with foam rubber and fitted across the seat if necessary.
- Many wheelchair seats are too short and do not support the patient's thighs sufficiently. The supporting surface should extend almost to his knees when his bottom is well back in the chair.
- The height and angle of the footrests need to be adjustable to attain a satisfactory position of the patient's legs. It will frequently help to maintain a good position of his trunk and his feet if his knees are extended a bit more than 90. For the patient whose feet tend to pull back off the footrests and under the chair, padded calfrests are useful attachments. It is not advisable to use a strap behind his legs to prevent them from pulling back as abrasions on his calves are often the result. Heelstops fitted to the footrests are also not recommended as his feet will tend to plantarflex over the front edge of the footplate.
- The small front wheels of the chair should not be air-filled and of the "balloon" type as these make the wheelchair heavier to push and difficult to turn or manoeuvre, particularly on carpeted floors. Their only advantage is a smooth ride when travelling along a rough surface outside.

Suggestions for Using Additional Support

Guided by her observation of the patient when he has been sitting for some time in a corrected position, the therapist can use additional material to support him if necessary.

1. For the patient whose trunk is always too flexed and who also tends to fall to one side: (Fig. 2.32a), a large, firm foam rubber block placed on the wheelchair table under his arms will facilitate more extension of his trunk and help him to control his head (Fig. 2.32b). The patient can also rest his head on the block when he feels tired, with it turned first to one side and then to the other (Fig. 2.32c).

Fig. 2.32a–c. Additional support for the patient's trunk in sitting. **a** The patient's trunk is too flexed and he falls sideways. **b** A padded block on the wheelchair table improves trunk extension. **c** When the patient is tired, his head is supported

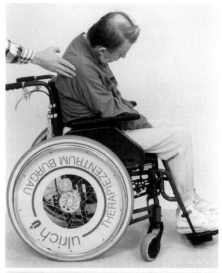

a

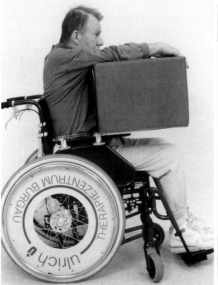

b

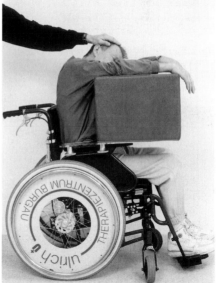

c

2. For the patient whose head and trunk push back into extension, a position often associated with his feet pulling back under the chair (Fig. 2.33a), a firm foam rubber wedge placed on the wheelchair table beneath his arms and in contact with his chest will help to maintain a good position (Fig. 2.33b). A padded board at his back stabilizes his trunk.
3. In the patient whose trunk is constantly displaced laterally with his pelvis shifted to the opposite side causing his legs to adopt a distorted position to-

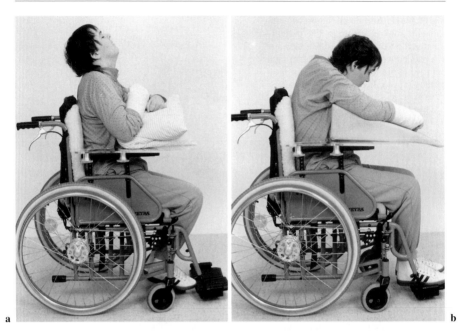

a   b

Fig. 2.33a. Patient's neck and trunk extend and her feet are pulled under the wheelchair. **b** A firm wedge against her chest corrects the problems

wards one side (Fig. 2.34a), the exaggerated "windswept deformity" of the pelvis and legs (Goldsmith et al. 1992) can become a fixed deformity and be detrimental for his walking later. In addition to the wheelchair table, a firm padded block is inserted between the side of the patient's side and the arm of the chair. A padded board is positioned along the outer side of his buttock and thigh, kept in place by the arm of the wheelchair (Fig. 2.34b). Another board reinforces the backrest and assists trunk extension (Fig. 2.34c). If the footrests are set more forwards, the patient's legs are less likely to push into the pattern of total extension as his feet are well supported from below and make better contact with the footplates.

4. For the patient whose legs are always widely abducted and press against the sides of the wheelchair, with his ankles supinating as a result: (Fig. 2.35a), firmly padded boards placed between the arms of the wheelchair and the lateral aspect of the patient's thighs will correct the position in the most satisfactory way (Fig. 2.35b). Not only will his legs remain in position but the pelvis and hence his trunk will be more symmetrical.

Many other ways of improving the individual patient's sitting posture will be discovered by the determined therapist who uses her ingenuity, and the time she takes to sort out the problems will be time well spent.

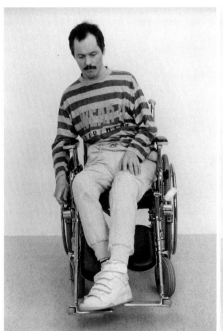
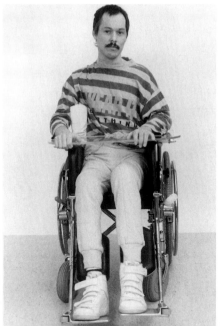

a

b

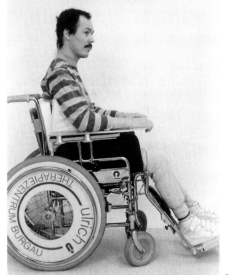

Fig. 2.34a. Patient with lateral shift of trunk and pelvis. **b** Position corrected with wheelchair table, padded block and boards. **c** Backboard and lateral block support his trunk

c

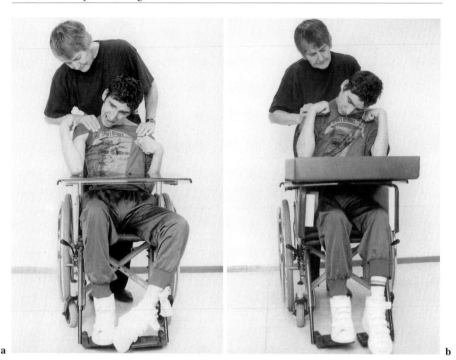

a   b

Fig. 2.35a. Patient with legs abducted and foot supinating. **b** Boards along the lateral aspect of his
thighs correct the position of the lower limbs

Adjusting the Patient's Position in the Wheelchair

It should always be remembered that no position, however good it may look at first,
can be maintained for hours on end. The patient will move, shift his weight or slide
down in the chair after a relatively short time and he should be helped to adjust his
position again without any irritation on the part of the staff. It is after all normal for
people to change their position in sitting frequently even if only by slight alterations in posture. It can be helpful for the staff to experience consciously the number
of times they or the others present alter their position during a team meeting for
example, and to realize how impossible it is to remain absolutely motionless for
any length of time.

   If the patient has slipped down in the chair with his seat moving forwards as
often happens, the therapist or nurse must correct the position at once to prevent his
sliding out of the chair onto the floor (Fig. 2.36a).

   Standing in front of the patient she presses her knees against his to stop him
from sliding any further and flexes his trunk as far forwards as possible with his
head underneath one of her arms (Fig. 2.36b,c).

   Placing her hands underneath the patient's trochanters the therapist leans back
to lift his seat off the chair by using her knees to extend his knees slightly and then
places his bottom well back in the chair (Fig. 2.36d).

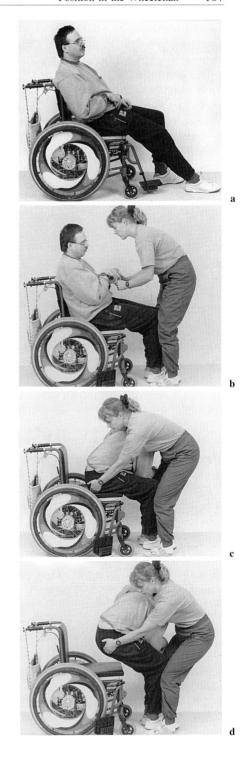

Fig. 2.36a–d. Lifting the patient back in the wheelchair. **a** Position after sliding down in the chair. **b** An assistant prevents further sliding with her knees. **c** Patient's trunk flexed well forward. **d** Lifting his seat to place it back in the chair

Lengthening the Time Spent in Sitting

In the early days, many patients will only be able to tolerate sitting for an hour or so before needing to be put back to bed. It is certainly preferable for them to lie down for a while between periods of sitting than to remain for hours on end in an abnormal posture in the wheelchair. The time which the patient spends in the wheelchair each day should be gradually increased according to how long he can tolerate the sitting position.

The length of time which he is able to spend in the wheelchair is also directly related to the amount of stimulation he receives when out of bed. For anyone, 2 h spent sitting completely still, alone in a room with absolutely nothing to do would seem like an eternity.

The patient's relatives, if carefully guided, can be of inestimable value with regard to providing appropriate stimulation. Some will automatically find ways to entertain the patient and hold his attention, but others will need help in this respect. It is often difficult to talk to someone who is unable to reply and who perhaps does not even appear to understand what is being said to him. Activities, such as those described in Chap. 1, where the patient's hands are guided when performing different tasks are a meaningful way in which his relatives can help him.

At no time should the patient be left sitting completely alone if there is the slightest danger of his falling out of the chair or fainting while in an upright position.

Propelling the Wheelchair Independently

A Standard Wheelchair

As soon as the patient has regained consciousness and is able to sit upright in the wheelchair which has been chosen for him the therapist can start teaching him how to push it himself. The method of propulsion which the therapist chooses will depend upon the individual patient's motor function, that is, which of his limbs he is best able to move actively. It is seldom that a patient can push the wheelchair in the way a patient with a spinal paraplegia does, using both his hands. Many, particularly those who fall within the ataxic group, will in fact not use their hands at all, but use their feet to propel the chair in all directions using a walking action. Others, whose symptoms are of a hemiplegic nature, can use the less affected hand together with the leg on that side to push and steer the wheelchair. In fact it is perfectly feasible for a patient to manage the chair using only one of his legs if the other has not regained sufficient activity and control. The therapist tries out the various possibilities with the patient, guiding the movement of his limbs in the way required to propel the chair forwards and to turn it in different directions. When she feels that he is taking over actively, she decreases the amount of assistance that she is giving. Not only does the therapist guide the patient while he is learning to push the wheelchair, but she also guides his hands when she is teaching him how to put on the brakes, remove the armrests and lift the footrests before transferring onto his bed or the toilet.

For the patient it is a big step forward when he is able to push his chair independently and go somewhere on his own, even if it is only along the hospital corridor at first. The patient should be encouraged to propel the wheelchair and to use it for various self-care activities because in all probability he will be independent in the chair long before he is able to walk around safely on his own. Some patients are unwilling to use the wheelchair because they have been led to believe that if they do they will never learn to walk again, a belief that is quite unfounded and certainly not true.

An Electric Wheelchair

When the patient first regains consciousness and is still dependent in the activities of daily living, it is unlikely that he would be able to manage an electric wheelchair safely. Some type of power-driven chair should however be considered for a patient who is unable to propel a standard wheelchair, not because of any perceptual difficulties which he may have, but because he has severe contractures in his arms and

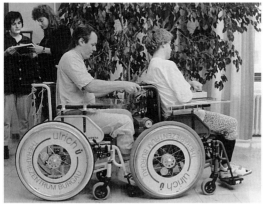
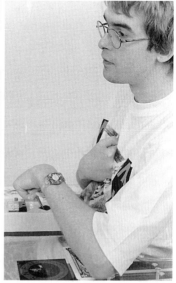

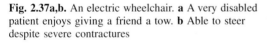
Fig. 2.37a,b. An electric wheelchair. **a** A very disabled patient enjoys giving a friend a tow. **b** Able to steer despite severe contractures

legs which make it impossible. Patients who cannot walk unaided due to marked ataxia which also prevents them from pushing a chair, but who are functioning at a high level when performing other complex tasks can also profit from being able to get around on their own in an electric wheelchair. Certainly they will enjoy the freedom it offers (Fig. 2.37a). Many types of driving mechanism are available and must be selected to suit the individual patient (Fig. 2.37b).

A Wheelchair with a One-Hand Drive Mechanism

Using a wheelchair with both wheels controlled by separate rims attached on the same side is extremely difficult for the patient with marked perceptual involvement. Most patients will not be able to cope with the complex mechanism but in specific cases the chair may be a help. A patient who has a total paralysis of one arm and due to some secondary problem is unable to use either of his legs for steering, may be able to manage the one-armed propulsion (Fig. 2.38). Even if he is unable to cover long distances or find his way alone, just being able to move about within the confines of his room and immediate vicinity is positive, or if someone is leading the way and he can follow. It can also be a great help for the person who is pushing the patient's chair if he can take over temporarily when she needs to use her hands for some other purpose. A good example is the situation where the patient is going home for the weekend and his wife is carrying his belongings as well as holding the door open for him.

The wheelchair should be considered as being a useful vehicle enabling the patient to move about or be moved easily from one place to another so that he is not always confined to the vicinity of his bed. It is also useful in that it allows

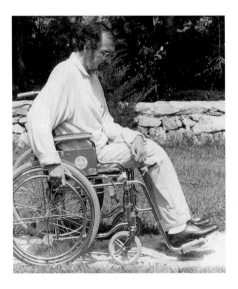

Fig. 2.38. Managing a wheelchair with a one-hand drive mechanism — patient with right leg amputation and left-sided paralysis

easier correction of his sitting posture with all the possible adaptations and supports which have been described As soon as his condition has improved sufficiently, however, he should be transferred to sit on a normal chair at mealtimes, with the table in front of him and also at other appropriate times when someone is working with him. Once the patient is able to walk without too much assistance, members of staff or his relatives should stand and walk with him as much as possible during the day. The therapist should instruct all those caring for him how they can facilitate a good walking pattern as well as how to help him to stand up from a chair, the bed or the toilet and sit down again correctly. She practises the correct handling with them until they feel confident.

Ways in which to assist the patient when he is walking are described in Chap. 8.

The Importance of Turning and Positioning the Patient

The need to turn the unconscious or paralyzed patient at regular intervals, day and night, is advocated in most nursing and physiotherapy textbooks and careful positioning in lying and sitting is advised. Although the necessity is recognized in theory, the relatively simple procedure is unfortunately not always carried out in practice. For the following reasons, turning the patient and positioning him correctly are an essential part of his overall treatment and should be most conscientiously carried out.

Preventing Contractures and Deformity

Most people have had the experience of sleeping soundly in one position for a long time and of finding on waking up that some joint feels stiff and rather painful. For example their elbow may hurt to straighten after being flexed underneath them for some hours. The symptoms are quickly relieved by a few brisk active movements.

The patient, however, who is left to lie in one position for hours on end is unable to move actively and the painful stiffness remains causing him to become fixed in a set position. Because a certain joint hurts, he will resist any attempts on the part of the nurse or therapist to move it passively. A vicious circle ensues in that the longer the joint remains in one position, the more it will hurt to have it moved and the limitation of movement increases. By turning the patient every 2–3 h and repositioning his limbs, the danger is avoided and the development of contractures with all their devastating consequences can be prevented.

Spasticity in stereotyped patterns can easily lead to muscle shortening because the limbs are held constantly in the same position by the dominant muscle groups. Correct positioning will help to reduce the hypertonus, as will the turning into different positions. The patient whose muscles are flaccid with very little reflex activity present will become fixed in the position in which he is left lying for long periods. Referring to spinal cord injuries, Hobson (1956) emphasizes the point strongly: "maintenance of the correct position is of the utmost importance, especially *in the early stages* after injury, to prevent the development of contractures and of pressure sores."

Avoiding the Development of Pressure Sores

Prolonged pressure on the skin and the underlying tissues will cause ischaemic necrosis with the formation of pressure sores as a result (Fig. 2.39). Any part of the body is vulnerable but those areas which have little or no padding are more prone to decubital ulcers, most commonly the sacrum, trochanters, knees, fibulae, malleoli and heels. The occiput and the elbows are vulnerable sites when the patient lies on his back for too long. Patients who are already sitting in the wheelchair will tend to develop sores over their ischial tuberosities if they do not relieve the pressure regularly, or over the area between their buttocks if they sit with their hips too extended. The patient who is left too long in a half-lying position in bed with the head of his bed elevated instead of sitting in a chair will frequently develop an open wound over the bony coccyx, which can take considerable time to heal. It is interesting to note that the Oxford dictionary defines "decubitus" as "the manner or posture of lying in bed" and "decubital" as "pertaining to or resulting from" same! Pressure sores should never be considered as an inevitable result of the head injury itself. They are a preventable complication. "It must be stressed that the formation of pressure sores should never occur if the patient is turned frequently during the early stages after injury" (Hobson 1956).

The treatment of the established pressure sore has been described by Sir Ludwig Guttman on many occasions as well as by many of those who had the privilege to

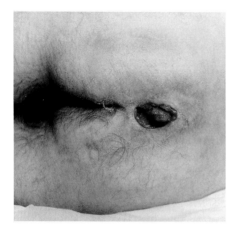

Fig. 2.39. Sacral sore caused by lying supine for prolonged periods, now healing through regular turning

study under him. "It does not matter what you put on the pressure sore as long as it is not the patient's own weight!" (Guttmann 1962). The patient is positioned carefully in such a way that the affected area is not in contact with the bed, for example by lying the patient only on his side or prone if the sore is over the sacrum and turning him at regular intervals. Patients who are already sitting out of bed when the sore develops should not be left sitting for long. Guttmann himself (1973) advises a period of total bedrest for the patient until the sore is completely healed. For the patient with brain damage, however, the detrimental effects of being kept in bed are so great that the therapist should adapt the seat cushion or backrest in such a way that the patient can sit for short periods without any weight on the sore. Apart from relief of pressure, which is usually sufficient if the skin has not broken down, there are many types of dressing which may help to speed up the healing process. In the presence of a severe infection, an antibiotic cream is necessary, but otherwise a nonstick cream or solution with a closed dressing is recommended. Important is that the open sore be kept meticulously clean and that the dressing is kept moist by regular changing. In the foreground however, is the maxim "if pressure is not relieved over the sore any other measures will prove unsuccessful" (Bromley 1976).

Plastic surgery may be required for a very large or deep pressure sore where there has been so much destruction of the soft tissues that healing it by conservative therapeutic measures would take too long and result in such scarring that there would be a danger of repeated breakdown of skin and underlying tissue in the future.

Improving the Circulation

Turning the patient will improve his circulation generally because of the movements it involves and because the change of position will prevent stasis due to prolonged pressure on the weight-bearing areas. The loss of any active muscle pumping activity in the paralyzed limbs, together with reduced vasoconstriction in the blood vessels themselves inevitably leads to poor circulation. Any procedures which assist the circulation will help to reduce the risk of thrombosis, lung embolus, pressure sores and oedema, and speed up the healing of open wounds or decubitus.

Maintaining Mobility of the Spine

When the patient lies on his back, his spine is extended, and when he lies on his side, there is slight flexion, rotation and even lateral flexion so that some joint movement is assured merely by the change in position. During turning procedures, the vertebral column moves as well so that there is less danger of it losing range of motion. Sitting the patient out of bed in the early stages after injury will certainly help to maintain mobility and prevent loss of flexion. When a patient has been nursed for long periods only in the supine position, it is common to find that his spine has become rigid and immobile in extension. There is a resultant loss of rotation (Davies 1990) the effects of which can be far-reaching in the later stages of his rehabilitation. The extended position of his lumbar and thoracic spine cause difficulties in regaining activity in his abdominal muscles, and it may well be a problem for the staff to bring him passively from lying to sitting at all. Certainly his own attempts to sit up actively from lying will be grossly handicapped if he cannot flex his trunk. If he has been nursed in a half-lying position on his back, as frequently happens, then the fixed flexion of his trunk will make it difficult to attain an upright posture in sitting or standing.

Receptors in the cervical spine play a prime role in maintaining balance, so much so that orthopaedic patients who wear a collar because of pain problems have an increased risk of falling and sustaining a fracture of the wrist. If the patient is positioned correctly on his side, the cervical spine remains mobile to enable him to balance when he starts moving against gravity again. The patient who has been nursed only in supine lying will often have a very stiff neck, which has the same effect as wearing a collar in that he will have great difficulty in maintaining his balance when he starts moving against gravity.

Improving Respiratory Function

Going hand in hand with the fixed position of the patient's trunk is a loss of ribcage excursion. The chest wall becomes fixed in a position of inspiration with the ribs elevated anteriorly, secondary to the extension of the thoracic vertebrae to which they are firmly attached and to the loss of tone and activity in the abdominal muscles below. Frequently, another typical deformity of the thorax can be observed with a decrease in its anterior/posterior diameter. The ribcage is flattened and has a wedge-shaped appearance laterally, with indentations anteriorly at about the level of the sternal angle. During inspiration, the hollows deepen and the lower ribs flare outwards. For optimal respiratory function and efficient activity of the muscles involved in respiration, in particular the diaphragm and intercostals, the ribs need to be freely mobile with the thoracic spine erect but not hyperextended. By positioning the patient on both sides the intrinsic flexibility of the ribs themselves is maintained through the weight of his body pressing the ribs downwards and medially on the underneath side. The sternocostal, costovertebral and costo-transverse joints remain more mobile through the regular alteration in their positions. The hyperextension of the spine so often associated with supine lying is inhibited in prone lying and side lying, so that the ribcage retains its normal contour and does not become distorted.

Adequate respiratory function is essential before the patient can learn to speak again, an ability which is of prime importance for him and for his relatives. Turning the patient and positioning him on his side, particularly if he has a tracheostomy or is unable to cough adequately on his own, is most beneficial because the drainage of secretions from the lungs is facilitated. Routine chest physiotherapy with assisted coughing or suctioning should be performed before and after the patient is turned. Once cerebral oedema is no longer a problem, the footend of the bed can be raised for the postural drainage to be more effective. Once the patient is able to lie prone, the position will also be useful for postural drainage.

Preventing Pain of Cervical Origin

The patient who lies flat on his back for prolonged periods with his neck in extension will be at risk of developing severe pain along the distribution of the cervical nerves. The likelihood will be even greater if his head is in addition rotated to one side, a common posture for patients who are being ventilated. The resultant intense headaches, facial pain or pain down the arm and in the hand are often misinterpreted and thought to be a direct result of the brain damage, when in fact they are equally common in patients who have no brain lesion but orthopaedic problems related to their cervical spine (Maitland 1986; Magarey 1986). When taking into account the mechanism of the initial trauma, sufficient to cause a head injury of such magnitude, it is easy to understand that the cervical spine would in all probability have suffered some degree of trauma at the time of the accident with a "whiplash" effect (Bower 1986; Jull 1986). Patients, including those with a lesion of nontraumatic origin, who have undergone lengthy brain surgery may already have lain in a pain provoking position of the cervical spine at the time of the operation with their neck extended and rotated to one side.

Correct positioning in bed, be it in supine with a pillow to support the head in some degree of flexion or in side lying with the head adequately supported, will prevent the symptoms from developing or increasing. Should the patient complain of pain in one of these areas later when he regains consciousness, a careful examination and assessment should be carried out, followed by appropriate treatment of the signs and symptoms (Maitland 1986).

The possibility of a cervical fracture or dislocation should always be considered before the patient's neck is mobilized in any way.

Reducing Hypertonicity

Reflex activity due to the influence of tonic neck reflexes as described by Magnus (1926) is thought to play a significant role in the development of spasticity. Their influence is intensified when the patient is lying supine with his neck extended (Bobath 1974). In a prone position the labyrinthine reflex decreases extensor tone throughout the body, while in side lying with less tendency for the cervical spine to be hyperextended or rotated, the influence of the tonic neck and labyrinthine reflexes is considerably reduced. Disturbances of perception, particularly those involving the tactile/kinaesthetic modalities, may have an even greater effect on muscle tone. The patient is in a continuous "where am I" state, with too little or only confusing information provided by his internal perceptual processes. In such a totally disorientated condition, he searches desperately for more information in various ways as has been described in Chap. 1; namely, by increasing the tension in the muscles themselves, by ramming the joints into end-of-range positions where a total resistance is encountered, by constantly moving parts of the body vigorously or by pressing hard against objects or surfaces in his immediate vicinity. When the patient is lying supine or sitting in a wheelchair without a table in front of him, extensor tone will increase as he searches for more contact with his surroundings by pressing back against the only surface available, either the bed or the backrest of the wheelchair, both of which are always behind him.

By turning the patient regularly and positioning him on his sides or in prone lying, the information from the surroundings makes contact with different parts of his body and prevents the marked increase of tone in one direction. The movement of his body when he is turned provides other information.

The bed with its special antidecubitus mattress provides little in the way of a firm surface to press against, so that instead the tone in the patient's muscles increases and his limbs or trunk either pull or push until coming up against an absolute resistance at the end of the range of possible movement. Such a resistance occurs when a joint is either fully extended or fully flexed or one part of the body approximates with another. The patient's legs (or arms), for example, may extend completely in the total extension synergy and he could be classified as having marked extensor "spasticity". The same phenomenon can be observed in relation to his trunk, involving the joints of the lumbar, thoracic and cervical spines.

A total resistance will also be met if the limbs flex maximally, a typical posture for the patient's arms and hands to adopt if he is said to have flexor spasticity. In the flexion synergy, the shoulder joint is not at the end of the mechanical range of adduction but the upper arm approximating with the side of the trunk provides the total resistance. More medial rotation in the glenohumeral joint itself would also be possible, but the patient's hands pressing against the chest wall prevent further movement in that direction. Without the appropriate treatment such flexor "spasticity" can easily lead to loss of shoulder elevation, abduction and outward rotation, elbow extension, and wrist and finger extension. When the patient's lower limbs pull up continually into a flexed position, flexion contractures of the hips and knees are a common sequela if adequate treatment measures are not taken to counteract the effect, one of which is prone lying. With correct positioning the effects of the extensor and flexor synergies can be counteracted and if the patient is turned routinely his limbs do not lie constantly in one stereotyped position.

The patient who moves himself continuously in bed receives additional information from kinaesthetic sources and usually does not exhibit hypertonicity to the same extent. He is, therefore, far less likely to develop contractures.

Preventing Any Peripheral Nerve Damage

The danger of damaging peripheral nerves through prolonged compression is eliminated by turning the patient every 2–3 h in the early stages following his accident. The lateral popliteal nerve as it passes around the fibula head is particularly vulnerable to such damage if the patient lies supine with his leg laterally rotated, and the ulnar nerve as it transverses the elbow is subject to pressure if his arms are flexed and inwardly rotated. Once he is in a wheelchair, the patient who is left sitting out of bed unattended for long periods may suffer a radial nerve palsy, caused by his arm hanging unnoticed over the side of the wheelchair and pressing against the armrest. Damage to the ulnar nerve has been described in cases where patients' flexed elbows have pressed down against the rim of a solid wheelchair table with additional weight on them due to the flexed trunk position.

It would indeed be a pity for a patient who has regained consciousness and function in his limbs to have to contend with the additional problems caused by a peripheral nerve lesion which a little time and trouble could have prevented.

Accustoming the Patient to Being Moved

Through turning, positioning and sitting out of bed in the early days following the accident, the patient is less likely to be afraid of being moved or moving in the later stages of his rehabilitation. Patients who have spent months in bed, lying in one position totally supported, are frequently terrified of moving at all or being brought to sitting or standing later. Such fear is most distressing for the patient and is extremely difficult to overcome. His rehabilitation may well take much longer as a result.

When taking into consideration how much time, effort and money is spent on caring for the patient in the intensive treatment stage following acquisition of a severe brain lesion, it would be illogical to omit the relatively simple procedures of positioning, turning and sitting out of bed. They are of immense benefit to the patient and are a means to prevent many devastating secondary complications.

A Case in Point

T.B. was 18 years old when he was involved in a road traffic accident on his way to school, shortly before taking his final examinations, and he suffered a severe traumatic brain injury. It was a terrible shock for all who knew this good-looking, intelligent, hardworking, friendly young man who was on the point of starting out on a career. While in hospital T.B.'s level of consciousness gradually improved, but for some inexplicable reason his physical condition was allowed to deteriorate to a horrifying degree. Extensive pressure sores developed over his

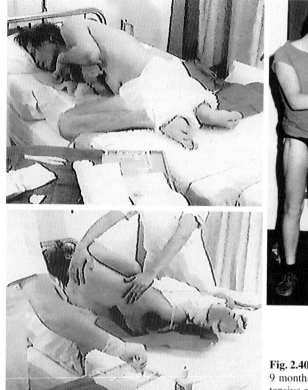

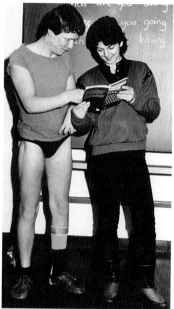

Fig. 2.40a. T.B. with contracted limbs 9 months after head injury. **b** Extensive pressure sores. **c** Learning English with a pretty teacher. (Archive photos from video films)

sacrum and both trochanters, his hips and knees became progressively more contracted in flexion, and his shoulders, elbows and hands had fixed flexion deformities of a marked degree (Fig. 2.40a,b). In addition, the lateral popliteal nerve sustained damage through compression, damage which has unfortunately proved to be of a permanent nature. Incontinent of both urine and faeces, he lay in bed for months on end, crying pitifully when any attempt was made to move him and begging the therapists just to leave him alone. His desperate parents did everything in their power to have their son moved to a rehabilitation centre, and eventually succeeded 9 months after the date of his accident. Once in the hands of the experienced and enthusiastic team at the centre, T.B. made rapid progress. He was sat up out of bed, his contractures were fully overcome through serial plastering and active therapy (Fig. 2.40c). The only surgical intervention required was plastic surgery for his pressure sores, which although greatly improved were not completely healed and were interfering with his rehabilitation. At a later time T.B. underwent surgery to free tendons which had been entrapped in a badly set forearm fracture. He was discharged from hospital completely independent and able to walk considerable distances with a cane, as well as being able to use public transport (see Fig. 6.63c). Sadly he was not able to continue with the career which he had previously chosen, but an alternative training was initiated.

T.B. suffered pain, demoralization and resignation during many long months in hospital, all of which he could have been spared by routine turning and positioning in conjunction with sitting out of bed and standing in the early stages. His rehabilitation took far longer and was more arduous because of the subsequent measures required to overcome the secondary avoidable complications.

3 Moving and Being Moved in Lying and Sitting

"To move is all mankind can do and for such the sole executant is muscle, whether in whispering a syllable or in felling a forest" (Sherrington 1947). In fact, we are moving some part or parts of our bodies during all our waking hours, and even during sleep the muscles of respiration and other vital functions continue to contract rhythmically to keep us alive. If we remain motionless for any length of time we feel stiff and uncomfortable, so that the first thing we do when we awake after sleeping soundly or rise after watching a long and absorbing television programme is to move and stretch ourselves. The patient who is unconscious or cannot move himself will need to be moved by others as his trunk and limbs will otherwise become stiffened in a fixed position, and he will not only be uncomfortable but will experience pain on being moved. If he is not completely mobile it will also be more difficult for him to learn to move actively when he starts to recover.

An action, a reaction or an interaction with the environment is only possible if a muscle contracts. As Kesselring (1992 b) explains, "the central nervous system translates into action information streaming in through very different channels from the inner world of the organism itself or from the world outside it; there is however only one effecter or output system: namely the musculature with its controlling organisation in the central nervous system." It is as if the motor systems were "servants" to the rest of the nervous system in that they can only respond or not respond depending upon the integrity of the different sensory systems and the integrative action of the system as a whole (Tuchmann-Duplessis et al. 1975).

Requirements for Efficient Muscle Action

For the muscles to perform their tasks efficiently, they must be able to shorten and lengthen with minimal resistance in all ranges of movement. Such economic and finely adjusted muscle contraction, apart from the accurate feedback and feedforward circuits provided by the nervous system, is also dependent upon the following:

1. The elasticity and complete extensibility of the muscles themselves. Any muscle shortening or increase in tone will interfere with the subtle interplay between agonist and antagonist required for normal movement.

2. Full painless range of motion in the joints involved in the movement. If joint mobility is restricted and painful, the pattern of movement will be altered and pain inhibition can cause a loss of muscle activity or a decrease in muscle strength. A good example of such inhibition is the loss of activity in the serratus anterior muscle with "winging" of the scapula, which is seen in association with a "frozen shoulder" of orthopaedic origin or the inability to activate the quadriceps following meniscectomy.

3. A freely mobile and extensible nervous system.

Adaptive lengthening or shortening of the nervous system is essential in order for a part of the body to move without restriction or resistance. Up until now, most treatment concepts have focused on normalizing muscle tone and preventing contractures in muscles and joints, but, as Butler and Gifford (1989) and Butler (1991a,b) have brought to the attention of therapists, when a part of the body moves, nerves are required to move as well, so that the integration of nervous system mobilization in treatment is equally important. The need for a mobile nervous sytem would seem to be obvious and logical when the path followed by various peripheral nerves is considered in relation to the line of pull of certain muscles in their immediate vicinity. For example, when the elbow flexes the ulnar nerve must lengthen while the median and radial nerves must adapt by shortening, and vice versa. The bed of the median nerve has been calculated as being 20% longer when the elbow and wrist are extended than when they are flexed (Millesi 1986).

The straight leg raise (SLR) test, in which the patient lies supine and his extended leg is lifted by the examiner to ascertain at what degree of hip flexion pain is felt or resistance encountered, has long been used in the examination and diagnosis of back problems. The SLR in fact moves and tenses the nervous system from the foot and along the neuraxis right up to the brain (Breig 1978). It has also been demonstrated that ankle dorsiflexion in the SLR position could tension the nervous system up to and including the cerebellum (Smith 1956). In the past, limitation of an SLR was often mistakenly considered to be caused by "tight hamstrings", because the examiner thought only in terms of muscles. The enormous difference in range created by dorsiflexing the foot, however, cannot be explained in terms of shortened muscles, because no muscle extends from the toes to the pelvis. The only structures which are put under more tension in this way are nerves and the connective tissue surrounding them. "Tension tests, and for that matter body movements, not only produce an increase in tension within the nerve but also move the nerve in relation to its surrounding tissue" (Butler and Gifford 1989).

Not only peripheral nerves have to adapt in length, but the spinal cord as well. "The spinal canal undergoes substantial length changes during movement" according to Breig (1978) and Louis (1981) as it must elongate by between 5 and 9 cm when the spine is flexed after being extended. From lateral flexion of the trunk from one side to the other the canal alters in length by 15%. Passive neck flexion has been shown to move the cord and put the meninges under tension as far down as the sciatic nerve tract (Breig 1978).

As the main function of the nervous system is impulse conduction, it is obvious therefore that adaptive lengthening, both centrally and peripherally, is essential in order to accommodate the enormous variety and extent of body movements and postures used in everyday life without impeding nerve conduction.

Possible Lengthening Mechanisms

The mechanisms of adaptation to movement are complex but it has been postulated that the nervous system adapts to lengthening in the following ways (Butler 1991 b):

- The corrugations of the axons unfold and straighten out, and the axons untwist.
- The nerve moves in relation to the tissues which surround it or within the nerve itself, and neural tissue elements move in relation to connective tissue. For example, a fascicle can slide in relation to another fascicle in peripheral nerves and in nerve roots, or the spinal cord move in relation to the dura mater.
- The nervous system can also adapt to elongation by the development of tension or increased pressure within the nerve, the dural sheath or in fact, within the entire nervous system.

The Importance of Mobilizing the Nervous System

Maintaining or Restoring Adaptive Lengthening of the Nervous System

After damage to the nervous system, the normal adaptive mechanisms are often disturbed or interrupted, a fact which could be responsible for or increase the severity of some commonly observed problems such as:

- Muscle shortening or contractures
- Abnormal muscle tone including spasticity and clonus
- Limitation of joint motion
- Loss or disturbance of sensation, including paraesthesia or anaesthesia
- Decreased muscle activity through peripheral nerve involvement
- Pain, including headache and facial neuralgia
- Circulatory disturbances and other autonomic nervous system signs such as increased sweating.

Techniques aimed at maintaining mobility of the nervous system should therefore be included in the treatment prophylactically right from the start, and where such symptoms are already presenting problems, the lost mobility must be carefully but determinedly regained.

The Tension Tests

Although any of the tests recommended by Butler (1991b) may reveal abnormal tension and the same tests be used as treatment techniques as well, experience has shown that the following are most useful for the differentiation and alleviation of related symptoms which commonly occur after brain damage.

For clarity, only the final position of maximum tension is given in the following descriptions of tension tests. Slow carefully graded progression with various components being added or left out is necessary before the full range of motion for each test can be achieved. A comprehensive description of the tests for both the upper and lower limbs with the sequences for adding the different components is clearly presented in Butler's own book (Butler 1991b). The therapist is advised to study the tests carefully and practise performing them on a normal subject before using them in treatment.

Upper Limb Tension Test 1 (ULTT 1). Depression of the shoulder girdle, abduction of the arm with lateral rotation and supination, elbow extension, wrist extension, finger extension, abduction/extension of the thumb.

Upper Limb Tension Test 2 (ULTT 2) with Median Nerve Bias. Shoulder girdle depression, lateral rotation and abduction of the shoulder, elbow extension, supination of the forearm, dorsal extension of the wrist and fingers, extension/abduction of the thumb.

Upper Limb Tension Test 2 (ULTT 2) with Radial Nerve Bias. Shoulder girdle depression, medial rotation and abduction of the shoulder, elbow extension, pronation of the forearm, flexion of the wrist with ulnar deviation, flexion of the fingers and thumb.

Upper Limb Tension Test 3 (ULTT 3). Shoulder depression, shoulder abduction with lateral rotation, elbow flexion, supination of the forearm, dorsal extension of the wrist, fingers and thumb. Pronation of the forearm may reveal more significantly increased tension than supination and can be useful for assessment and treatment in such cases.

> When the shoulder girdle is depressed during the ULTT, full abduction of the shoulder is mechanically no longer possible.
> The addition of lateral flexion of the neck towards the contralateral side will further increase tension to a marked degree.

Lower Limb Tension Test 1 (LLTT 1). Trunk supine, hip flexion, knee extension, dorsal flexion of the foot. For testing and for treatment purposes various additions and variations can be most useful, namely hip adduction or abduction, plantar inversion of the foot, simultaneous ULTT 1.

Slump Test. Sitting position with thighs supported, and knees together. Neck and trunk flexion , knee extension, dorsiflexion of the foot. Abduction of the hip is a useful addition for treatment.

Prone Knee Bend (PKB). Prone lying, the head turned towards the therapist. Knee flexion. Hip extension may be added.

> Warning: The prone knee bend test should only be performed if the patient is conscious and able to protest vocally when pain is elicited.

The extreme variation in the normal range of extensibility of the rectus femoris muscle together with the powerful leverage provided by flexing the lower leg could otherwise lead unwittingly to soft tissue damage with the concomitant danger of heteroectopic bone formation (see Chap. 6). With the patient lying prone, it is difficult for the therapist to observe early nonverbal signs of pain, and the position makes voluntary muscle activity to prevent the test movement impossible. Performed with care the PKB is, however, a useful treatment technique, particularly in the later stages of rehabilitation to overcome extensor hypertonus in the lower limbs and to facilitate the initiation of the swing phase of walking.

The Nervous System Is a Continuum

"The peripheral and central nervous systems need to be considered as one since they form a continuous tissue tract" advises Butler (1991b) and goes on to describe the system as a continuum, one of the reasons being that the connective tissues are continuous. It becomes easier to understand why a change in part of the system will have repercussions for the whole system. Because of the arrangement of the nervous system with a network of connections both horizontally, i.e. from one side of the body to the other, and vertically, i.e. from head to foot, if one arm is placed in such a position that neural structures are tensed, then there will usually be increased tension in the arm on the other side as well, or even in the contralateral leg for that matter. Likewise in the SLR position, when the foot is dorsiflexed the brainstem may be tensed, or raising the extended leg may prevent full extension of the elbow when the arm is abducted (Fig. 3.1).

The therapist, therefore, cannot treat one part of the patient's body in isolation but must ensure that all parts are incorporated in the treatment programme. It may appear, for example, that the patient's legs are far less affected than his arms and as a result might receive little attention in the overall treatment. Examination could, however, reveal that his SLR is dramatically reduced and that the adverse neural tension is affecting the return of useful function in his hands.

In the Bobath concept of treatment, the value of moving the patient proximally to reduce distal spasticity has long been recognized and emphasized because the strategy is so obviously effective, even though the reason has never in fact been convincingly explained. After devoting 50 years of her life to unravelling the mysteries of spasticity and finding better ways to treat it, Bertie Bobath herself admitted "I still don't know why rotating the trunk inhibits spasticity in the

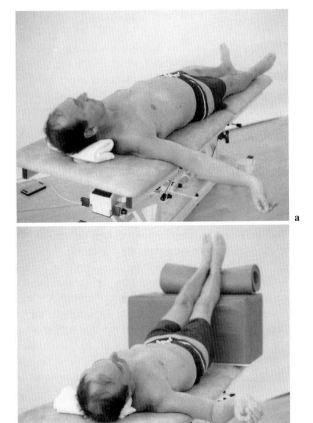

Fig. 3.1a,b. A patient with right hemiplegia. **a** His abducted arm lies relaxed in extension. **b** With legs raised his arm is tensely flexed

limbs, I only know that it does!" (B. Bobath, personal communication). The explanation could well be that the trunk rotation and many of the other ways which Bertha Bobath discovered to inhibit spasticity were in fact mobilizing adverse tension in the nervous system. Analysis of the successful inhibitory patterns of movement inherent in her teaching would certainly be compatible with such an hypothesis. Within the Bobath concept, there are already many activities which do in fact mobilize the nervous system, and which can do so even more effectively if certain movement components are added or postures altered.

Causing Pain Is Not The Aim

For the patient who has significantly increased neural tension, passive mobilization will be painful in positions which place the nervous system under more tension, especially if "stretching" techniques are applied. As Butler (1991a) so rightly pointed out, "to hurt the patient is not actually the aim of the treatment, you know!" In fact, eliciting pain would be counterproductive because there would be a reflex increase in tone in those muscles which oppose the movement, and the patient will actively resist if he is in a position to do so. The therapist should avoid pain as much as possible, mobilizing the structures in gradually increasing painfree ranges of motion, instead of stretching them in extreme end of range positions. She should always keep a picture in her mind of the mechanisms by which nerves elongate, and try to facilitate the unfolding and straightening out of the axons. Her aim should be to re-establish the easy gliding motion between the nerve and its surrounding tissues or between the nerve fibres and their connective tissue by using gentle repetitive movements. The information which the patient provides regarding the degree of pain he is experiencing guides the therapist as to how soon and how far she can increase the range of passive movement. If the patient indicates that something is hurting him, the therapist reacts immediately either by lessening the range or, in the case of adverse neural tension, releasing one component so that tension is reduced; for example, when she abducts his extended arm with the wrist and fingers dorsiflexed, he may say that he has a pain in his shoulder. Releasing the distal component of dorsal flexion may make full, painfree movement of the glenohumeral joint itself possible.

Warning: Particular care must be taken when treating a patient who is unable to communicate verbally or nonverbally that a movement is causing pain, for instance, a patient who is still unconscious, on a respirator, heavily sedated or too paralyzed. Without the protection provided by the patient's pain response, sensitive tissues and vulnerable structures around the joint may easily be damaged with the possibility of serious consequences.

Any marked resistance which the therapist feels when moving a limb should be respected and not overcome by force. A sudden reflex withdrawal of a part could likewise be a reaction to pain and should be treated as such. Other warning signals such as changes in heart or respiratory rate and profuse sweating should also be carefully observed and the treatment altered accordingly.

Because individuals have such very different mechanical ranges of movement in their joints and muscles, it is not sufficient for the therapist to be guided by the mean average range possible for each part of the body as stated in various text books.

Persistent Pain of Undiagnosed Origin

Abnormal tension in the nervous system can cause pain in bizarre distribution which does not seem to fit in with any known diagnosis. A patient who complains of persistent pain in areas not compatible with joint stiffness or nerve root symptoms may be unjustly labelled as having a low pain tolerance and thought to be making a fuss about nothing. On the other hand he may be inappropriately diagnosed as having "thalamic pain", a term often loosely applied to any painful condition which is not clearly understood by the team or for which no obvious cause can be found. In actual fact, "lesions of the CNS rarely cause pain in previously painfree individuals" (Fields 1987) and approximately half the patients diagnosed as having thalamic pain following a cerebrovascular lesion do not have lesions involving the thalamus at all (Boivie and Leijon 1991). As Wall (1991) describing the difficulties in finding a satisfactory explanation of neuropathic pain so pertinently states, "in addition we are faced with a similarly challenging fact that chronic pain is never present in 100% of the cases with the pathology to which the pain is commonly attributed." In a study of 27 patients with intermittent or persistent pain following a stroke, only three patients had identified haemorrhages affecting the thalamus (Boivie and Leijon 1991). Because their results show that only a minority of patients had thalamic lesions, the authors are of the opinion that the term thalamic pain is in many cases inappropriate. With computerized axial tomography revealing that in so many cases the lesion is not in the thalamus (Agnew et al. 1983; Bowsher et al. 1984) the condition is now called *central post-stroke pain* (CPSP) (Bowsher 1991), although it can follow not only classical "stroke", whether from infarct or haemorrhage, but also surgically treated subarachnoid haemorrhage, tumour removal and even head injury.

The term "sympathetically maintained pain" would seem most apt (McMahon 1991). Certainly, "the cortex is not the pain center and neither is the thalamus. The areas of the brain involved in pain experience and behaviour are very extensive" (Melzack 1991). In the recent literature there are well-documented cases showing that lesions located in any of the rostrocaudal parts of the neuraxis can result in CPSP (Boivie and Leijon 1991).

Sensory disturbances must be closely related to the development of such persistent, sympathetically mediated pain as it occurs independently of any other neurological symptoms common to all the patients, with the exception of sensory abnormalities which are always present, particularly in regard to pain and temperature. Patients "characteristically report neuropathic pain as an unfamiliar or strange sensation" (Fields 1987) and the pain is always felt in a region of sensory deficit. The pain intensity fluctuates considerably during the day in all patients and can be brought on or increased by a variety of factors such as movement, walking or touch, even by emotions such as sudden fear and joy and by loud noises (Garcin 1968; Riddoch 1938).

Perhaps difficult to understand is that the pain first appears at such different intervals following brain lesions. "The time from stroke to onset of pain varied from no delay up to 34 months" (Boivie and Leijon 1991), with the onset sometimes coinciding with improvement of the experienced sensory abnormalities.

Both these findings could, however, indicate that as the patient becomes more aware of his body and limbs, the "strange feelings" are intensified, and because they are so unpleasant the patient interprets them as "pain". Basmajian (1980) indeed once defined pain as being "a feeling of great discomfort based on individual experience."

Whatever the cause, the unpleasant feeling of pain is most disturbing for the patient and can delay his progress in all areas of rehabilitation. Its development should be avoided whenever possible because of its self-sustaining nature, caused by repeatedly abnormal sensations and abnormal afferent input (McMahon 1991). "The capacity of nociceptive afferents to induce a state of central sensitization has important consequences for pain management. Effectively it means that attempts should be made to prevent the initiation of central sensitization if possible. The best treatment for pain appears to be therefore that treatment is initiated before the pain is experienced" (Woolf 1991).

By moving the patient right from the start, ensuring more normal input and avoiding painful stiffness or overstretching, the development of persistent neurogenic pain syndromes can usually be prevented altogether. In the same way, if pain is already present, then a graduated programme of movement and activity should be commenced. "As disuse and loss of normal function appear to play an important part in the genesis of the clinical problem, it follows that resumption of activity is essential to sustain relief and promote ultimate resolution" (Charlton 1991).

Patients previously diagnosed as having "thalamic pain", "thalamic syndrome" or "CPSP" (Bowsher 1991) have in fact responded so well to mobilization of their nervous system that the symptoms have disappeared completely, when the mobilization was used in conjunction with an active and positive treatment programme. It should also be taken into account that, "fear, anxiety and stress contribute to all painful experiences and manoeuvres to reduce them should form part of a comprehensive management plan" (Goldman and Lloyd-Thomas 1991).

Important Movement Sequences

When treating patients either in lying and sitting, the following sequences should always be included to maintain full elasticity and extensibility of muscles, range of joint motion and the adaptive lengthening properties of the nervous system, as well as to improve circulation and respiration. The activities will help to keep the patient in as good a condition possible until he regains consciousness and is able to move himself actively once more. Many of the movements will serve to mobilize the nervous system to some extent, but require certain additions and some alterations in posture if full range is to be maintained or regained because the nervous system forms such a complex mesh throughout the body.

In addition to the movements described in the following, any other activities or movement sequences which the therapist finds to be beneficial for a patient can naturally be included as well, as long as they fulfil the criteria of maintaining range, normalizing tone, facilitating normal movement and not causing pain or possible injury. All the tension tests can also be used as additional treatment techniques in the later rehabilitation stage to overcome specific residual problems.

Moving the Head

The neck plays a key role in maintaining balance through information provided by receptors in the cervical region, and tonic neck reflexes influence muscle tone throughout the body. "In summary, the cervical area of the body appears to be the pivotal point upon which many of man's gross and fine sensorimotor functions depend" (Moore 1980). It is therefore of prime importance that the neck be kept fully mobile right from the start by correct positioning and passive movements. The effects of adverse tension in the nervous system arising as a direct result of the lesion itself or due to secondary injuries or immobility can be observed even in the early stages. The head is frequently pulled to one side and the shoulder girdle elevated, with the distance between the point of the shoulder and the neck markedly shortened (Fig. 3.2). The tensed position may well be bilateral, and the muscles and joints of the upper limbs feel stiff.

The head is moved gently in all directions but particularly important is lateral flexion of the neck. The therapist holds the shoulder girdle down with one hand while using her other to ease the patient's head over towards the opposite side and then moves round the bed to repeat the procedure from the other side (Fig. 3.3).

It is far easier to support the patient's head and move his neck if the headboard is removed and the therapist stands at the head end of the bed (Fig. 3.4a). In fact, the board is not necessary at all. Removing it and leaving it off from the start will facilitate many other procedures as well.

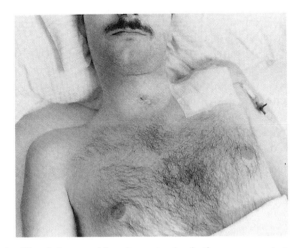

Fig. 3.2. Position of head and shoulder girdle caused by adverse tension in the nervous system following a head injury

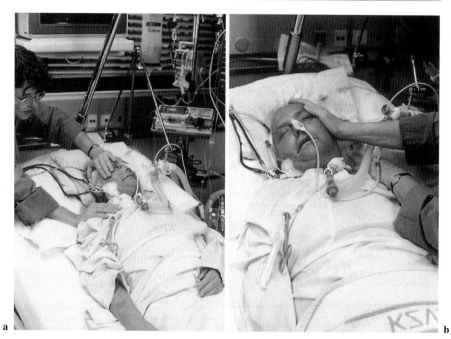

Fig. 3.3a,b. Mobilizing tension in the neck of an unconscious patient. **a** Depressing the shoulder girdle. **b** Moving the head while holding the shoulder down

From her position at the end of the bed, the therapist is better able to mobilize the lateral flexion of the neck while preventing elevation of the patient's shoulder girdle (Fig. 3.4b). Alternatively, with her hands in the same position, she can hold his head still and mobilize the tension through depressing his shoulder girdle instead, using gentle, rhythmic movements.

If skull fractures, open wounds or surgical incisions make it difficult for the therapist to hold the patient's head firmly in her hands in the acute stage, she can lift the pillow on which his head is supported and move his neck passively into flexion, rotation or side flexion (Fig. 3.5).

Care must be taken to ensure that flexion of the upper cervical spine remains free and that all the movement is not taking place at the level of the lower cervical vertebrae.

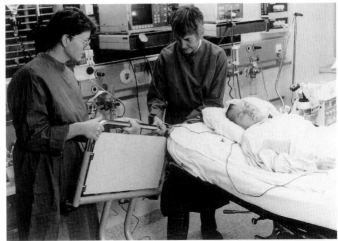

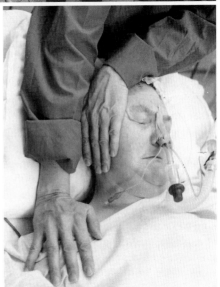

Fig. 3.4a. Removing the headboard facilitates therapeutic procedures. **b** Lateral flexion of the neck with depression of the shoulder girdle

Moving the Ribcage

With their many articulations and muscle insertions, the ribs can easily stiffen in a fixed position if the chest wall is not moved passively. Not only do the joints lose their range of motion, but the intrinsic flexibility of the ribs themselves is decreased. Normally the range of excursion of the ribcage is maintained by the movements of respiration as well as by the many movements made by the thoracic spine as it flexes, extends and rotates in everyday life. The shallow breathing of the

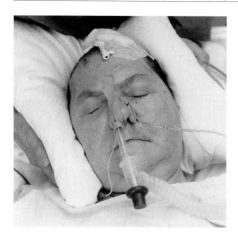

Fig. 3.5. Moving the patient's head on a pillow

patient in bed, perhaps assisted by a ventilator, and in addition, little or no trunk activity in sitting or standing makes it incumbent upon the therapist to maintain mobility of the ribs. A fixed posture of the ribcage reduces respiratory function and causes difficulties in regaining selective activity in the abdominal muscles later (Davies 1990).

With the patient lying supine, the therapist places her hands one on top of the other over his sternum just below the level of the sternoclavicular joints. Leaning her weight forwards, she presses the sternum with its rib attachments firmly down and in the direction of the umbilicus, timing the movement to coincide with the patient's expiration (Fig. 3.6a). The therapist allows the chest wall to elevate during the next inspiratory period before applying pressure in a downward direction again.

To maintain the lateral movement of the chest wall as well as to assist full expiration, the therapist moves the ribs downwards and medially with overpressure while the patient is lying on his side. She stands behind him on a level with his shoulders and with her hands over the lateral aspect of his ribcage moves his ribs in the required direction, i.e. towards his umbilicus, by transferring her weight forwards (Fig. 3.6b). As before, one of her hands is placed over the other and the movement is carried out smoothly and comfortably by weight passing through her extended arms. If she extends and flexes her elbows in order to move the patient's ribs, or his sternum for that matter, the movement is less flowing, tending to start and end abruptly and be rather jerky as a result. The full expiratory excursion will often cause secretions in the lungs to be moved sufficiently to elicit a cough reflex, and the therapist can immediately change the position of her hands to make the cough more efficient, so that the secretions are expelled actively or can be more easily suctioned. To assist coughing, she places one of her hands on either side of his lower chest and, as the patient starts to cough, she presses them forcefully towards each other, imitating the activity of the abdominal muscles during normal coughing (Fig. 3.6c). Movement of the lateral chest wall and assisted coughing are of great value in keeping the patient's lungs clear and should be carried out routinely before and after he is turned onto his side.

Fig. 3.6a–c. Mobilizing the ribcage. **a** Pressing the sternum down and towards the umbilicus. **b** Moving the ribs medially downwards. **c** Coughing assisted by compression of the ribcage

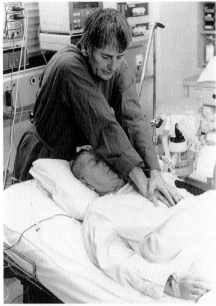

a

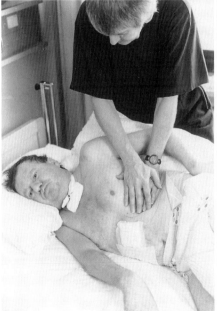

b

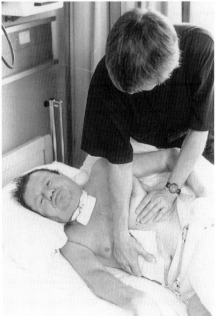

c

Rotating the Upper Trunk

In order to prevent loss of mobility in the thoracic spine the therapist flexes and rotates the patient's upper trunk, the movement required later for using the hands to either side of the midline and for a normal gait pattern. Flexion with rotation will prevent the thoracic spine from becoming stiff, which it will tend to do when the patient is still lying in bed for the greater part of the day or sitting immobile in the wheelchair with his back supported.

With the patient lying supine, the therapist stands at his side and reaches across him to place her hands behind the scapula on the opposite side. Shifting her weight sideways in the direction of his foot, she draws the patient's shoulder forwards, so that the upper part of his body turns towards her (Fig. 3.7).

The patient's head stays on the pillow, but should turn to face the therapist as his trunk rotates. If his back stays stiffly extended, the therapist moves one of her hands away from his scapula and uses it to facilitate flexion by pressing down over the lower part of his sternum.

The movement is repeated passively until no resistance is felt. If the patient is able to participate actively he can be asked to stay in the position, and the therapist gradually reduces the amount of support she is giving with the hand behind his scapula. When he holds the rotated position of his trunk actively with his head lifted off the pillow his abdominal muscles will be activated.

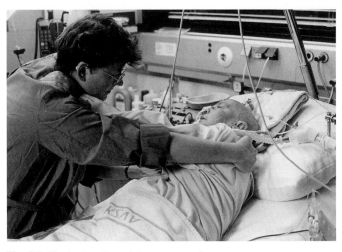

Fig. 3.7. Flexion/rotation of the upper trunk

Maintaining Full, Painfree Range of Motion in the Upper Limbs

Until the patient is able to use his arms and hands for activities of daily living, the therapist must move them for him in such a way as to prevent any limitation of movement. Painful contractures can delay or inhibit the recovery of functional activity as well as causing the patient to suffer unnecessarily. Due to the enormous variety and range of movement normally possible in the upper limbs, they are particularly prone to loss of range if great care is not taken.

In the acute stage, the patient's arms should be moved daily if not twice daily, and certainly on Sundays and holidays. Patients admitted to hospital following an accident just before a long weekend or on Christmas Eve, for example, could be in danger of painful restriction of movement if commencement of such treatment were to be delayed for 3–4 days. Mobilization of the neck and trunk should always precede passive mobilization of the arms because the proximal movements will inhibit distal hypertonus preparatorily.

Elevation of the Shoulder Through Flexion

Standing at the head end of the bed, the therapist lifts the patient's extended arm above his head, using one of her hands to support the shoulder joint in its normal alignment as she does so (Fig. 3.8). She moves the arm gradually further until elevation of the shoulder has been achieved.

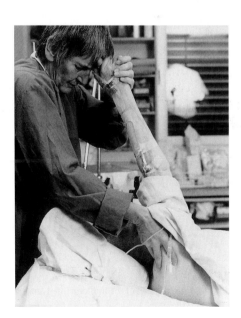

Fig. 3.8. Supporting the shoulder joint when the arm is lifted

PROBLEM SOLVING

An Infusion in the Arm. The presence of an infusion should not deter the therapist from moving the patient's arm. With modern catheters, the arm can be moved freely without jeopardizing the drip as long as due care is taken. Use of the sub-clavicular vein for intravenous feeding is recommended, not only to facilitate therapeutic procedures but also to avoid the all too common problem of distal oedema caused by fluid escaping into the tissues of the hand or in the region of the elbow, which can in some instances have serious repercussions.

Elevation of the Shoulder Girdle. Due to imbalance in muscle tone and activity and/or adverse tension in the nervous system, the patient's shoulder girdle may lie in an elevated position, with the distance from his ear to the point of his shoulder visibly shortened (Fig. 3.9a). Because the joint is mechanically out of alignment, flexion of the shoulder will cause pain unless the position is corrected before the arm is lifted. In the uncorrected position, the pain stems from the humeral head impinging against the acromion process and thereby compromising sensitive structures between the two bony surfaces. The therapist literally holds the head of the humerus in her hand by encircling it with her fingers and eases it away from the contours of the fossa and the inferior aspect of the acromion above. The scapula is

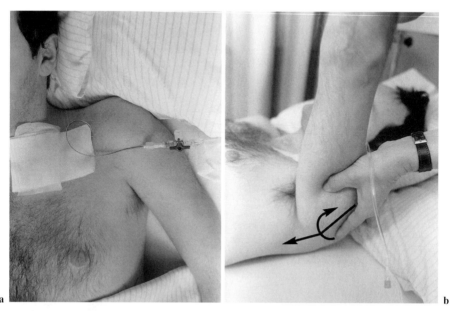

a   b

Fig. 3.9a,b. Correcting alignment of the shoulder during passive movements. **a** The scapula is elevated with the head of the humerus sited anteriorly. **b** Moving the scapula and humerus head into a normal position

rotated posteriorly and caudally , as is the humeral head which must in addition be rotated laterally to be repositioned and move freely in the glenoid fossa (Fig. 3.9b).

Depression of the Scapula with Subluxation of the Shoulder. Particularly in the early months following the lesion, the scapula may be depressed and so rotated that the glenoid fossa slopes downwards, with loss of the passive locking mechanism of the shoulder joint as described by Basmajian (1979, 1981). The integrity of the glenohumeral joint then depends almost exclusively on the rotator cuff muscles and, should these be hypotonic, the head of the humerus will displace downwards when the patient is brought into an upright position (Fig. 3.10). The subluxation is in itself not painful, but the shoulder without its normal muscular protection is very vulnerable and can be easily traumatized if the therapist moves the arm without first correcting the alignment of the joint (Davies 1985).

While moving the arm into elevation with one of her hands, the therapist corrects the alignment of the shoulder by relocating the head of the humerus in the glenoid fossa with her other hand. With her fingers she eases the humeral head in an anterior direction away from the posterior rim of the fossa and also prevents any contact between it and the acromion process (Fig. 3.11a). The gentle lifting of the humeral head draws the depressed scapula into the correct amount of elevation and

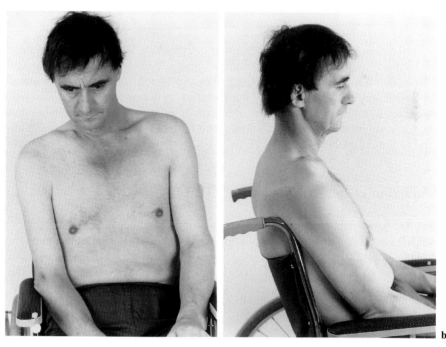

Fig. 3.10a,b. Subluxation of the shoulder. **a** Loss of the passive locking mechanism. **b** Hypotonic rotator cuff muscles

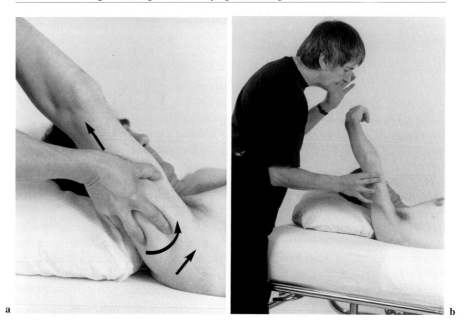

Fig. 3.11a,b. Correcting shoulder alignment. **a** Relocating the humeral head in the glenoid fossa. **b** Stimulating muscle activity

forward rotation to allow free movement of the shoulder, and by laterally rotating the humerus the therapist ensures that the greater tuberosity does not impinge against the coracoacromial arch. Once the arm is felt to be moving without any resistance, it is important for the therapist to encourage active control of the muscles of the upper limb particularly those around the shoulder. For example, while supporting the patient's arm above his head she can ask him to lift his hand to touch her chin (Fig. 3.11b).

Abduction of the Arm including ULTT1

Standing beside the patient, the therapist moves his extended arm from a position of 90 flexion of the shoulder gradually into horizontal abduction with the shoulder laterally rotated, the forearm supinated, the wrist and fingers in dorsal extension and the thumb extended and abducted (Fig. 3.12a). It is most important that she undress the patient sufficiently as she may otherwise fail to see when antalgic positions are occurring, for example elevation of the shoulder girdle, and erroneously believe that she has achieved full range of movement.

If the shoulder girdle is held firmly down in place however, there is often a marked increase in resistance to elbow extension when the wrist and fingers are extended (Fig. 3.12b). The therapist must be aware that in the presence of

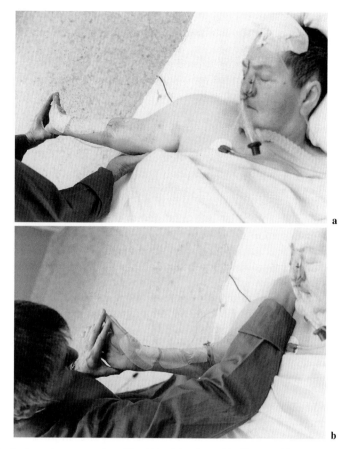

Fig. 3.12a,b. ULTT 1 in the intensive care unit. **a** Shoulder abduction with elbow and hand extension free. **b** Shoulder depression tenses elbow and wrist

adverse neural tension, depression of the shoulder girdle can cause the movement to become suddenly very painful and that the pain may be experienced not only at the elbow but anywhere along the whole length of the upper limb right up to the neck.

PROBLEM SOLVING

When the Addition of Another Component of Movement Causes Pain. As has been explained above in "The importance of mobilizing the nervous system", the therapist must react immediately on any expression of pain on the part of the patient, whether verbal or nonverbal.

The problem of pain during treatment to reduce abnormal tension is best dealt with by applying what Butler (1991 a,b) describes as "component thinking", i.e. the therapist does not consider the whole limb, in this case the arm, as one long lever to be moved directly into an end of range position, but thinks instead of how best and in what sequence she can mobilize its various subdivisions in order to reach the same goal. She may succeed more easily by starting with a distant component, one far removed from the most stiff or pain provoking part, or begin by mobilizing a distal segment such as the wrist, instead of starting proximally as she usually does. Moving the neck on its own may relieve tension in preparation before she even starts to include the arm itself. Certainly mobilizing the shoulder girdle by moving it between elevation and depression would seem to help in many cases, making the subsequent path to the desired end position far smoother and less painful.

The principles apply equally well when it is the leg that is being treated alone or in combination with other limbs and/or the trunk and neck, the axiom being always to move and not to stretch.

For Elevation and Lateral Shortening of the Shoulder Girdle. When the arm is moved into abduction at an angle of 90 to the trunk, the movement often appears to be full and painfree, but the shoulder is seen to be pulled upwards and closer to the patient's head (Fig. 3.13a). The distance between his ear and the point of his shoulder is significantly reduced. As there is no muscle which by its shortening could cause the phenomenon, the logical explanation could well be increased tension within the nervous system or loss of its propensity to elongate.

The therapist allows the elbow to lie in a flexed position and then presses her fisted hand against the surface of the bed or plinth in such a way that her forearm is holding the patient's shoulder girdle firmly down in place, preventing any elevation. With her other hand she maintains dorsal extension of his wrist and fingers and abduction of his extended thumb (Fig. 3.13b). She then moves his arm back and forth gradually increasing the amount of elbow extension until full range becomes possible again (Fig. 3.13c). Another possibility would be for the therapist to relax the position of the patient's hand and mobilize the elbow component before slowly adding wrist and finger extension. Achieving full mobility may take days if not weeks of patient, carefully graded treatment. Tension and immobility in the nervous system which have possibly been developing over weeks or months cannot be expected to disappear after one to two quick sessions with the therapist.

When the Patient's Head Is Pulled to One Side. When the patient's arm is fully abducted, his neck may laterally flex towards that side to decrease the amount of tension, the position being particularly obvious when the contralateral arm is lying in abduction as well (Fig. 3.14a,b). The therapist continues to stabilize the shoulder girdle, but shifts her arm so that she can at the same time use her forearm to prevent the patient's head from being pulled sideways (Fig. 3.14c). When preventing the compensatory lateral flexion of the neck she will at first have to release some of the tension in other components.

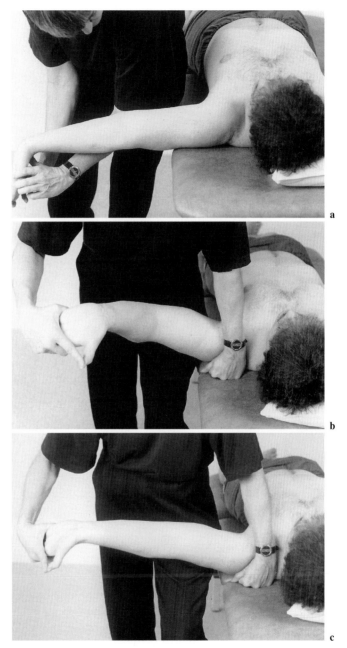

Fig. 3.13a. Distance from shoulder to neck markedly shortened. **b** Therapist holds shoulder girdle down and allows elbow flexion. **c** Gradual mobilization into full range of movement

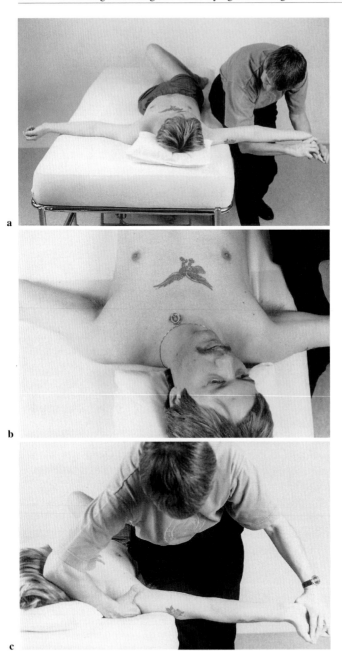

Fig. 3.14a. ULTT 1 with both arms abducted. **b** Neck pulled into lateral flexion. **c** Preventing side flexion of neck and shoulder girdle elevation

Incorporating ULTT1 Mobilization in Other Activities

It can be more effective to combine mobilization of the nervous system with other treatment activities, particularly if the patient is unable to tolerate the somewhat painful procedure in isolation. The inhibition of distal hypertonus through moving proximally can also be a help.

Turning the Upper Part of the Body

With the patient lying on his side, the therapist holds his undermost arm against her body, keeping his elbow as straight as is comfortably possible. She places her other hand on his opposite shoulder and moves the side of his trunk slowly backwards and forwards, gradually increasing the range of movement (Fig. 3.15a,b). As soon as she feels that the resistance is decreasing she emphasizes the turning backwards more and can even mobilize his chest wall when his thorax is almost supine by giving gentle pressure over the upper ribs on the side furthest from her (Fig. 3.15c). Once the arm is completely relaxed, the therapist holds his hand in dorsiflexion, keeps his shoulder girdle down and asks the patient to lie flat on his back with both his legs out straight without letting his arm pull into flexion (Fig. 3.15d). As he rolls onto his back she encourages him to turn his head away from her as well.

Rolling to One Side and Back Again in a Normal Pattern

Learning to roll over in bed in a normal way incorporates many useful active movements. The head rights, the trunk rotates and the abdominal muscles are activated, and as the uppermost leg lifts and moves forwards the same muscles are activated as are required later to take a step when walking. Once the patient is able to roll over in bed with ease, he will be able to turn himself at night without the help of the nursing staff.

The early facilitation of rolling over onto one side has been described in Chap. 2, and the patient has learned to do so in a normal way without pushing off with one foot behind him or pulling himself over with the help of one hand. Once the movement is possible without any undue effort he can concentrate on leaving his undermost arm lying relaxed on the bed as he turns from supine to side lying and back again, until he is able to do so, even when lying flat on his back with his other arm also abducted and extended. The therapist gives help when and where it may be necessary to facilitate or correct the movement (Fig. 3.16a–c).

Rotating the Trunk in Sitting with Arm Support Sideways

The patient sits on the edge of his bed or a plinth with one of his arms extended sideways and the hand flat on the supporting surface. The therapist stands behind him and helps him to maintain his balance and to keep his elbow extended while facilitating the trunk rotation in both directions (Fig. 3.17). The patient brings his

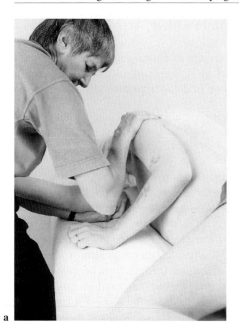

a

Fig. 3.15a–d. Trunk movement to mobilize arm abduction. **a** Side lying with
uppermost scapula forward. **b** Supporting
underneath arm with trunk rotated back.
c Pressing ribcage posteriorly on
contralateral side. **d** Complete range of
ULTT 1 attained

other hand first towards the supporting hand and then away out to the opposite side,
holding his arm in 90 abduction and moving it back as far as he can. By repeating
the movement, tone is inhibited and he is able to move further back each time so
increasing the amount of lengthening required of the nerves supplying the upper
limb. He is in fact mobilizing neural structures in the ULTT 1 as well as inhibiting
flexor spasticity in his arm and learning to take weight through it.

Mobilizing Abduction of the Arm in Sitting

When the patient is able to maintain his balance confidently in a sitting position
with his legs over the side of the bed, the therapist can mobilize his arm in abduction and outward rotation very effectively. Spasticity is inhibited and all components of the ULTT 1 can be incorporated in the activity and easily controlled.

The therapist stands or kneels behind the patient and supports his abducted arm
on the thigh of her leg nearest to him. Her thigh ensures that the shoulder joint itself
is kept in normal alignment and protected from being traumatized in any way
during the activity. She extends the patient's elbow, supinates his forearm and
holds this hand in full dorsiflexion (Fig. 3.18a). The patient can move his trunk
by flexing and extending his spine or by shifting his weight laterally from one side
to the other while the therapist keeps his arm in position. Alternatively, the therapist can place one of her hands on top of his shoulder girdle and move it gently and
rhythmically in a downward direction while the patient stabilizes his trunk. Should

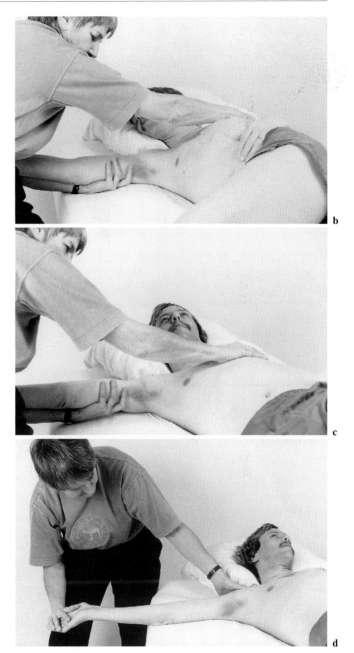

Fig. 3.15b–d

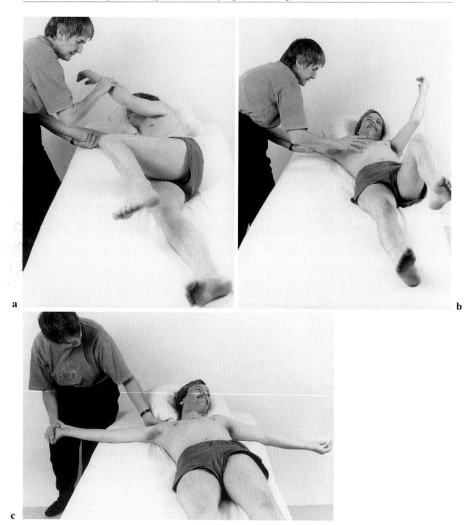

Fig. 3.16a–c. Rolling to mobilize upper limb tension. **a** Turning towards the affected arm. **b** Arm maintained in abduction as patient rolls back to supine. **c** Full abduction of both arms possible after repeated rolling

his head be pulled sideways, the therapist prevents the lateral flexion of his neck by pressing her forearm against the side of his head. When the structures are sufficiently mobile, she can increase the range by leaning his head towards the opposite side, the pressure of her forearm facilitating the lateral flexion (Fig. 3.18b). A further progression is included if the patient's other arm is also held in abduction and lateral rotation with the wrist and fingers extended. Because of horizontal structures within the nervous system, the degree of tension or amount of adaptive lengthening required will be increased (Fig. 3.19a), even more so if the patient is

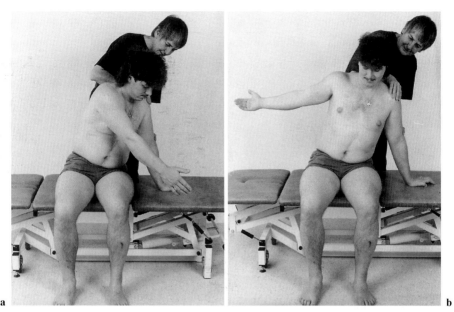

Fig. 3.17a,b. Inhibiting upper limb spasticity in sitting. **a** Rotating the trunk forwards with the arm supported sideways. **b** Trunk rotated back with contralateral arm abducted

asked to lean his head first to one side and then to the other while the therapist prevents compensatory elevation of his shoulder girdle (Fig. 3.19b). With the nervous system under tension and muscles fully elongated, care must be taken that the patient's trunk or limbs are not being pulled into unwanted postures which the body automatically adapts to escape or relieve the tension (Fig. 3.19c). If, for example, his trunk is translated sideways, the therapist can press her knee against his ribs to prevent or correct their lateral shift. Frequently when all deviations in posture are prevented, the patient complains of pain and tries to move out of the position. The therapist at once reduces the tension by releasing one or more of the components of movement. Depression of the shoulder girdle is a key component, and if a slight degree of elevation is allowed the pain is usually relieved instantly. However, the full range of depression must be regained as it is most important for function. It may be necessary for the therapist to mobilize it in isolation first, with all other components in nontensioned positions and then gradually include them again, one after the other in varying orders and increasing degrees.

For the patient who is already walking independently, mobilization of the upper limb in abduction can be combined with standing. The patient stands with one of his arms stretched out sideways, the palm of his hand supported against a wall. The therapist stands behind him and holds the hand in place while at the same time helping him to keep the elbow extended as he reaches towards the wall with his other hand and then turns away again. The patient keeps his arm extended and laterally rotated when he moves it at shoulder level away from the wall

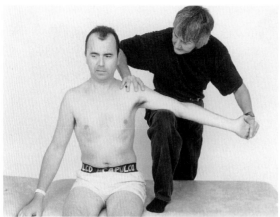

a

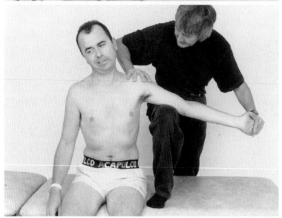

b

Fig. 3.18a,b. ULTT 1 in sitting. **a** Therapist's knee supports the abducted arm. **b** Neck side flexion to opposite side

and out to the side in abduction (Fig. 3.20). Turning his trunk away from the wall as well increases the effect still further. The therapist must ensure that the shoulder girdle is prevented from elevating during the movement.

Including ULTT 2 and ULTT 3 in the Treatment

ULTT 2

Although ULTT 2 is not usually as limited by abnormal tension as ULTT 1 following a lesion of the central nervous system, it should be carefully performed to check for any restriction. Some patients have shown significant improvement after mobilization to overcome even slight abnormal tension as revealed by means of the test.

ULTT 2 can be performed in two different ways, one with a median nerve bias the other biased towards the radial nerve (Butler 1991b). The therapist is advised to

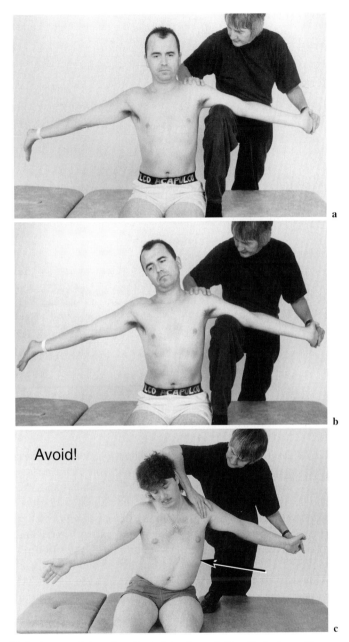

Fig. 3.19a–c. ULTT 1 with both arms abducted. **a** Contralateral arm held actively in position. **b** Active lateral flexion of neck. **c** Ribcage shifts laterally to relieve tension

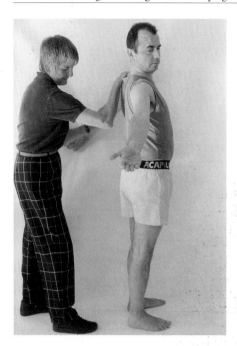

Fig. 3.20. Reducing upper limb tension in standing. The therapist maintains the patient's arm in position, his hand and fingers held flat against the wall

study the two variations carefully and practise their exact execution on a normal subject before using them in a treatment situation.

ULTT 2 with Median Nerve Bias. The therapist stands beside the patient with her thigh against his shoulder caudally. With the hand nearest to him she holds his elbow from the inner side and with her other hand she takes his wrist from above. She uses her thigh to depress the patient's shoulder girdle firmly but carefully and then straightens his elbow. After laterally rotating the arm, the therapist slides her lower hand down to extend the patient's wrist and fingers and abduct his extended thumb (Fig. 3.21a). Maintaining the position of his arm and hand she moves the whole limb away from his side by slowly abducting his shoulder. Although the therapist may feel little resistance the abduction may increase pain through tension quite suddenly and should therefore be undertaken very slowly within a small range of movement. Abduction is in any event normally only possible up to 40–50° with the shoulder girdle depressed.

ULTT 2 with Radial Nerve Bias. The therapist starts the movement as she did for ULTT 2 with median nerve bias, but once the patient's elbow is extended she medially rotates his arm and pronates the forearm. His wrist and fingers are then flexed (Fig. 3.21b). Adding flexion of the thumb will increase the sensitivity still further as will ulnar deviation of the wrist.

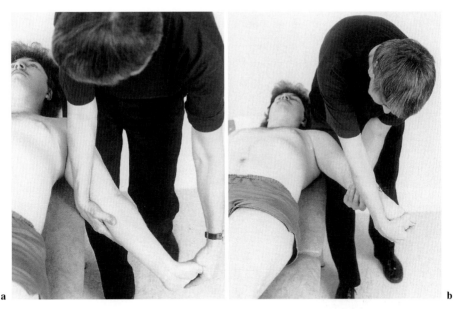

a   b

Fig. 3.21a,b. Mobilizing ULTT 2. **a** With median nerve bias. **b** With radial nerve bias

ULTT 3

Mobilization using ULTT 3 can be especially useful for a patient whose elbow resists passive or active flexion and whose fingers are difficult to straighten when his wrist is extended. Immediately after the mobilization it may be easier for him to extend his fingers actively.

With Supination. Standing at the patient's side, the therapist supports his flexed elbow on her upper thigh as she extends his wrist and fingers and supinates his forearm (Fig. 3.22a). Still maintaining the position of the other parts, the therapist flexes his elbow fully and, with her fisted hand pushing down against the bed to keep the shoulder girdle depressed, she transports the patient's arm up into abduction with lateral rotation of the shoulder (Fig. 3.22b). With his elbow still supported on her thigh, she continues to move his arm by shifting her weight towards the head end of the bed until his hand lies flat over his ear (Fig. 3.22c,d). The effect of the mobilization is increased when the therapist includes lateral flexion of the patient's neck by moving the pillow towards the opposite side (Fig. 3.22d). It is important to ensure that the lateral flexion occurs particularly in the lower cervical region. The therapist holds the patient's hand in place with one of her hands, releasing the other to move the pillow supporting his head towards the opposite side (Fig. 3.23a,b). With the patient's neck remaining in the side-flexed position she can once again include depression of his shoulder girdle (Fig. 3.23c).

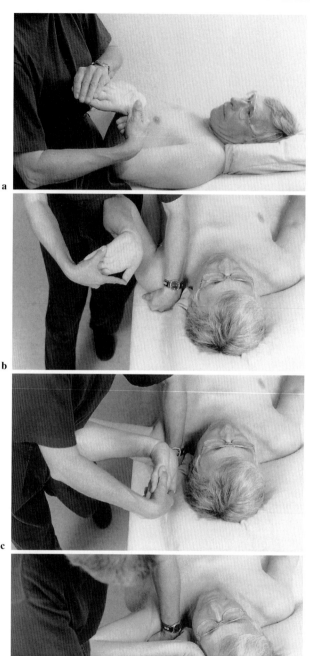

Fig. 3.22a–d. ULTT 3 with supination. **a** Wrist and fingers in dorsiflexion. **b** Forearm supinated with shoulder held down. **c** Therapist supports patient's elbow with her thigh and moves arm into abduction. **d** Extended hand placed over his ear

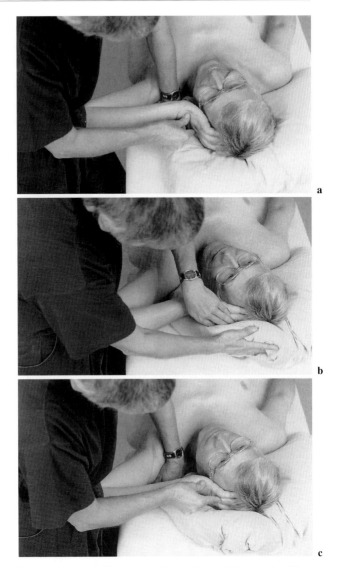

Fig. 3.23a–c. Adding the cervical component. **a** Keeping hand in position. **b** Moving the pillow sideways. **c** Depressing the shoulder girdle

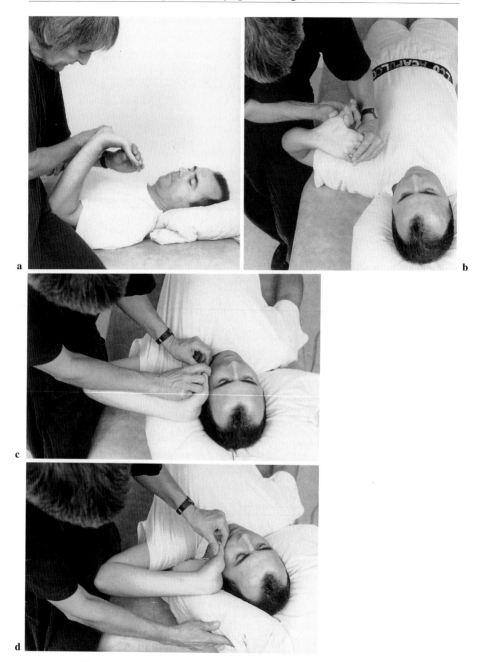

Fig. 3.24a–d. ULTT 3 with pronation. **a** Wrist and fingers extended. **b** Forearm pronated with elbow supported. **c** Hand placed against patient's head. **d** Adding lateral flexion of neck

With Pronation. The movement is performed in the same sequence but the therapist pronates the patient's forearm from the start with his elbow supported in flexion (Fig. 3.24a,b). In the final position, the patient's hand is once again placed flat over his ear but with his fingers pointing down towards his chin (Fig. 3.24c). When the position can be easily achieved, the therapist mobilizes tension still further, by adding lateral flexion of the lower cervical spine which she does by moving the pillow on which the patient's head is resting towards the contralateral side (Fig. 3.24d).

Regaining Active Control of the Arm

As the patient starts to regain consciousness, active movements of the arms should be attempted after mobilizing the trunk and using the ULTTs as treatment techniques. For example:

- The patient moves his hand to touch the top of his head and tries to leave it in a position with the palm and fingers in contact with his hair. The therapist facilitates a small movement as if he were rubbing his head (Fig 3.25a). She can also guide his hand down to touch his face or to lie over his mouth.

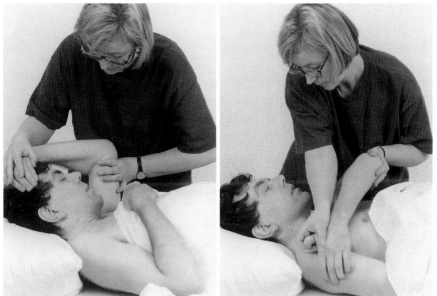

a   b

Fig. 3.25a,b. Initiating active movement of the arm. **a** Patient's hand rests on his head. **b** Patient rubs his opposite shoulder

- A useful way of facilitating movements with the patient's elbow flexing is for the therapist to help him to bring his hand to the opposite shoulder and use it to massage the outer side of his arm lightly by flexing and extending his elbow (Fig. 3.25b). The same can be done with his hand massaging his chest or abdomen.
- The patient who is at a more advanced stage can actively extend and relax his elbow selectively while the therapist holds his wrist and fingers in extension and moves the arm gradually sideways from a position vertically above his shoulder (Fig. 3.26a,b). The patient continues to move his elbow while his arm is being brought further and further into abduction with lateral rotation (Fig. 3.26c).

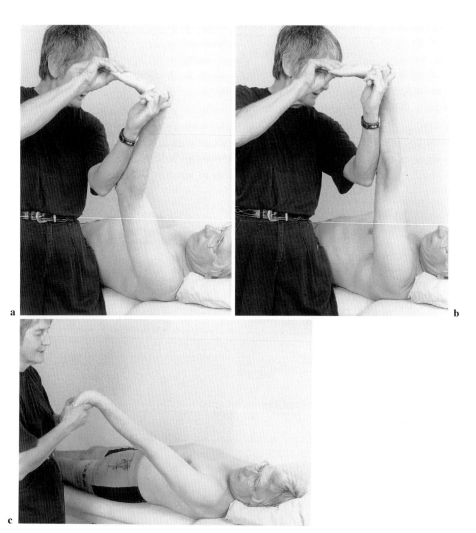

Fig. 3.26a–c. Selective extension of the elbow. **a** Allowing the elbow to flex. **b** Active assisted extension. **c** Elbow extension with the arm abducting

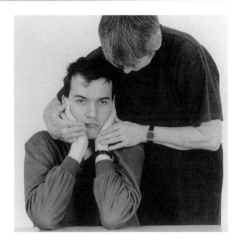

Fig. 3.27. Selective elbow flexion

- Sitting in a wheelchair with his arms supported on a table in front of him, the patient can be helped to bring his hands to his face, or to rest his chin on his hands (Fig. 3.27).

As has been explained in Chap. 1, such movements will be easier and provide a greater learning effect if they are combined with performing an actual task, such as the patient washing his face, applying aftershave lotion or drinking from a cup.

Mobilizing the Trunk and Lower Limbs

Instead of moving the legs passively from their distal end, it is far safer and more meaningful to combine their mobilization with movements of the trunk, particularly with regard to the hip joints and the structures surrounding them.

Moving the Lower Trunk

The patient's lumbar spine will tend to become extremely stiff during the acute stage, even more so if he is nursed in a supine position for long periods. Associated with the rigid extension in the lumbar area is a loss of pelvic mobility and often significantly increased extensor tone in the lower limbs. Right from the start, the therapist should mobilize flexion/rotation of the patient's lower trunk, either prophylactically or to overcome already existing stiffness, and certainly every day before she moves his legs.

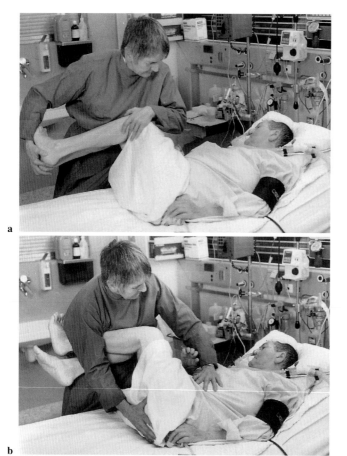

Fig. 3.28a,b. Flexion/rotation of the lower trunk. **a** The patient's flexed legs totally supported by the therapist. **b** Tilting the pelvis up in the front

With the patient supine, the therapist flexes both his legs in the air and rotates his trunk towards her until his knees and shins are resting against the front of her body with his hips flexed to an angle of 90 and not more (Fig. 3.28a). She continues to hold his legs in place with her hands, adjusting her position until she feels that the lower legs are totally supported by her body, before bending her knees a little to increase the amount of rotation occurring in the patient's lumbar spine. As only a small amount of rotatory movement is mechanically possible in the lower trunk, the therapist must be careful that the rotation is not tending to take place in the thoracic region instead, which it will do if the patient's legs are turned too far to the side.

The therapist places a hand directly over the patient's sacrum with her fingers pointing in the line of his vertebral column and holds his legs in position by pressing them against her body with her arm. Her other hand is positioned at about the level of the sternal angle with the thumb and fingers spread out to enable her to ease both sides of the patient's lower ribcage down towards his pelvis.

Transferring her weight towards the head end of the bed, the therapist tilts the patient's pelvis up in the front with a small movement as if she were drawing his sacrum forwards between his legs while at the same time moving his ribs in a downward direction so that the flexion is localized in the lumbar region (Fig. 3.28b). Shifting her weight back over her other leg she allows the pelvis to return to the starting position before repeating the movement sequence.

When flexing the lumbar spine with rotation the degree of hip flexion should not increase at all, but the original angle of 90 should be maintained constantly.

Mobilizing Flexion of the Trunk and Lower Limbs

After flexing and rotating the patient's lumbar spine, the therapist brings his hips into more flexion and flexes his whole spine (Fig. 3.29a). She includes neck flexion, which reduces the hypertonus in the extensors, and brings him up to a crook-sitting position with his arms forward around his knees (Fig. 3.29b,c). She waits for

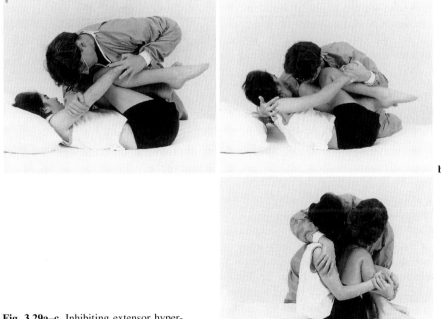

Fig. 3.29a–c. Inhibiting extensor hypertonia. **a** Both legs flexed. **b** Neck and trunk flexion combined. **c** Patient brought to crook-sitting

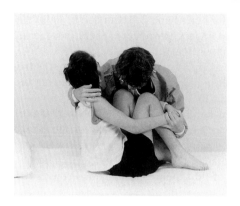

Fig. 3.30. Rocking gently back without extensor spasticity elicited

the patient to relax before attempting to ease his head forward to touch his knees. Crook sitting is one of the best positions for achieving an equal distribution of flexion throughout the whole spine and to overcome the problem of hypertonus in the hip extensors.

Once the patient is comfortably in the position, the therapist can move him slowly back towards lying, rocking gently back and forth only as far as is possible each time without his head, trunk or legs pushing into extension and with his arms remaining in place around his knees (Fig. 3.30). Eventually it should be possible for the patient to be moved right down to the starting position and back up again without any loss of flexion, first passively and later actively as well.

Trunk Flexion in Sitting

To prevent the patient's trunk from stiffening in extension, the therapist can from a very early stage onwards, sit him up over the side of the bed with his feet flat on the floor and help him to lean forwards to touch his toes. When the patient is still not able to move actively, she stands in front of him holding his knees in place with her knees to prevent him from slipping forwards off the bed as she supports his trunk while flexing it forwards (Fig. 3.31a).

She then kneels in close proximity so that she can guide his hands towards his feet, going further down each time the movement is repeated until the aim is achieved (Fig. 3.31b). When he leans forward in this way, the patient's spine flexes easily with gravity, and his hips are automatically flexed as well.

The therapist does not let him remain in a flexed position for long but brings his trunk to an upright position again with as much assistance as is necessary (Fig. 3.31c). The patient's heels must remain in contact with the floor throughout the procedure.

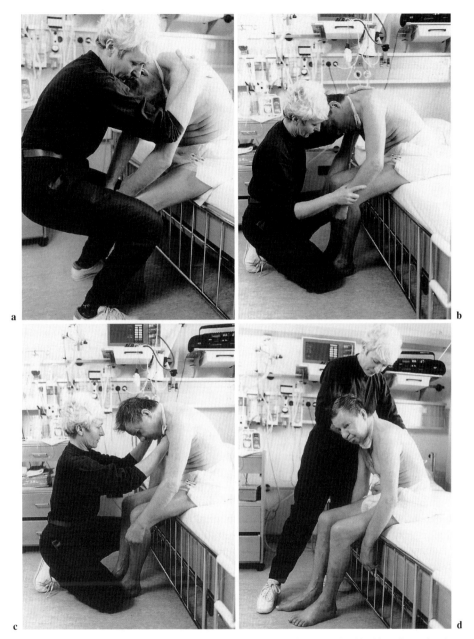

Fig. 3.31a–d. Trunk flexion in sitting. **a** Bending forward with therapist blocking the patient's knees. **b** Hands down towards feet. **c** Assisting return to an upright position. **d** Assisting extension of the thoracic spine

Once the movement can be performed without too much effort on the part of the patient or the therapist, she stands next to him and facilitates trunk extension as the first step towards attaining an upright sitting posture. With one hand over his sternum to give counterpressure in an upward direction, the therapist uses her other hand to extend the patient's thoracic spine by pressing down and forwards (Fig 3.31d). At the same time, one of the patient's relatives can call on him to look up at her in order to provide a stimulus for active extension.

Flexing and Extending the Trunk in Sitting

Flexion and extension of the patient's trunk in sitting will not only mobilize the intervertebral and lumbosacral joints but will also improve the patient's sitting posture. Later the ability to move the lumbar spine selectively will be important for a normal walking pattern. The process of regaining the movement can be commenced as soon as the patient starts to sit out of bed.

When the patient is sitting in a wheelchair with his arms supported on a table in front of him, the therapist stands beside or behind him and, with one arm placed round the front of his chest and the other over his upper thoracic vertebrae, she flexes his trunk. The arm in front of his body draws the lower ribs down and away from the table while her other hand eases his shoulders forward. If the backrest of the wheelchair is removable the therapist can position herself so that she use more of her own body in contact with the patient's to increase the amount of flexion in the whole spine (Fig. 3.32a).

After giving the patient time to relax in the flexed position, she moves her hands so that she can extend his trunk as much as possible. With one hand over his sternum and her arm in contact with the anterior aspect of one of his shoulders, she extends the patient's upper trunk, while her other hand eases his thoracic spine forward so moving his lower ribs nearer to the table (Fig. 3.32b).

As the patient's balance in sitting improves, he should be transferred to sit on a normal, upright chair without armrests at various times during the day, and the same activity can be practised in different situations but still with a table supporting his arms, for example, at mealtimes or in the occupational therapy department prior to performing other tasks. The therapist encourages the patient to flex and extend his whole spine as fully as he can, using her hands to increase the range of movement in both directions (Fig. 3.33a,b).

Once he is able to flex and extend his trunk freely in a total pattern of movement, the patient must learn to move his lower trunk selectively while stabilizing his thoracic spine. The therapist places one of her arms in front of him and brings his ribs on both sides towards the midline with some compression to help him keep his thorax still while he is flexing and extending his lumbar spine. With her other hand she indicates the part which should be moving and teaches him to localize the movement to only that region (Fig. 3.33c,d).

As his ability improves, the patient practises the selective flexion and extension of his lumbar spine sitting with his arms held loosely at his sides or resting on his

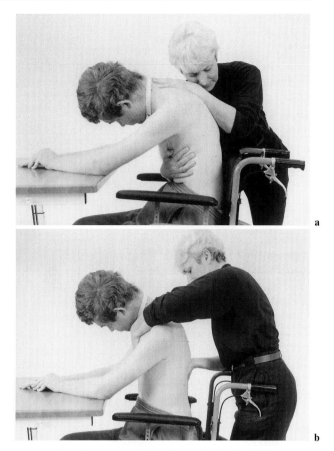

Fig. 3.32a,b. Passive flexion and extension of the trunk. **a** Mobilizing flexion. **b** Achieving extension

knees (Fig. 3.34). Without the help of the table in front of him, the activity is far more difficult because he has to stabilize his thoracic spine actively in an upright position despite the weight of his arms and the freely movable shoulder girdle. The therapist facilitates the correctly localized movement by using one of her hands as a point of reference for the stationary thorax and her other hand to help him tilt his pelvis back and forth rhythmically.

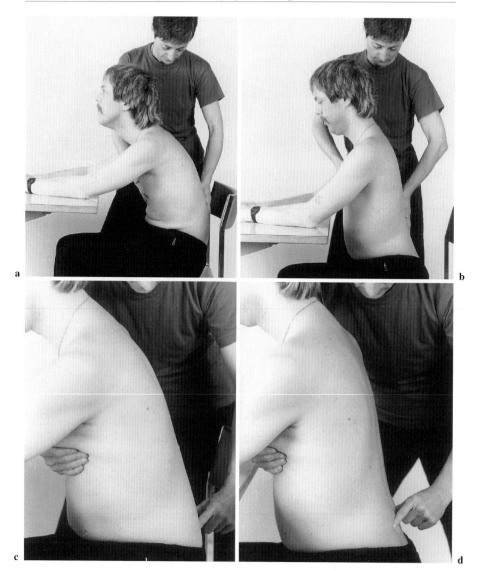

Fig. 3.33a–d. Flexing and extending the trunk actively with arms supported. **a** Assisting total flexion. **b** Encouraging active extension. **c** Facilitating selective flexion of the lumbar spine. **d** Selective extension with thoracic spine stabilized

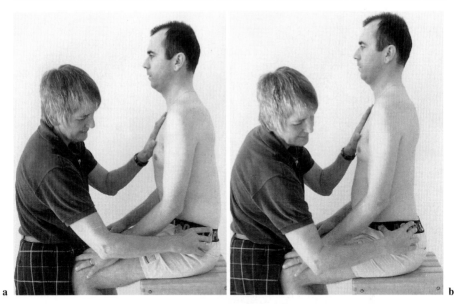

Fig. 3.34a,b. Selective trunk flexion and extension with arms free. **a** Thoracic spine stabilized during lumbar spine flexion. **b** Active extension of lumbar spine

Mobilizing the Trunk and Hips in Cross-Sitting

Cross-sitting is a useful position for mobilizing the hips and trunk, because with the legs in the total pattern of flexion, hypertonus of the lower limb extensors is inhibited. This enables the therapist to flex the hips and trunk more easily as well as to adjust the position of the pelvis. The movement of the trunk proximally mobilizes the hips in abduction with outward rotation.

It is advisable for the therapist to inhibit extensor hypertonus before attempting to bring the patient into a cross-sitting position. She does so by using the inhibitory movement of lumbar flexion with rotation until she feels that his legs have relaxed (Fig. 3.35a).

Maintaining the flexion of the trunk and limbs, she crosses his ankles and gradually abducts the patient's hips, using one hand to press his knees apart while supporting his feet in position with her other hand (Fig. 3.35b). When his knees are sufficiently abducted, the therapist places one arm behind the patient's shoulders and brings him up to sitting, moving at once to kneel on the bed behind him.

Keeping her body in close contact with the whole length of his back she eases his trunk forwards, moving his arms further and further out in front of him (Fig. 3.35c). With her head the therapist guides the patient's head into position. If the patient's arms pull up strongly into flexion, the therapist inhibits the spasticity by placing his hands flat on the bed behind him with his elbows extended and

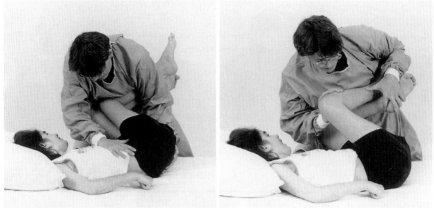

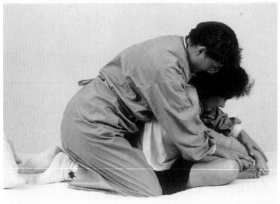

Fig. 3.35a–c. Moving to cross-sitting. **a** Inhibiting extensor spasticity. **b** Abducting the legs in flexion. **c** Easing the knees apart and increasing hip flexion

the arms laterally rotated so that his fingers are pointing backwards (Fig. 3.36). In this position, she moves his trunk in all directions while his arms remain in place, thus inhibiting the distal hypertonus by proximal movement.

The therapist places her hands over the patient's shoulders and draws them back to retract the scapulae and facilitate trunk extension. She uses her forearms and elbows to help him to keep his arms extended (Fig. 3.37a). With her hands in the same position the therapist moves the scapulae into protraction and helps the patient to flex his trunk forward (Fig. 3.37b).

In order to extend the patient's whole spine with increased hip flexion, the therapist stands behind him and lifts his laterally rotated arms above his head and supports them underneath her arms. Her hands grasp the inferior borders of his scapulae so that she can take the weight of his trunk as she elongates his spine, without pulling on his shoulder joints. She presses her knees gently forwards against the patient's lower thoracic spine to ease it into extension (Fig. 3.37c). By moving his whole trunk forwards, the degree of hip flexion is

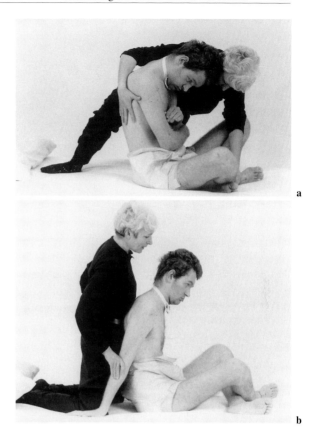

Fig. 3.36a,b. Sitting cross-legged with extended arms. **a** Upper limbs pulled into flexion. **b** Therapist supports arms in extension and outward rotation behind patient

increased. The therapist then asks the patient to relax his trunk into flexion before helping him to extend his spine fully again. Maintaining the extended position, she can also use her knees to transfer his weight from one side to the other.

Mobilization in Long-Sitting

Patients who have suffered a central nervous system lesion usually have extreme difficulty in sitting up with their legs extended in front of them and in moving their hands towards their feet (Fig. 3.38a). A considerable resistance to the movement can be felt and the patient experiences pain usually behind his knees and thighs. Dorsiflexion of the feet or even of one foot increases the difficulty significantly and will often cause the patient's neck to extend in order to relieve tension (Fig. 3.38b). Previously the problem was interpreted as being due to short or tight hamstrings, but it is obvious that dorsiflexion of the foot does not change the length of the hamstring muscles themselves, and neither can neck flexion which also reduces

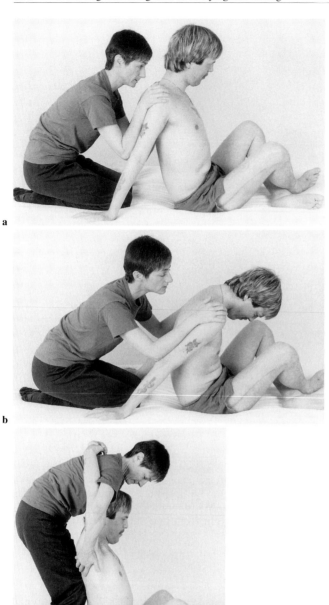

Fig. 3.37a–c. Trunk flexion and extension in cross-sitting. **a** Extension with arms supported. **b** Trunk flexion with scapula protraction. **c** Trunk extension with increased hip flexion

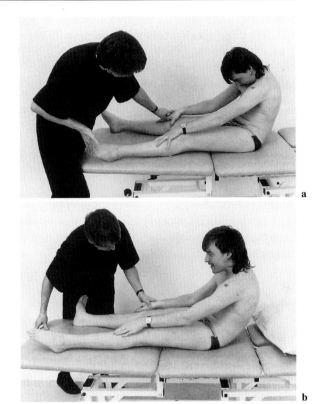

Fig. 3.38a,b. Difficulties experienced in long-sitting. **a** Patient unable to move his hands to his feet. **b** With right foot in dorsal flexion trunk further back and neck extended to relieve tension

the range of movement and increases the degree of pain. A more logical interpretation is that the position tenses the nervous system and the presence of abnormally increased tension prevents full range of movement. The position is in fact that of the slump test in long-sitting as described by Butler (1991b), with tension increasing from the foot right up to the cerebellum. It is most important that the loss of range be prevented by early mobilization or overcome if the problem already exists, because the increased nervous tension will cause other difficulties which limit function. Some examples of movements limited by such tension are sitting up in bed, sitting in the bathtub, and walking. The patient cannot take a step of normal length because at the end of the swing phase when the knee must extend to carry the foot forward before heel-strike the tension prevents the movement. The knee remains flexed and the step length is reduced. If the knee does extend, the ankle plantarflexes so that the ball of the foot reaches the ground first.

The abnormal tension causes the foot to plantarflex and the toes to flex, the increased resistance preventing active dorsiflexion when the knee is extended. Ankle clonus may develop and interfere with standing up from sitting or weight-bearing on a plantigrade foot. The knee flexors become hypertonic particularly when the hips are flexed as they are in a half-lying position or in sitting. In the wheelchair the patient's feet will be pulled back off the footrests and under the chair. Flexion contractures can easily develop at the hips and knees, and the Achilles tendon shorten.

Movement Sequence for Mobilization

The therapist brings the patient into cross-sitting as described above and waits until the patient has relaxed in the position (Fig. 3.39a). From her position kneeling behind him, she slowly straightens out first one leg and then the other allowing the legs to remain slightly flexed and laterally rotated (Fig. 3.39b). The therapist then slowly extends the patient's knees with her hands and corrects the rotation of his legs to a midposition. With her body in close contact with his, she leans forwards to bring his hands towards his feet (Fig. 3.39c). In the acute stage she will need another person to hold the patient's feet in dorsiflexion while she moves his trunk backwards and forwards to mobilize the tight structures and slowly increase range (Fig. 3.39d).

PROBLEM SOLVING

If the abnormal tension is so marked that it is not possible for the therapist to straighten the patient's legs when he has been brought to sitting although he has no actual flexion contracture of his knees, it is imperative that a solution be found (Fig. 3.40a). The patient's legs can be held in extension by splints made of plaster of Paris which are bandaged on when he is lying on his back. The therapist kneels behind him and moves his trunk repeatedly up and down within a relatively small range by extending and flexing her knees, bringing him a little further forwards each time. The keyword here is "move"; the therapist must not try to overcome the resistance with force (Fig. 3.40b,c). An assistant moves the patient's feet up and down with an increasing range of dorsiflexion, supporting one foot against her thigh while moving the foot furthest from her with her hands (Fig. 3.40d).

It is often far easier in such a case to stand the patient up with the knee-extension splints bandaged firmly in place and then flex his trunk forward towards a table in front of him (see Fig. 4.22, showing the same patient in action). When the patient is in standing, dorsiflexion of his feet can be maintained and the amount increased by placing a rolled bandage beneath his toes.

Using LLTT 1 as a Treatment Technique

In order to maintain the adaptive lengthening of the nerves and neural tissues of the lower limb and lumbar region, the therapist can mobilize the LLTT 1 using the same procedure to regain any lost range of motion. After mobilizing the lumbar spine in flexion and rotation, she kneels at the foot end of the bed and places the patient's lower leg on her shoulder, sitting back on her heels so that his knee can

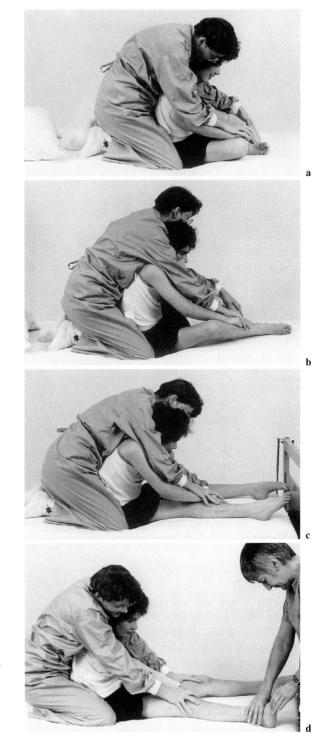

Fig. 3.39a–d. Early mobilization of long-sitting. **a** Cross-sitting reduces extensor hypertonia in the lower limbs. **b** Gradually extending one leg. **c** Both legs extended. **d** Dorsiflexion of foot added

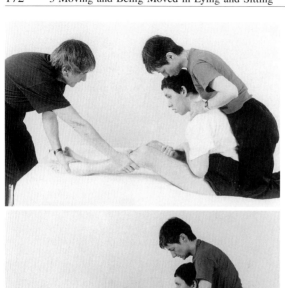

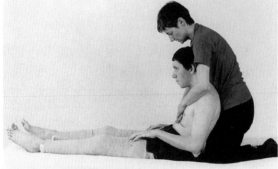

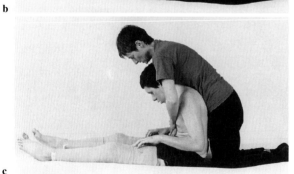

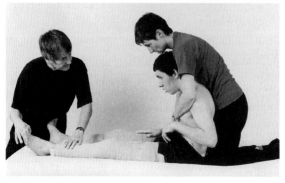

Fig. 3.40. a Patient's legs cannot be extended in long-sitting. **b** Legs held in extension by plaster splints. **c** Moving trunk gradually further forward. **d** Helper adds distal component by dorsiflexing feet

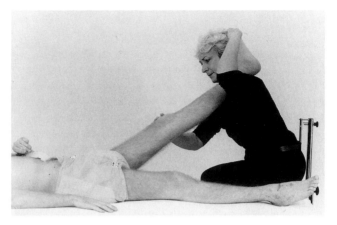

Fig. 3.41. Flexing and extending the knee in the straight leg raise (SLR) position

relax in full extension without discomfort. With one hand the therapist reaches up and holds the patient's foot in full dorsal flexion while her other hand extends his knee before moving it into slight flexion again and repeating the movement (Fig. 3.41). If the patient is able to participate, he can perform the movement actively with as much assistance as is necessary. He extends his knee actively and then allows it to flex again. As the leg relaxes, the therapist gradually increases the amount of hip flexion by extending her hips and knees appropriately in order to raise the height of her shoulder to the right level. Should the patient's contralateral leg lift off the bed, the therapist holds it in place with her knee pressing on his thigh.

For some patients, the possibility of using LLTT 1 with the foot plantarflexed and inverted should be considered, particularly if pain in the limb is the main problem or if an Achilles tendon lengthening has been performed and the foot habitually pulls strongly into dorsiflexion.

Using the Slump Test to Mobilize the Nervous System

Using the slump test as a treatment technique is a very effective way of mobilizing the nervous system as a whole. It not only helps to reduce tension in the lower limb but will often influence the tone in the upper limbs positively as well. The trunk becomes more flexible and scapula retraction is inhibited.

The patient sits with his legs over the side of the bed or a plinth, sufficiently far back to ensure that his thighs are well supported. The therapist places one hand over his thoracic spine to prevent his falling backwards as she lifts one of his feet from the floor and extends his knee. One of her hands holds his foot in dorsiflexion and her knee pressing on his thigh keeps his leg in place on the bed (Fig. 3.42a). The patient's trunk is then moved forwards over his knees and back towards the upright position, his arms hanging loosely at his sides. The therapist tries to in-

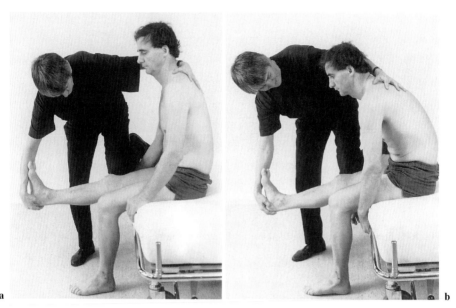

a

b

Fig. 3.42a,b. The slump test as a treatment technique. **a** Maintaining knee extension and ankle dorsiflexion. **b** Moving the trunk forwards

crease the forward inclination each time by giving gentle overpressure with her hand behind his back and shoulders, flexing the spine only as far as the patient can tolerate easily (Fig. 3.42b). At first she leaves his neck in extension, but as the range of movement improves she tilts his head forward as well.

Alternatively the movement can be performed with the leg being the moving lever instead of the trunk. While the patient's feet are still resting on the floor, the therapist first flexes his trunk and neck with her arm placed right round behind him so that her hand rests on his furthermost shoulder to enable her to bring both sides forward symmetrically and keep his head down too (Fig. 3.43a). Still maintaining the position of his trunk, the therapist holds the patient's foot in dorsiflexion with her other hand and lifts it to extend his knee as far as is possible without causing too much discomfort. She lowers and raises the foot repeatedly, trying to increase the amount of knee extension as she feels the resistance lessening (Fig. 3.43b). It is sometimes advisable to mobilize the patient's leg first with the foot left free, and to add the distal component of dorsiflexion only when the knee is moving easily.

It may well be that the patient's spine is stiffer in some parts than in others and the movement into flexion is not evenly distributed throughout the vertebral column. Through close observation, the therapist will notice should too much motion be occurring in one section while at another level the smooth normal curve appears flattened. The flattened area may be localized to a few vertebral segments or may extend over the entire lumbar or thoracic region. In order not to place too much stress on the more mobile areas, the therapist can position a firm padded roll against the front of the patient's trunk so that it is directly beneath the stiffened

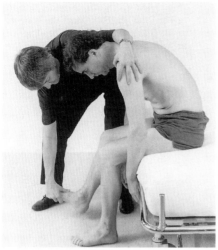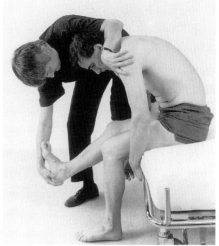

a   b

Fig. 3.43a,b. Using the slump test to mobilize the nervous system. **a** Patient's trunk and neck flexed. **b** Lifting his foot to extend his knee

section when he flexes forwards. Pillows can be used to adjust the height of the roll exactly the right amount. With his feet still on the floor, the patient bends forwards as far as he can and in the flexed position, the therapist mobilizes his spine, his ribs and his scapulae, the roll providing a stable counterpressure from below (Fig. 3.44a). Extending one of his knees as she did before with the foot dorsi-flexed, the therapist moves the patient's trunk forwards and back again with his arms relaxed over the top of the roll, at first with his head left free (Fig. 3.44b). When she feels that there is less resistance to the movement, she adjusts the position of her arm which is round behind him so that she can use her forearm against the back of his head to move his neck into flexion as well (Fig. 3.44c). Once again it may be preferable to hold the patient's trunk in the flexed position with the roll correctly placed and then lift and lower his foot, moving the distal components for the mobilization instead of the proximal.

The Slump Test with the Legs Abducted

Patient's whose movements are hampered by adductor hypertonus frequently benefit from mobilization of the slump test with hip abduction. The sitting position must be adapted, however, because most patients will not be able to prevent the contralateral leg from being pulled inwards when one leg is being mobilized in abduction.

After working to inhibit adduction and extension of the lower limbs in cross-sitting, the therapist draws the patient's legs apart and lowers one down on either side of the plinth with the knee flexed placing a pillow on the inside of each thigh to prevent discomfort through pressure against the hard edge. Sitting astride the

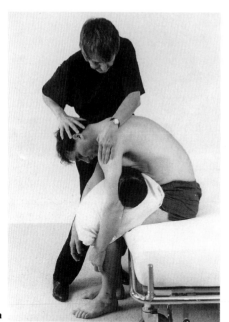

Fig. 3.44a–c. Localizing spinal flexion. **a** Firm roll placed beneath the stiffened area. **b** Leg extension with head up. **c** Neck flexion included

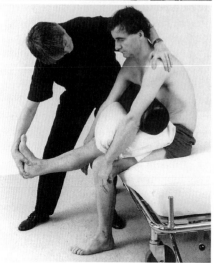

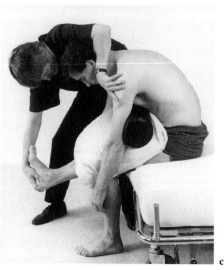

plinth, the patient flexes his trunk and brings his forehead down to touch the supporting surface in front of him. If he is unable to keep his hands actively in place on the plinth as he moves, he clasps them together and rests his forehead on his crossed thumbs. With the patient's trunk flexed, the therapist dorsiflexes his foot and extends his knee. Mobilization can be carried out either by the patient moving his trunk back and forth while his leg is held in extension, or by the therapist flexing and extending his knee without his changing the position of his head and trunk (Fig. 3.45).

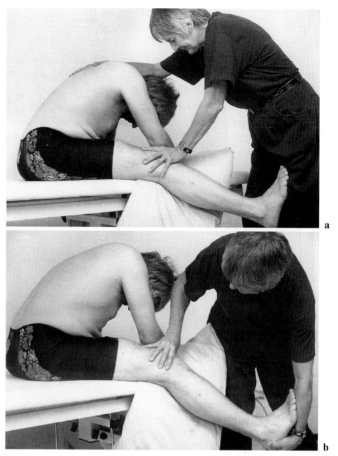

Fig. 3.45a,b. The slump test with legs abducted. **a** Therapist maintains knee extension and ankle dorsiflexion during repeated trunk flexion. **b** Patient keeps trunk flexed while leg is moved repeatedly

Conclusion

The more the patient moves or is moved, the less he will be likely to develop complications associated with long periods of immobilization. If he is moving actively, the therapist is guided by the quality of the movement which provides her with information about the suitability of the activity, the tone of the muscles and the appropriateness of the support she is giving. Should a movement be performed in an abnormal pattern, the therapist must carefully analyze the reasons for the deviation and adjust her treatment and facilitation accordingly. Any movement which takes place in an abnormal way with too much effort or an increase in tone should not be repeated without alteration because the patient will otherwise only experience an abnormal input and through repetition, store an incorrect motor engram.

Mobilization of adverse mechanical tension in the nervous system is of great value in preventing the development of painful stiffening or limb contractures. Active functional movements should always follow the passive mobilization techniques to make use of the freedom of movement and improved sensation resulting from such mobilization. Improvement of the patient's motor function is possible even years after the initial lesion when mobilization of the nervous system is included in the treatment programme.

A Case in Point

R.B. was 11 years old when he was knocked off his bicycle by a car on his way to school. He sustained a severe head injury and was in coma for more than 3 weeks before slowly starting to regain consciousness. Fortunately for R.B., he had informed therapy from the start so that full range of movement was maintained and marked spasticity had not developed by the time he started active rehabilitation. He was, however, unable to use his right arm for any function and when walking required a brace to maintain his foot in dorsiflexion. Any attempt to move his arm or hand resulted in side flexion of his trunk and an increase in flexor tone in his whole upper limb particularly in the wrist and hand (Fig. 3.46a).

With intensive outpatient treatment over the next 2 years, R.B. became completely independent in the activities of daily living, attended a normal school and could walk safely at a relatively good speed. At 14, however, R.B. was not able to use his hand functionally, still required the brace for walking and was having difficulties with spelling and grammar at school despite his obviously high level of intelligence.

He and his family decided to spend their summer vacations so that he could combine the holiday with periods of intensive therapy at a specialized centre. Despite the unwillingness of the insurance to pay for further treatment after 5 years, R.B. continued to have some sessions with his steadfast therapist at home, and worked every weekend to earn money to pay for the additional intensive therapy during his summer vacations.

One innovation in his treatment allowed him to discard the brace and regain good motor activity in his arm, although sadly not in his hand (Fig. 3.46b), while a second helped to improve his academic performance. The motor improvement followed the inclusion of selective trunk activity in the treatment with specific ball activities included in his home exercise programme (Davies 1990). Therapeutic guiding as described in Chap. 1 was introduced and diligently carried out at home as well as with the therapist. The guiding appeared to solve the cognitive problems because at the age of 18, R.B. finished school with flying colours. However, his

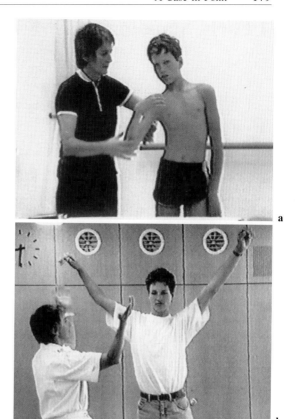

Fig. 3.46a. R.B. aged 12 attempting to move his arm actively. **b** R.B. aged 17 lifts both arms actively (Archive photos from video films)

hand continued to be frustratingly inactive despite all therapeutic efforts, and he still walked with a limp, with steps far too short for his exceptional height, 1.96 m.

To the surprise of everyone, mobilization of the adverse tension in his nervous system at last allowed his hand to start moving actively. Following the use of the slump test as a treatment technique, particularly when his left leg was mobilized, R.B. could for the first time in 7 years move his fingers in extension. He was shown how to perform automobilization at home in addition and at the age of 20 could walk at a normal speed and was able to fulfil one of his dreams — he learned to windsurf (see frontispiece).

4 Early Standing

It is imperative that every patient who has suffered a significant brain lesion with resultant paralysis be helped to stand in a fully upright position, even if he is still unconscious or totally unable to move actively himself. Assisted standing should commence in the early days following any cerebral lesion, whatever its cause may be. There are very few real contraindications to standing, and the team should discuss fully and try to circumvent any complications which could prevent the patient from being brought into an upright standing position. It was ingenuity on the part of the staff, for example, which enabled a young patient to stand despite a complicated fracture of his tibia that was sustained at the same time as his head trauma. A platform was placed beneath his other foot so that he could stand without any weight being taken on the injured leg.

From the time that the patient's medical condition permits standing and the position has been achieved, supported standing should be continued on a daily basis until such time as the patient is able to stand up and walk on his own. The erect bipedal posture is part of man's heritage and affords a feeling of physical well-being, energy and alertness. After sitting for extended periods in a flexed position or lying in bed for too long, perhaps as a result of illness, everyone has a strong urge to stand up straight, stretch cramped limbs and move again. Similarly the brain-damaged patient's psychological and physical condition improves through standing upright and feeling the earth beneath his feet again.

The Importance of Standing the Patient

It is of the utmost importance for the patient to stand upright for the following reasons:

- The development of the all too common contractures in the patient's legs can be avoided altogether, eliminating the need for surgical or conservative correction at a later stage. The patient is spared an incalculable amount of pain and suffering and the end result of his rehabilitation is optimized. When a patient has marked spasticity in the plantar flexors of his foot, standing him upright is often the only way in which the therapist can maintain the range of dorsiflexion of the ankle and prevent shortening of the Achilles tendon. It is often not possible to maintain the range of motion in the lower limb by passive movements alone if excessive hypertonicity is a problem.

- Spasticity in the lower limbs is dramatically reduced even in patients with spinal lesions.
- While the patient is standing, movements can be performed which mobilize adverse tension in the whole nervous system and prevent any abnormal tension which may already have developed from increasing still further.
- Osteoporosis with the concomitant danger of spontaneous fractures in the lower limbs and spinal column is reduced or even prevented altogether.
- Clinical observations have revealed that once patients start to stand not only does their motor performance improve but their ability to perform other tasks as well. Clinically, the comatose patient appears to be less deeply so when standing and it is just possible that the period of unconsciousness may be shortened as a result.
- The patient who has stood in the early stages is less likely to be afraid while standing and walking when his level of consciousness improves. Patients who have been immobilized in bed for long periods following onset of coma are often terrified when brought into an upright position later.
- Standing brings improved circulation and relief of pressure over vulnerable areas, which help to prevent the development of pressure sores and speed up the healing process of any that may already be present.
- Bladder function improves, particularly bladder emptying, once the patient stands regularly.

Children with traumatic brain injury or other severe brain lesions must be stood every day including Sundays and holidays, to ensure normal bone growth in the lower limbs through weight-bearing.

It would be a pity if a child who later recovers function sufficient to enable him to enjoy a normal lifestyle were to be burdened by having marked shortening of his legs. Fortunately it is far easier to stand with a child than it is with an adult patient!

Considerations Before Standing the Patient

At first the therapist will require assistance when bringing the patient into a standing position from his bed or from the treatment table. The patient's relatives can provide invaluable help in this respect if they are encouraged and carefully trained from the start. They should not be sent out of the room when therapy is being carried out but should become an integral part of the rehabilitation team. If they know what to do, they will be more than willing to help in any way they can.

Cooperation and teamwork between the physiotherapist and nursing staff is, of course, essential. In the ideal situation, be it during the intensive care stage or later, the nurse can help the therapist to bring the patient out of bed and into the correct standing posture. She can then, for example, make the patient's bed while the therapist is supporting him in standing.

There are various ways in which the comatose or severely paralyzed patient can be helped out of bed and supported in a standing position. All of them require time and considerable effort on the part of the staff, but for the patient's future it is certainly more than worth such effort, and the time is indeed well spent.

Whichever method is used, until the patient is completely continent once more, it is advisable for him to wear an incontinence pad in order to avoid frustrating and time-consuming accidents. Disposable padded shorts are easy to apply and provide in addition a modicum of decency for patients when they are first brought out of bed. Once a patient has left the intensive care unit and can sit out of bed for longer periods, he will in any event be dressed in his own clothes.

Standing the Patient Upright

The patient can be supported in different ways while standing:

1. Using knee-extension splints.
2. Using a standing frame.
3. Using a tilt table.

Using Knee-Extension Splints

The method of choice for standing the patient is with his knees held in extension by firm splints bandaged on behind his knees. Standing behind the patient, the therapist is able to move him easily in all directions. She can control the position of his trunk, move his trunk and shift his weight from one side to the other or forwards and backwards. With the therapist supporting him, the patient can be encouraged to participate actively. Particularly if the patient is still in the intensive care unit where the available space is limited, an additional advantage of using knee-extension splints is that no other equipment is needed.

The splints, which should reach from about 8 cm below the patient's ischial tuberosity to 4 cm above his malleoli, are in the form of a firm posterior shell made of plaster of Paris or some other hard material (Fig. 4.1). Another type of support is the so-called keystone splint which is made of canvas covering longitudinal metal struts. The material is wrapped around the patient's leg and then firmly fastened in place. Air-filled splints are not recommended because by their nature they offer little stable tactile information and reduce the amount of input the patient receives through contact with his surroundings. The therapist is, for example, not able to stimulate activity by tapping the patient's knee extensors, or to indicate the correct location with her fingers.

Plaster of Paris splints in the form of back slabs are made by the therapist or orthopaedic nurse for the individual patient, ensuring an exact fit in the same way as recommended for para- and tetraplegic patients (Bromley 1976). How this type of splint can be quickly and easily made even if the patient is still in the intensive care unit is described in Chap. 6. The other splints can be ordered through a firm of orthopaedic suppliers or an orthopaedic technician and usually come in three sizes, small, medium or large and are so designed as to fit either leg.

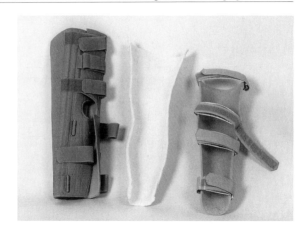

Fig. 4.1. Knee-extension splints in the form of (from left to right): wrap-around canvas with metal struts, plaster of Paris back slab, and a posterior shell of hard plastic material

Bandaging on the Splints

Whichever type of knee-extension splint is used, it will need to be bandaged in place with two 10 cm wide crepe bandages in order to give adequate support and maintain an optimal position of the patient's leg. The bandages should have only a slight degree of elasticity as the patient's knee will otherwise tend to sag forwards in flexion despite the back slab. Even those custom-made supports which have fitted straps with a fastening device will need to be bandaged on more firmly in addition.

The patient lies supine and the therapist bandages on the splints in such a way as to correct any inward or outward rotation of the limb.

To Correct Outward Rotation (Fig. 4.2a). If the patient's leg lies laterally rotated, the therapist starts bandaging at the level of his knee, pulling the bandage firmly from the lateral side towards the medial (Fig. 4.2b). In order to prevent the splint from rotating as well, the therapist uses one of her hands to press down on its outer edge at the same time as she pulls the bandage medially over the top of the patient's leg with her other hand (Fig. 4.2c). Two bandages are required so that the whole length of the splint is covered. When the splint is applied in this way it is often possible to correct the asymmetrical rotation altogether (Fig. 4.2d).

To Correct Inward Rotation. The patient's knee will often tend to turn inwards (Fig. 4.3a) and will even do so when placed in a splint with the attached straps fastened (Fig. 4.3b). To correct the rotation, the therapist pulls the bandage from the medial side towards the lateral instead, while holding the inside edge of the splint down in place. The effect is greater if a piece of foam rubber is placed directly over the knee beneath the bandage to give more purchase, allowing a complete correction of the abnormal posture of the knee prior to weight-bearing in standing (Fig. 4.3c–e).

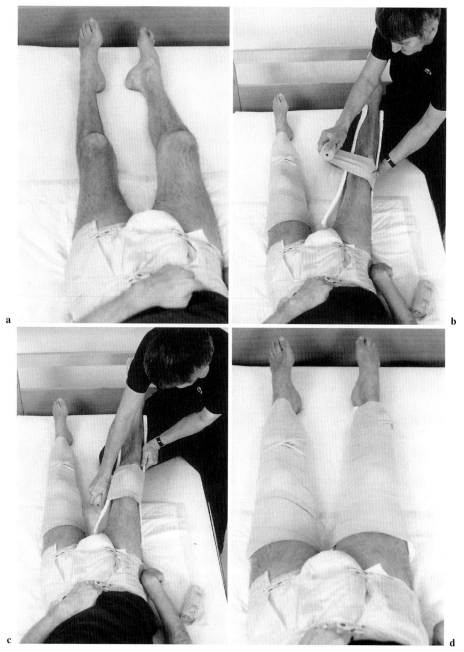

Fig. 4.2a–d. Bandaging to correct lateral rotation. **a** Leg outwardly rotated. **b** Bandage applied from lateral to medial. **c** Holding down the outside edge of the splint. **d** Rotation corrected

To Overcome Knee Flexion Spasticity. It is essential for patients whose legs constantly pull up into flexion in bed to stand every day if contractures are to be avoided. Often a resistance to full knee extension can be felt, and if the patient experiences pain he will tend to hold actively against any attempts to straighten his knee passively.

The therapist uses an extra bandage or two to achieve full knee extension without causing pain. She first places the patient's leg in the splint but does not press down on his knee in order to straighten it. Instead, as she bandages the splint into place, she gradually increases the pressure over the knee with each subsequent turn of the bandage. The patient's leg slowly straightens down into the splint and, when his knee is fully extended, the therapist continues to bandage the rest of the splint in place.

Bringing the Patient from Lying to Standing

When the splints are firmly in place, the therapist and an assistant bring the patient to a half-sitting position with his legs over the side of the bed and his feet on the floor. Great care must be taken that the patient's feet do not slide forward which they will tend to do when his knees are extended in the splints. Either the therapist must have her knees pressed against the patient's knees to prevent his seat from slipping forwards off the bed or the assistant must be stabilizing his feet from below (Fig. 4.4a). The assistant can be a nurse, one of the patient's relatives or a student, as long as he or she has been told beforehand exactly what to do.

With her hands behind the patient's back, the therapist uses her body weight to bring his buttocks off the bed (Fig. 4.4b). She moves one of her hands down behind his buttocks and draws his pelvis forwards until his weight is vertically over his feet.

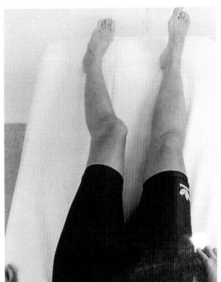

Fig. 4.3a–e. Bandaging to correct medial rotation. **a** Leg inwardly rotated.

a

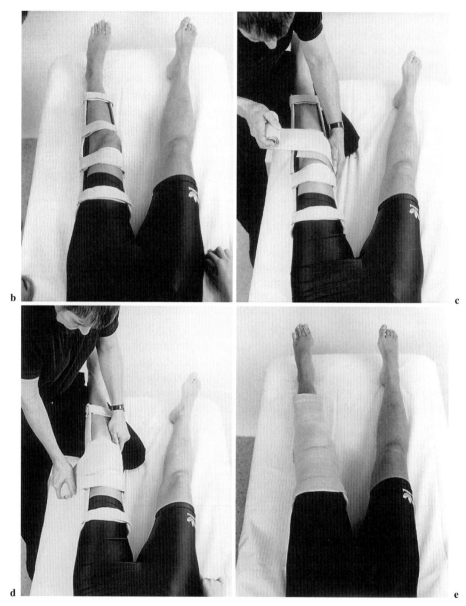

Fig. 4.3b–e. Bandaging to correct medial rotation. **b** Knee still turns inward despite the fastened straps. **c** A piece of foam rubber placed over the knee and the bandage applied from medial to lateral. **d** Counterpressure applied over inside edge of splint. **e** Rotation corrected (compare with **a**, previous page)

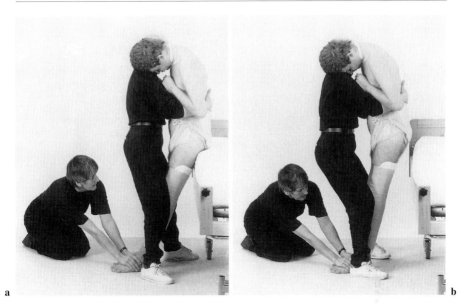

a   b

Fig. 4.4a,b. Starting position for standing the unconscious patient. **a** Feet held firmly to prevent forward sliding. **b** Buttocks lifted from the bed

Once his weight is directly over his feet, they will no longer be in danger of sliding forwards and the assistant is freed from her stabilizing task to help in other ways (Fig. 4.5a). Always keeping one of her hands in front of the patient's chest to prevent him from falling forwards, the therapist manoeuvres herself round one side of the patient so that she can support the patient from behind (Fig. 4.5b). Standing directly behind the patient, the therapist adjusts his posture by moving his buttocks forwards with her body to extend his hips and bring his weight forward over his feet (Fig. 4.5c). With one of her hands constantly in front of his chest she continues to correct his position until his ankles are dorsiflexed and she feels that there is no pressure against her hand anteriorly nor from his buttocks posteriorly.

A heavy table or an additional hospital bed placed in front of him will provide him with more information as to where he is in space (Fig. 4.6). The patient's thighs or some other part of his body should be in firm contact with the table.

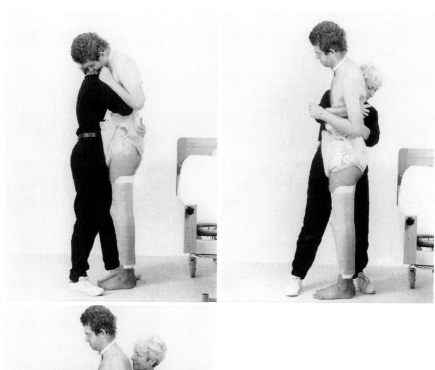

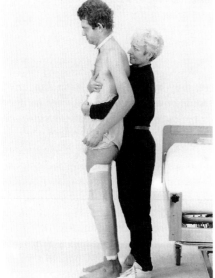

Fig. 4.5a–c. Supporting the patient in standing. **a** His weight brought forward over his feet **b** Therapist moving round behind him. **c** Hips and trunk extended

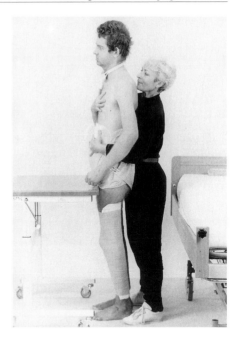

Fig. 4.6. A table in front of the patient provides a point of reference

Lifting the Patient Back onto the Bed

In order to bring the patient back into a lying position after he has been standing for a while, the therapist moves round to stand in front of him again (Fig. 4.7a).

The assistant stabilizes the patient's feet securely once again as the therapist lowers the patient's seat slowly onto the bed behind him (Fig. 4.7b).

Once the patient is safely supported by the bed, the assistant stands up and moves so that she is in a position to grasp his shoulders from behind as the therapist lifts his feet; together they then place him back into bed (Fig. 4.7c).

Using a Standing Frame

The patient can be supported in an upright position by a solid frame which has a a padded strut in front of his knees to keep them extended and a broad strap behind his hips to prevent them from flexing. Using the standing frame may be useful when the patient has regained consciousness and is able to extend his trunk actively, because it is then possible for him to stand for longer periods with the help of his relatives, or even alone if he is in the position to occupy himself in some way. Once he is out of the acute stage and no longer having therapy at weekends and on holidays, the standing frame can enable him to stand with the help of a relative or

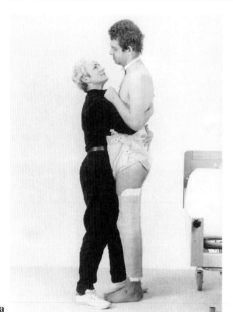

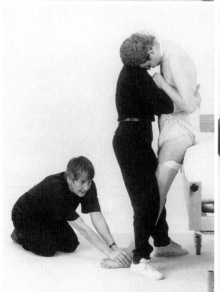

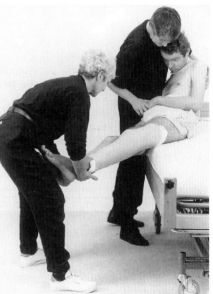

Fig. 4.7a–c. Lifting the patient back into bed. **a** Therapist moves to stand in front of the patient. **b** Lowering his seat to the bed with feet stabilized. **c** Supporting his trunk as legs are lifted

a

b

c

nurse, even at times when the therapist is not present. Standing supported by the frame should, however, never replace the more therapeutic standing with the therapist facilitating active movement and mobilizing the patient while he stands upright, but should be regarded as an additional opportunity for suitable patients to stand more often, time and available help permitting.

Before using the standing frame, the following points should be carefully considered by the therapist:

- The frame is cumbersome to move about from place to place so that for the patient who is still in intensive care or not able to be transported to the physiotherapy department its use would be too time consuming. The time would be better used moving the patient instead.
- Mechanical factors make it extremely difficult, if not impossible to bring an unconscious or totally paralyzed patient into a standing position within the frame. Struggling to do so could easily traumatize him or the therapist in some way.
- Standing in the frame is very static because of the nature of the fixation and little progression is therefore possible. Because the patient is strapped firmly in place, the position is rather passive and cannot be easily adjusted when spasticity is inhibited and an increased range of movement thus becomes possible. For example, the amount of dorsal flexion at the ankle cannot be increased because the relationship between the stabilized knee and the feet remains constant. The patient would need to be returned to a sitting position, his feet brought further from the knee support, and then stood up once more or alternatively his feet pulled back forcefully while he still has weight on them.
- Because the patient is supported by the frame in such a way that he cannot fall, it is tempting for busy therapists to leave him standing alone for a short period while they hasten to carry out some other task. They naturally intend to return to him in just a minute or two, but may easily be delayed on the way by something unforeseen happening, such as a doctor asking about another patient's progress or a colleague needing help. The patient strapped in his standing frame with nothing to do droops dejectedly forwards onto the table in front of him (Fig. 4.8), or becomes bored and restless and starts calling repeatedly for help, much to the irritation of others working nearby, both staff as well as fellow patients. After a few such experiences, he begins to dislike being placed in the frame in a position which is often uncomfortable for him and protests vehemently, which may easily lead to his becoming unpopular and being unfairly labelled as uncooperative and not motivated.

If the patient is not accustomed to standing or has persisting vasomotor problems, there is a very real danger of his fainting while held upright by the frame. The consequences could be serious unless someone notices what has happened and brings him quickly down into a lying position.

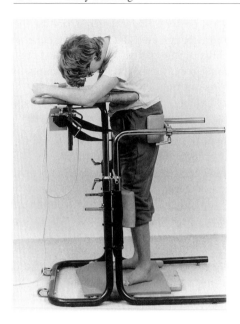

Fig. 4.8. When using a standing frame, the patient should not be left alone. An appropriate stimulus for activity must be provided

Using a Tilt Table

The use of a tilt table to bring the severely disabled patient into an upright position has gained popularity in recent years. Its lightweight construction makes it easy to bring to the patient's bedside and, with the help of nursing staff, to slide the patient across onto its adjacent surface. After the patient has been strapped firmly into place, the therapist can bring him to an almost vertical position mechanically, simply by inclining the table. Although it can be said that any standing is better for the patient than not standing at all, there are certain disadvantages inherent in standing the patient on a tilt table. It should, therefore, only be used if for some reason standing more therapeutically with the aid of knee-extension splints is not feasible. The situation might arise, for example, when an inexperienced therapist has weekend duty and does not feel confident enough to stand the patient in this way or if the nursing staff stand him routinely at other times during the day.

The following disadvantages are associated with using a tilt table:

- Being brought directly from lying to standing without the customary hip and knee flexion is a strange and rather alarming experience, as any therapist who has tried it out for herself will know. It evokes the sensation that the table will incline too far forwards and tip over even when it has not yet reached the vertical. In the same situation, the patient's feet plantarflex strongly so pushing his heels off the supporting surface, and his toes claw in flexion (Fig. 4.9). The

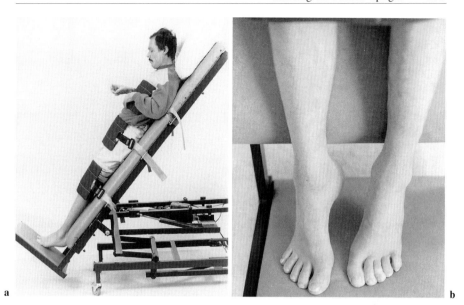

a   b

Fig. 4.9a,b. Using a tilt table. **a** Patient afraid of coming vertically upright. **b** Feet plantarflex strongly

overactivity of the plantar flexors is still further increased by the balls of his feet pressing against the footboard (Fig. 4.9b). The so-called positive supporting reaction is elicited causing increased tone in the mass pattern of extension in the whole lower limb (Magnus 1926; Bobath 1990). It is often impossible for the therapist to correct the position of the patient's feet in such a situation and any attempt to do so will elicit pain (Fig. 4.10). Using any force to bring the patient's heels down is contraindicated because he could easily sustain a soft-tissue or bony injury as a result.

- If for some reason a tilt table is being used for standing the patient, then it is preferable to use one which supports him anteriorly instead of from behind. The patient is placed prone on such a table and the straps fastened firmly before the table is tilted to bring him into the upright position. With the supporting surface in front of him, the patient feels more confident and as a result the plantarflexion of his feet is less marked and can be corrected more easily (Fig. 4.11).

- The perceptually disturbed patient pushes back in extension against the surface of the table behind him because there is only an empty space or at most a small table in front of him, which all adds to the problem of the already hypertonic extensors.

- Standing supported by the tilt table tends to be very passive for the severely disabled patient because the therapist will not be able to control the weight of his trunk from her position in front of him, or when standing beside him. She is not able to stand behind him in order to prevent his trunk from falling

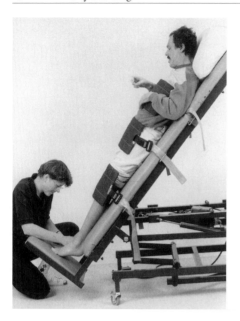

Fig. 4.10. With the tilt table inclined, the position of the patient's feet cannot be corrected

forwards when movement is attempted, and all the straps will need to be fastened to hold him safely in an upright posture, which will therefore be quite static.

- As it is when using a standing frame, the danger of the patient fainting unnoticed is a very real one. The attendant may be only a few feet away from him, attending to some piece of his equipment or his records, secure in the knowledge that he cannot fall and injure himself, but he is unable to call for help and the back of the table can easily block her view. Patients who have fainted and remained in an upright position not only may lose consciousness but if not brought down immediately into a lying position can suffer a cardiac arrest.

PROBLEM SOLVING

Whichever method is being used to stand the patient, certain problems will need to be solved for optimal treatment benefit. It is particularly important to move the patient whenever he is in an upright position and to use the valuable time for the treatment of other difficulties particularly those associated with disturbed perception because by so doing some of the problems can be avoided before they even arise.

Fig. 4.11a.b. A tilt table for prone support. **a** Decreased spasticity in the plantar flexors. **b** with anterior support the feet are easier to correct

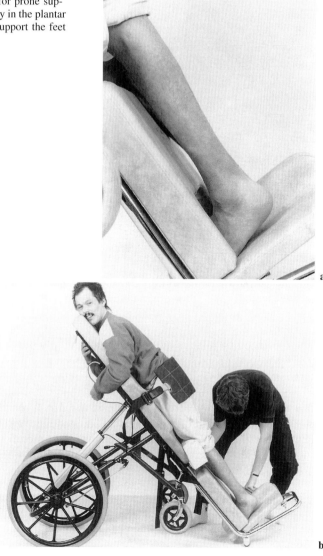

For the Patient Who Does Not Extend His Trunk Actively. A patient who is brought out of bed and stood upright in the very early stages will often be comatose still or almost so and his whole body droops forward (Fig. 4.12a). Instead of trying to pull him up and hold him in the erect position the therapist can guide the patient during an appropriate activity as described in Chap. 1 to try and stimulate his active participation (Fig. 4.12b,c). Frequently, if the stimulus is right, he will lift his head spontaneously and even extend his trunk to perform the task (Fig. 4.12d).

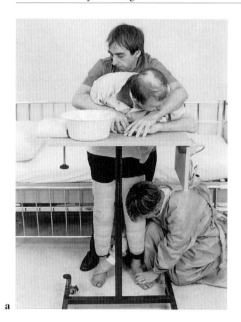

a

Fig. 4.12a–d. Stimulating activity in standing. **a** A barely conscious patient droops forward over the table. **b** A task is presented, and his wife watches. **c** During guiding he lifts his head. **d** Active neck and trunk extension as he washes his face

The presence of a relative in the guiding situation is very positive and in addition enables whoever is present to learn how they too can guide the patient during other tasks in the future.

For the Patient Whose Heels Remain in the Air. If the patient's heels are only slightly raised off the floor when he is standing upright with knee splints (Fig. 4.13a,b), the difficulty can often be overcome merely by placing a solid table in front of him, which approximates with his thighs when he is in the upright position, and then waiting for a few moments for the heels to sink down slowly (Fig. 4.13c). The therapist's quiet voice speaking to him and her calm manner will also help him to relax.

If, however, the patient's feet push so strongly into plantarflexion in sitting that he would be almost on his toes if brought into a standing position (Fig. 4.14), a different strategy must be used. The recommended method will almost always be successful as long as there is no actual shortening of the Achilles tendon, or only a slight loss of range. When such excessive plantarflexion is present, two assistants may be required to hold the feet in position while the patient is being brought into a standing position (Fig. 4.15a).

Once the patient has been brought into the upright standing position, if his heels remain in the air (Fig. 4.15b) the therapist then shifts his weight over to one side so that the assistant can lift his other foot off the floor. She moves it either out to the side or backwards so that the patient has all his weight on one leg. Within a very short time the heel of the weight-bearing leg will sink down and make contact with the floor (Fig. 4.15c).

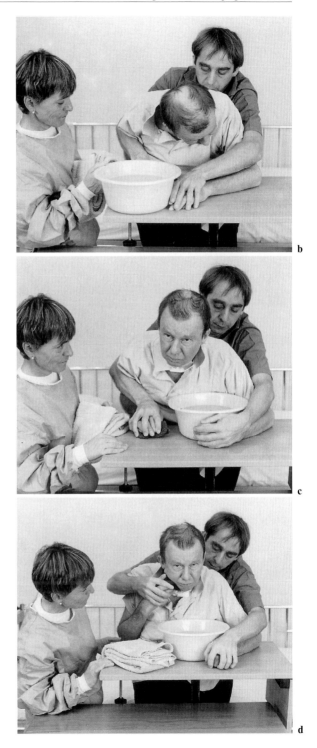

Fig. 4.12b–d

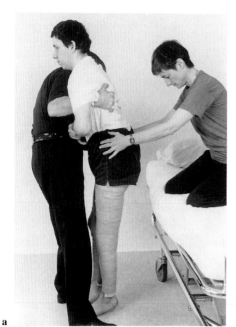

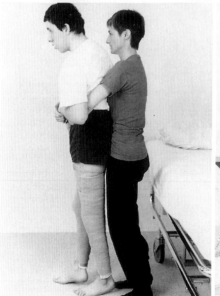

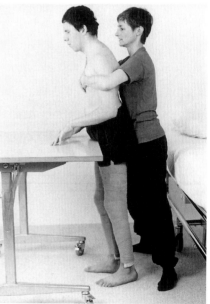

Fig. 4.13a–c. Overcoming plantarflexion in standing. **a** Bringing the patient upright with knee-extension splints. **b** Heels off the floor. **c** With a table in front, his heels gradually sink down

a

b

c

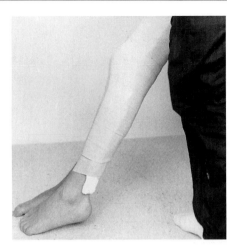

Fig. 4.14. Marked spasticity in the plantar flexors

The same procedure is then carried out towards the opposite side, with the patient standing on the leg which was previously being held in the air. When the heel on that side is also right down on the floor, the assistant places his feet in line with one another and the therapist moves him back to the middle so that he is taking weight through both his legs (Fig. 4.15d).

The patient's feet may invert once his heels are down with weight taken only through their lateral aspect as quite often occurs (Fig. 4.16a). The assistant uses one of her hands to press downwards and medially over the top of his foot (Fig. 4.16b). At the same time she will need to control the position of the patient's knee by turning it outwards with her other hand as the therapist shifts his weight over that leg. If she only pushes the medial side of the foot down towards the floor, the patient's hip will be adducted through the pressure which she is having to apply in that direction and his knee will rotate inwards.

If the therapist is using only the standing frame or tilt table to bring the patient into a standing position and finds that it is increasingly difficult or even impossible to correct the position of his feet, then standing with the knee extension splints instead will usually solve the problem and be sufficient to bring his heels down onto the floor.

Regular standing in the correct position will maintain range of dorsal flexion of the ankle joint sufficient for walking when the patient reaches that stage but if he has not been stood out of bed from the beginning, his Achilles tendon may have shortened already. By standing him daily in the knee splints with one foot held off the floor by an assistant, it may be possible to regain the lost range of motion to an astonishing degree without having to resort to other measures. Should the problem persist, however, then it will be necessary to correct the position of the foot by means of serial plastering, as described in Chap. 6.

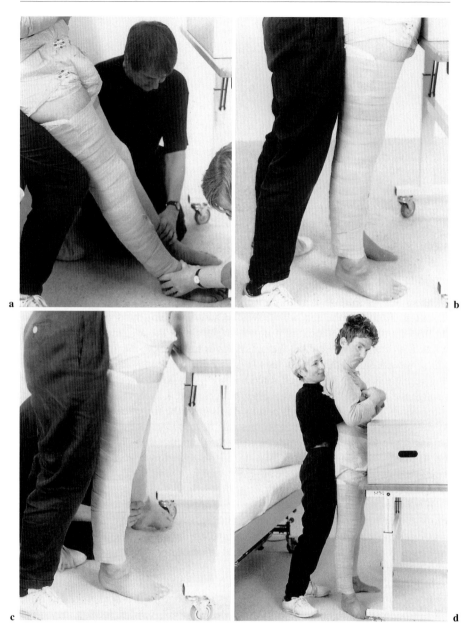

Fig. 4.15a–d. Preventing shortening of the Achilles tendon. **a** Two assistants support feet. **b** In standing, both heels are off the floor. **c** Lifting one foot into the air. **d** Feet flat on the floor

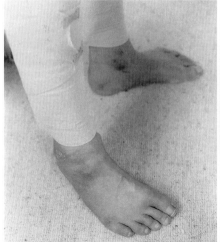

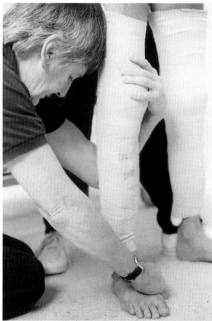

Fig. 4.16a. Heels down but feet inverting.
b Correcting the foot posture

For the Patient Who Can Only Stand for a Very Short Time. If the patient is not used to standing, or if he is still not at the stage where he can exercise actively because he realizes that it will help him to learn to walk again in the future, he will often beg to be allowed to sit down again almost as soon as he has been helped to stand erect, particularly if the standing frame is being used to support him. If he is left standing without any activity or treatment, he will either droop over the table in front of him and sleep (Fig. 4.17a), or become very agitated and shout for someone to help him to sit down. Many will ask repeatedly to be allowed to sit down as they claim to feel so tired. A patient who is unable to speak will show signs of distress or may cry pitifully. As soon as the therapist guides some activity with the very same patient, however, he is no longer tired or distressed and can remain standing as long as he is working at the appropriate level (Fig. 4.17b).

Other stimuli which hold his attention can also be presented by his family, friends or other patients. For example, hitting a balloon back and forth to another person or throwing and catching a ball can serve as a useful distraction and encourage the patient to stay upright, but with the purely motor activity there will be no other learning effect. It can, however, be enjoyable for the patient, and enable him to stand for a longer time.

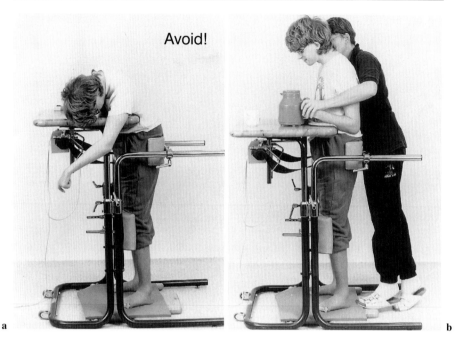

Fig. 4.17a,b. Active participation in standing. **a** Without a task, the patient dislikes standing in a frame. **b** A guided task encourages activity

For the Patient with Some Loss of Hip and Knee Extension. If for some reason slight flexion contractures have developed in the patient's hips and knees, they can usually be overcome within a short time by standing him upright every day with the help of plaster back slabs to hold his legs in extension. The therapist will need to make the back slabs to accommodate for the degree of loss of knee extension. Before making the slabs, she first treats the patient using inhibitory techniques in order to gain the maximum amount of extension, and then lies the patient in prone while smoothing the plaster into place and allowing it to set firmly. Should it not be possible for the patient to lie prone, she can make the splints with the patient lying supine, but it is rather more difficult from a technical point of view (see Chap. 6).

Once the plaster has set firmly and is completely dry, usually on the following day, the splints are bandaged firmly into place using an extra bandage over the knee to ease it slowly down into position. The therapist stands the patient up and uses her body to ease his seat forwards and gain as much hip extension as possible. A table in front of the patient is a great help as a point of reference because she can ask the patient to try and touch it with his thighs. The table should be strategically placed near enough to allow him to succeed and then gradually moved further away after each successful attempt. Activities which incorporate extension are then guided, or if the patient is sufficiently conscious to participate actively, he can be encouraged to extend his legs and trunk voluntarily.

Lying prone is used in conjunction with the daily standing routine, to avoid constant flexion of the hips and knees during the rest of the day. The time which the patient spends in prone each day is gradually increased according to how long he can tolerate the position. If the range of extension does not improve rapidly during the next few days it will be necessary to commence serial plastering of the patient's knees to prevent the contractures from increasing further and becoming a serious problem (see Chap. 6).

Moving While Standing

While the patient is in a standing position, many movements can be performed, either passively by the therapist if he is still not sufficiently conscious or with the appropriate amount of assistance as soon as he is able to participate actively. The activities which are chosen can include neck movements in all directions, inhibition and facilitation of the arms, weight shifts to both sides as well as forwards and backwards and trunk rotation or lateral flexion.

One movement is, however, so important that the activity should be incorporated in the treatment of all patients from the beginning and used continually until the later rehabilitation stage has been reached and the patient has started walking, namely, flexion of the trunk.

Flexion of the Trunk in Standing

The patient, with knee-extension splints bandaged firmly in position, stands with his thighs is contact with a table, a plinth or a bed which is directly in front of him. With his head on his hands, he flexes his trunk forwards until his elbows touch the table and then returns to the upright position. The therapist facilitates the movement so that the patient does not have to struggle to regain the vertical and uses her hands to prevent deviations from the normal direction of the movement and to correct evasive or compensatory postures. While the patient is flexing and extending, the quality and pattern of movement will need to be observed carefully, as will the position which his body adopts when he is flexed forwards. To facilitate the movement, the following steps are taken:

- The therapist stands behind and slightly to the side of the patient, her hand on that side supporting his clasped hands from below and her other arm right around his waist until her hand is approximately over his diaphragm (Fig. 4.18a).
- Keeping his thighs firmly in contact with the edge of the table with her body, the therapist flexes the patient's trunk forwards while taking some of its weight with

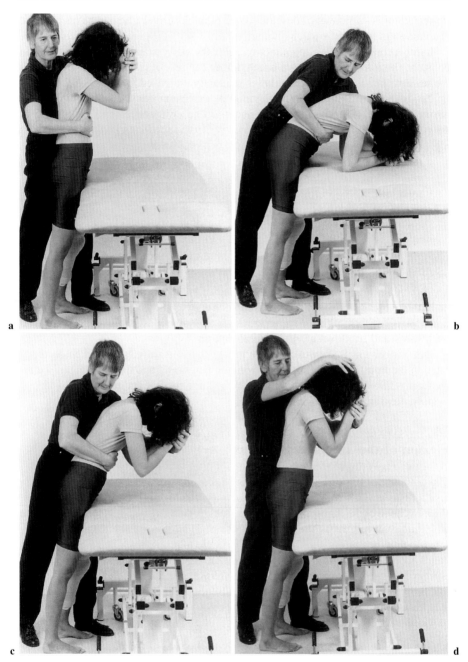

Fig. 4.18a–d. Mobilizing the nervous system in standing. **a** Forehead rests on clasped hands. **b** Bringing elbows down to touch the table. **c** Returning to an upright position with help. **d** Neck remains flexed

the arm which is around his waist and controlling the speed and direction simultaneously with the help of her other hand which is underneath his clasped hands (Fig. 4.18b).

- As soon as his elbows and head have touched the table, the therapist immediately helps the patient to stand up again, facilitating the movement with both her hands (Fig. 4.18c). During early attempts, remaining in the flexed position for any length of time is avoided, because a resultant increase in flexor tone can sometimes make it difficult for him to return to standing.
- Should the patient lift his head off his hands, his neck extending strongly in his efforts to come upright, the therapist guides it forward again with one hand, at the same time helping him to bring his trunk into an erect position by giving more support underneath his arms with her other hand (Fig. 4.18d).
- To correct any abnormal posture which she has observed when the patient's trunk is flexed and his elbows have reached the table, the therapist stands behind him and "moulds" his body into a more symmetrical position or increases the amount of flexion if his back appears to be too flat (Fig. 4.19). Any tension in the muscles of the back can be eased, and often mobilization of the ribs unilaterally will be required to restore the normal contour of the thorax. The therapist can only treat the patient in the flexed position once she has ascertained that flexor tone will not increase to such an extent that standing up again becomes a problem afterwards.

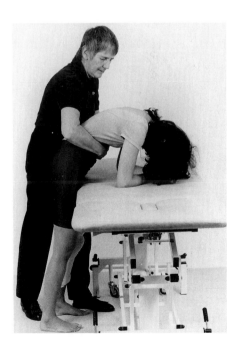

Fig. 4.19. Mobilizing flexion of the whole spine

As the patient's ability to flex and extend his trunk in standing improves, the effect of the activity can be increased further in three different ways:

1. By lowering the height of the table to increase both the amount of forward flexion and the extensor activity required to stand up again.
2. By placing one of the patient's legs behind him so that all his weight is taken on the other leg as he bends down and returns to the vertical (Fig. 4.20). The pelvis remains parallel to the table as he moves back and forth. Performed unilaterally, the activity will further inhibit flexor tonus in the weight-bearing leg as well as increasing active extension of that hip. Particularly remarkable is the inhibition of hypertonus in the plantar flexors and toe flexors, including the disappearance of ankle clonus which can otherwise be such a problem when standing or walking with the patient. The inhibitory effect on the muscles of the calf and the flexors of the toes can be further increased if a rolled bandage is placed beneath the patient's toes to hold them in extension.
3. By standing the patient on a wedge-shaped board, his heels on its lower end when he is moving his trunk through flexion to bring his head down to the table (Fig. 4.21).

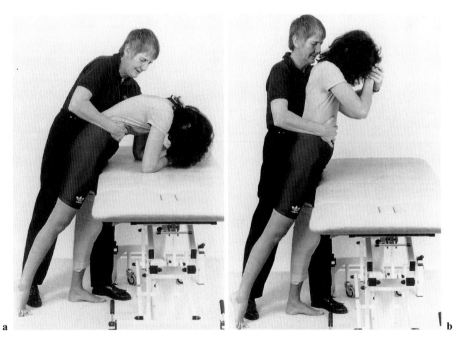

a   b

Fig. 4.20a,b. Normalizing tone and retraining active hip extension. **a** Trunk flexion with weight on one leg. **b** Returning to an upright position

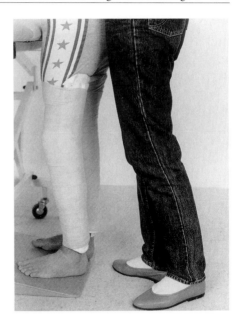

Fig. 4.21. Standing on a wedge to increase dorsal flexion of the ankle

Therapeutic Value of Trunk Flexion in Standing

The sequence of movement involved in trunk flexion in standing with the knees held in extension by dorsal splints is of great benefit for all patients with an upper motor neurone lesion. It will prevent problems from occurring, it will maintain mobility and it will overcome problems that have already arisen. It should, therefore, be used at all stages of rehabilitation, from the early days following a lesion of the central nervous system onwards:

- Spasticity in the lower limbs is reduced to a remarkable degree and the full length of the knee flexors and the plantar flexors of the foot is maintained (Fig. 4.22).
- Active movement can frequently be observed in the toes and ankle immediately following the procedure.
- The spine does not stiffen in extension, or if it already has, mobility is quickly regained allowing the selective activity of the abdominal muscles to be retrained. Rotation of the trunk, necessary for walking as well as using the arms functionally, becomes possible again once the thoracic spine is no longer locked in extension.

The significant effect is in all probability due to the mobilization of neural structures throughout the nervous system, as the sequence performed in standing incorporates the components of the lower limb tension test 1 (ULTT 1) and the "slump" test in long sitting (Butler 1991 b), which have been described in detail

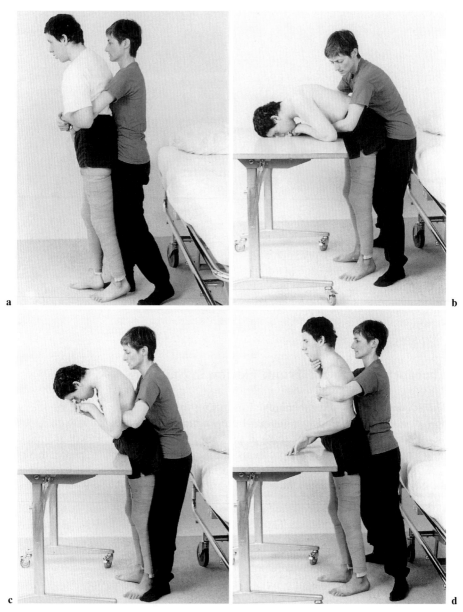

Fig. 4.22a–d. Inhibiting spasticity in the lower limbs. **a** Knee extension splints control knee flexion spasticity. **b** Trunk flexion. **c** Trunk extension with assistance. **d** Plantar flexors relaxed and fully lengthened

in Chap. 3. Since the nervous system is a continuum, the effect can be observed as an overall reduction of hypertonus; for example, the patient's hands may be less spastic and his mouth and tongue more relaxed afterwards, without inhibitory measures specific to these areas having been used.

Conclusion

Because standing is so beneficial for the patient and because numerous problems can be prevented from arising through the therapeutic procedure, not to include it automatically in the treatment programme would be illogical and irresponsible. It is still not possible with absolute certainty to predict how long a patient will remain unconscious or to what extent he will recover his mental and physical ability. Against all statistical odds many patients have made amazing recoveries. Why some patients do so much better than others is at present unknown. All that is certain is that if the patient's body is maintained in as good a condition as possible during the "wait and see" period, he will suffer less pain and misery, the length of his rehabilitation will be shorter, and the final result will not be jeopardized by secondary complications.

A Case In Point

Beautiful, vivacious and enjoying life to the full, E.S. was 17 years old when she sustained a severe head injury in an accident involving her motorcycle and another vehicle. She was rushed to hospital unconscious and despite emergency operations remained in coma for nearly 4 months. Although her level of consciousness started to improve slowly, her physical condition was allowed to deteriorate steadily for reasons which to this day remain unclear. It would seem that internal disagreement about the type of therapy to be used and a degree of negativity instilled by the severity of her brain injury with a statistically poor prognosis for recovery combined to make the therapy perfunctory and passive. E.S. was not positioned and turned regularly, never lay prone, did not sit out of bed nor was she stood up with the help of knee-extension splints. In the ultramodern hospital with all facilities available including an adequate physiotherapy staff complement, her legs and arms developed appalling contractures, her spine became rigid in extension with the medial borders of her scapulae retracted so strongly that they overlapped one another. Her bed in the acute hospital was urgently required, but finding an alternative placement proved to be very difficult. A period in the only rehabilitation centre in her area willing to take her in proved unsuccessful. Attempts to mobilize her limbs by means of passive range of motion exercises were so painful that in-

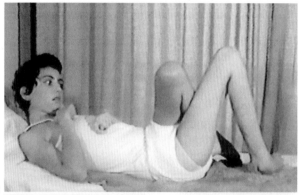

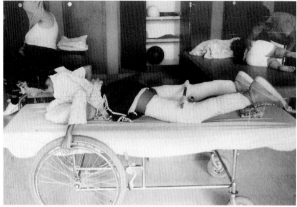

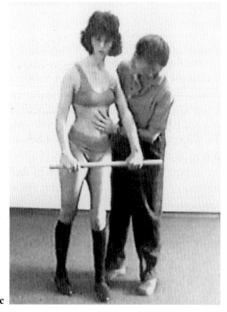

Fig. 4.23a. E.S. with severe contractures
of all her limbs. **b** Correcting lower limb
deformities with serial plastering and
prone-lying. **c** Learning to walk again.
(Archive photographs printed from video
films)

creasing doses of sedatives were given to the point that she suffered a circulatory collapse with loss of consciousness which necessitated an emergency transferral back to the original acute hospital.

Thanks to the incredible efforts made by her father, E.S. was at last admitted to a rehabilitation centre which specialized in the treatment of brain-damaged patients. On admission, 6 months after the accident, she had severe flexion contractures of her upper limbs, which included the shoulders, elbows, wrists and fingers. Her left biceps had been torn, presumably by overzealous stretching, and the upper arm was hot and swollen. Her legs were fixed in flexion of the hips and knees and her feet were plantarflexed to the extent that the dorsal aspect of the toes of her left foot were pressed against the bed (Fig. 4.23a). X-ray examination revealed a secondary dislocation of the left hip caused by the prolonged position in adduction with medial rotation, and both hips showed a marked osteoporosis. Treatment as described in Chap. 6 commenced immediately and, after the contractures and hip dislocation had been overcome, E.S. was able stand up again and start learning to walk and to use her hands for independent self-care activities (Fig. 4.23b,c). Due to the severity of the deformity of the left foot, surgical intervention was deemed advisable and a lengthening of the Achilles tendon with division and reinsertion of the tibialis anterior muscle was performed. E.S. continues to improve, despite persisting problems with short-term memory, thanks to further treatment in a rehabilitation centre near her home (Fig. 4.24).

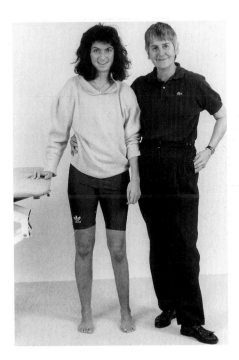

Fig. 4.24. Four years after her head injury, E.S. continues to make progress

From an outsider's point of view the rehabilitation can be considered as having been amazingly successful, but it should never be forgotten that all the above-mentioned problems could have been prevented by correct positioning and early mobilization with standing included during the acute phase. E.S. suffered terribly both physically and mentally as a result of the secondary complications, and her rehabilitation has been long and arduous. She had to spend a year in the rehabilitation clinic, which was far from her family and friends, before she could return home. The correction of the deformities was at times so painful that an implant for the regular administration of intrathecal morphine was carried out and later removed. Serial plastering needed to be continued for more than 2 months before her legs were straight and her feet plantigrade, and additional plastering with her legs held in abduction was required to reduce the dislocation of the hip (see Fig. 4.23b). Other forms of splinting were used to straighten out her hands, and for many months her left leg had to be supported by a full leg brace when she walked.

Long-term physical limitations remain which interfere with her further progress. The foot which underwent surgery has been pulled somewhat out of shape by the resultant muscle imbalance, and the activity necessary for a normal walking pattern is not possible. Her stiff thoracic spine and retracted scapulae continue to cause difficulties.

5 Reanimating the Face and Mouth

The face and mouth play a significant role in the lives of all of us, both young and old alike. They are the means by which we express our feelings and our wishes verbally and nonverbally, and they enable us to share our thoughts with others. How we look is important to us, a fact clearly shown by the flourishing cosmetic trade with its numerous advertisements for aids to beauty and the maintenance of a youthful appearance or the always busy hairdressing salons. The mouth, with the wonderfully agile tongue, allows us to eat and drink whatever we please, quickly and all too easily, not only to fulfil our daily needs but also for the pleasure it affords. So sensitive is the mouth that even the slightest change in sensation is magnified. A dental filling, although perhaps only a millimetre too high, which prevents normal mouth closure can lead to a sleepless night and an emergency appointment the next day! The unilateral loss of feeling following local anaesthesia for a dental procedure can make drinking or rinsing out the mouth with the pink liquid a major problem.

It seems strange, therefore, that although after brain damage the patient's face and mouth often suffer a considerable sensorimotor disturbance, they frequently receive far less attention and intensive treatment than do his arms for example. The reasons for the comparative neglect of such a vital area are not clear. Perhaps there is a certain inhibition to handling another person's face or touching the inside of a stranger's mouth, a reason which has been expressed by students participating in postgraduate courses on the rehabilitation of the face and oral tract. Possibly the face and mouth fall into a sort of "no man's land" with regard to treatment, and in the end no-one undertakes responsibility for specific therapy; the nurses carry out the task of ensuring intake and output and attend to basic oral hygiene, the occupational therapists deal with the adaptations required for food to reach the mouth or with establishing an alternative form of communication, and the physiotherapist usually treats the body only as far as the neck.

It is often taken for granted that the speech therapist will automatically deal with the problems because they concern the mouth, but in most acute hospitals such specialists are in short supply, and tend to concentrate on patients with language difficulties. In any event many speech therapists have had little training or experience in the management of severe dysphagia and are justifiably reluctant to assume full responsibility. It could well be that the members of the team simply do not know that the treatment of the complex problems is not only possible but can be amazingly successful and as a result, the problems observed in the area are accepted as being inevitable and insuperable.

Whatever the reason or reasons may be, every effort must be made to ensure that intensive orofacial treatment is carried out on a regular basis. Team discussion, organization, allocation of time, in-service teaching and cooperation from all staff members will soon eliminate any difficulties. Although one professional group may take responsibility for carrying out the actual treatment, each and every member of the team as well as the patient's relatives should understand and be involved in the treatment approach so that they are able to assist the patient appropriately during the different therapies or at mealtimes.

It is essential that the mouth and face be treated right from the beginning and that further treatment for any residual difficulties be included in the total rehabilitation programme because the problems are extremely disabling and distressing for the patient and those who care for him. The face and voice in fact form an integral part of the individual's whole personality and in the true sense of the word rehabilitation, every effort must be made to restore them to their previous state if the patient is to be his own "self" again.

Common Problems and Their Treatment

Problems

The most common difficulties experienced by the patient are the following:

- The patient's neck is held constantly in a fixed position and as a result there is a loss of the social head movements and postures which usually complement or even replace speech during everyday conversation. If the neck is too extended, swallowing becomes difficult, if not impossible, and the tension on the anterior structures hampers the production of a normal voice. With the neck pulled strongly to one side, saliva will tend to escape from the lower corner of the mouth as will fluid when the patient tries to drink from a cup. During eating attempts, food particles will fall into the space between his teeth and cheek, and he will not be able to keep the solids in place for chewing.
- Abnormal tone and sensation cause the patient's face to be mask-like, often with wide open eyes and constantly raised eyebrows, giving an alarmed or surprised impression. His facial expression does not change in order to be appropriate for the situation in which he finds himself. In the presence of hypotonia his face may droop, causing others to think that he is sad or depressed. Due to abnormal reflex activity or muscle imbalance his face may be permanently held in a particular expression which has nothing to do with what he is really feeling and lead to his being wrongly interpreted. For instance he may appear to be snarling because his upper lip is pulled back or frowning sullenly, both of which would make others unwilling to approach him.

- Facial asymmetry, which becomes particularly obvious when the patient smiles, can be very upsetting. The overactivity of the less affected side increases the asymmetrical effect.
- There may be very little movement in the upper two-thirds of the patient's face, causing his eyes to lose all expression. He may be unable to open or close one or both eyes.
- The patient's mouth may be permanently open with the jaw depressed and retracted. The problem is often made worse by the fact that his tongue movements are reduced and he is therefore unable to cope with his saliva.
- Little or no active movement of the tongue is a frequent problem for the patient who can only move his tongue slowly and clumsily in mass patterns. His tongue may thrust forwards inappropriately or be strongly retracted. Involuntary uncoordinated movements including tremor may be present.
- Some patients will have difficulty in opening their mouth, the teeth tightly clenched together with perhaps an exaggerated bite reflex in addition. Adequate oral hygiene is not possible and there is a danger of broken teeth if attempts are made to open the patient's mouth forcibly.
- Dribbling or drooling, with saliva or food escaping from his mouth is an embarrassment for both the patient and his relatives.
- Eating and drinking may be difficult for the patient or only possible in an abnormal pattern. He may be unable to take food by mouth at all.
- Frequent choking when swallowing solids or liquids or even his own saliva can be most unpleasant and even dangerous for the patient.
- The inability to chew or not being able to chew adequately with the normal rotatory movements can mean that the patient's diet is very restricted causing health problems and certainly a loss of enjoyment.
- Inadequate or absent closure of the soft palate during eating leads to an increased risk of choking as well as food or fluid entering the nasal cavity. When the patient is speaking he sounds abnormal because air escapes through his nose or he has a nasal tone of voice.
- The patient may be unable to produce sounds at all or can only phonate with inspiration. His voice if he can speak, sounds strange, may be uncontrolled so that it suddenly becomes very loud or unexpectedly changes pitch while lack of any modulation or melody is very tiring for the listener.
- The patient may be unable to articulate clearly, with difficulty in forming consonants.
- He may speak very quietly perhaps with sudden bursts of volume, or in short telegraphic sentences, possibly only able to utter one or two words per breath.
- The patient's teeth may not be clean, having a coated appearance and possibly early evidence of caries. His gums are often in poor condition with signs of bleeding and infection, and his mouth may have an unpleasant odour.

Such problems, whether they are very obvious and disabling to a marked degree, or could be termed "slight" if compared to other more handicapped patients, will be most distressing for the patient, his family and his friends. They will also alter the way other people behave towards him, making his return to living and being accepted in the world outside the clinic more difficult. Any problem in the area of the face and mouth, will detract from the patient's quality of life in some way because they either cause him to look less attractive than before, limit his facial expression, prevent him from speaking normally, or diminish his enjoyment in eating and drinking (Fig. 5.1). Assessing, treating and overcoming the difficulties should therefore be considered as a priority in the treatment programme.

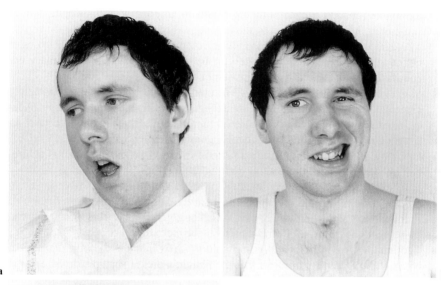

a

b

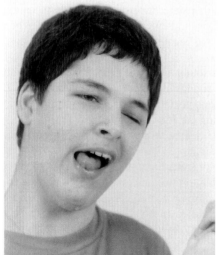

c

Fig. 5.1a–c. Severe problems of face and mouth diminish the patient's quality of life. **a** Unable to close his mouth. **b** Asymmetry accentuated when smiling. **c** Sensorimotor difficulties prevent eating and speaking

Prevention and Treatment

The face and mouth cannot be treated in isolation but are very much influenced by the patient's posture, his muscle tone generally and the mobility of other parts of his body. It would be impossible, for example, to regain normal mouth closure or start oral feeding if the patient is still being kept in bed all day, lying supine with his neck extended and has not yet been transferred into a wheelchair and helped to achieve a good sitting position (see Fig. 2.1). Similarly treatment for the neck, face and mouth will help to improve his condition as a whole. The rich innervation of the area makes stimulation most effective.

Handling Hints

Useful Grips

When assessing or treating the patient's face and mouth two useful basic grips are recommended:

GRIP A
The therapist stands beside the patient and puts her arm round behind his head until her hand is within easy reach of the lower part of his face. She holds his chin between her index and middle fingers while her thumb rests lightly against the side of his face approximately on a level with the middle of his ear (Fig. 5.2a). With her index finger the therapist can facilitate mouth opening with a slight pressure downwards and forwards or, when the patient's mouth is closed, help him to bring his lips together. Because of the circular form of the orbicularis muscle, the facilitation from beneath the lower lip will also assist closure of the upper lip.

The therapist can use her middle finger, below the patient's chin, to help him to close his mouth by moving his jaw upwards and forwards. With her middle finger, the therapist can also facilitate movements of the tongue either forwards or backwards. She flexes her finger slightly to fit into the space between the two bony rami of the jaw where the lower aspect of the muscular tongue can be felt, and while applying an upward pressure can move the patient's tongue with her finger in the required direction, either upwards and forwards or upwards and backwards (Fig. 5.2b). The therapist's thumb provides her with information as to changes in muscle tone in the cheek or possible subluxation or lateral movement of the temporomandibular joint when the jaw moves to open or close the mouth or during chewing.

It is most important that the patient's head is in the correct position, tipped slightly forwards. With her upper arm or shoulder, the therapist elongates the back of the patient's neck with a lifting movement and prevents his head from pressing back into extension.

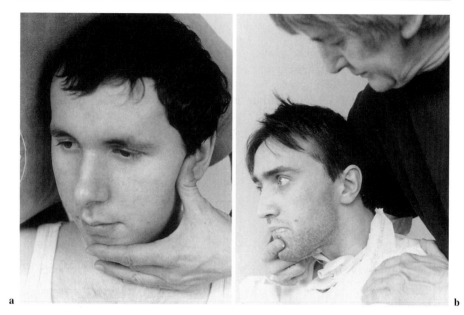

a   b

Fig. 5.2a,b. Grip A for assessing and treating the mouth. **a** Index and middle fingers assist mouth opening and closing. **b** Middle finger beneath chin moves tongue from below

Grip A is particularly useful for the following:

- When treating a patient who is in a side-lying position in intensive care (Fig. 5.3a).
- When the patient is unable to control the position of his head in sitting during assessment and treatment (Fig. 5.3b).
- When assisting the patient during functional activities such as eating, drinking or teeth cleaning (Fig. 5.3c).

GRIP B

When using grip B the therapist is positioned directly in front of the patient and can observe his whole face and the inside of his mouth more easily. She will need to sit on a low stool or adopt a kneeling position, because if her face is higher than that of the patient, he will automatically look up at her with his neck in too much extension which makes movements around and within the mouth even more difficult. The therapist places her thumb lightly on the patient's chin with her index finger resting on his cheek. Her middle finger is flexed sufficiently to fit comfortably into the space between the rami of the lower jaw beneath his chin (Fig. 5.4a). Her finger so placed enables her not only to feel and influence the tone of the muscles forming the floor of the mouth, but also to facilitate movements of the tongue and swallowing.

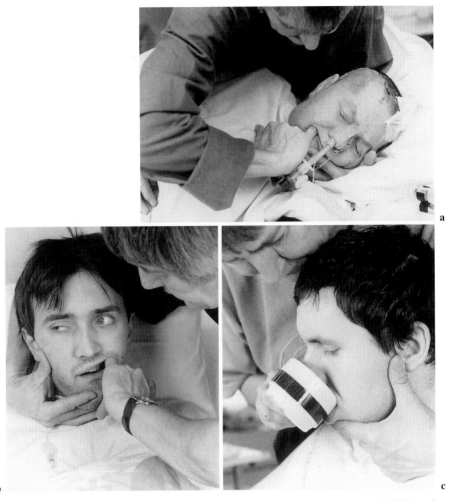

Fig. 5.3a–c. Grip A when patient is still unconscious in intensive care unit (**a**), cannot hold his head in position (**b**), and requires help with drinking (**c**)

With her thumb on the patient's chin, the therapist can help him to open his mouth, being careful not to push the jaw back as she does so. The jaw must in fact protract from the temporomandibular joint to enable it to glide downwards and with a simultaneous movement of her middle finger from below the therapist guides the chin forwards to facilitate mouth opening.

If the patient is unable to close his mouth, the therapist assists the movement by lifting his jaw with her middle finger. Her thumb eases the lower lip up towards the upper to achieve lip closure.

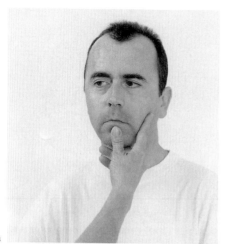

Fig. 5.4a. Grip B allows patient to observe therapist's face. **b** Used for a patient whose head needs support

a

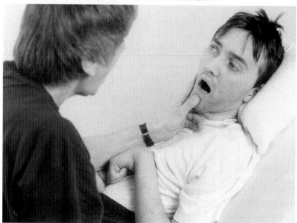

b

Grip B is particularly useful for the following:

- When re-educating active movements of the face and mouth with patients who are able to maintain a good position of their head without difficulty. If the patient is unable to hold his head in the correct position or can only do so with great effort and concentration, the therapist can use the same grip but with the patient well-supported in half-lying, either in bed or on a plinth (Fig. 5.4b).
- When treating patients who have difficulty in understanding verbal instructions. The therapist can show the patient what is expected of him and when looking directly at her face he is better able to follow her commands.

Illuminating the Inside of the Mouth

Using Daylight. Placing the patient so that he faces a window at the correct angle will usually ensure sufficient light for the therapist to observe and treat the structures within his mouth and pharynx, and has the advantage of allowing her to use both her hands freely without having to manipulate a torch at the same time.

Using an Angle-Poise Lamp. A standard lamp can be placed and adjusted so that light shines into the patient's mouth. The disadvantage is that the lamp can easily be knocked over and requires constant adjustment whenever the therapist changes her position. It is preferable to have an angle- poise lamp fitted to the wall, so that the therapist can move it easily with one hand into any position as required.

Using a Torch. If the therapist is holding a torch to provide light in the patient's mouth, she will have only one of her hands free for other tasks. Should she need to use a spatula as well as support his head, for example when observing or stimulating activity in the soft palate, difficulties arise. An ingenious device is available which does much to solve the problem. A small pocket torch has an attachment which allows a normal disposable spatula to be slid into place and held there firmly, so that the therapist is able to manipulate both with one hand (Fig. 5.5). A secondary advantage is that the torchlight is always directed to the appropriate area.

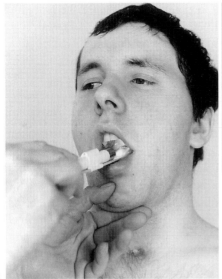

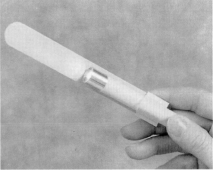

b

a

Fig. 5.5a. Torch with spatula attached leaves one hand free for facilitation when examining the mouth. **b** Torch with disposable tongue depressor

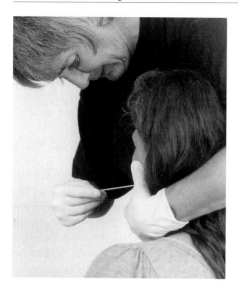

Fig. 5.6. Wearing rubber gloves to prevent cross-infection

Wearing Rubber Gloves

Many therapists prefer to work without gloves and claim that they can then feel and manipulate sensitive structures better. Wearing protective, rubber surgical gloves is, however, essential if either the patient or the therapist has a diagnosed or possible transferable infection in order to eliminate any danger of cross-infection through the intimate contact within the mouth (Fig. 5.6). It requires only a short time to become accustomed to wearing gloves, and the quality of the therapy need not suffer in any way. Dentists and dental hygienists have adopted the procedure without loss of skill, just as surgeons for many decades have carried out delicate procedures with their gloved hands.

Therapeutic Procedures

Although specific treatment to prevent or overcome individual problems is described, the procedures used for each of these will have a beneficial effect on the other parts as well. For example, assisted movements of the tongue will influence the activity of the soft palate, and facilitating better eating patterns can be the first step towards speaking more clearly. Likewise, stimulating activity in the muscles of facial expression will improve eating and drinking patterns.

Mobilizing the Neck

Before attempting to treat the patient's face or mouth and before facilitating eating or speaking, the therapist should always mobilize his neck to ensure an optimal starting position. The mobilization may be carried out in lying (see Fig. 3.4b), in half-lying or in sitting and it may be necessary to normalize the tone and posture of the trunk prior to moving the neck. Free movements of the cervical spine will be extremely difficult to achieve if the trunk is too flexed or too extended. The patient's head should be moved in all directions but lateral flexion of the neck and flexion of the upper cervical spine are usually significantly limited.

Mobilizing Lateral Flexion

With the patient sitting erect, if necessary with his arms supported on a table, the therapist stands at his side and uses one of her hands to draw his head towards her. She stabilizes his trunk with her body against his nearside shoulder to prevent it from moving sideways as well. With her other hand, she presses downwards over the contralateral shoulder girdle to localize the movement to the patient's neck (Fig. 5.7a). The therapist uses her voice to encourage the patient to relax and try not to resist the movement with words such as, "Just let your head move easily," and " Let it lean against me". Even if he is unable to understand the words themselves, the soothing tone of her voice will be a help. When moving his head towards the opposite side, the therapist may prefer to stand on the patient's other side and carry out the same procedure, or she can change the position of her hands and ease his head away from her (Fig. 5.7b).

Achieving Flexion of the Upper Cervical Area

The therapist stands behind the patient and places one hand on each side of his head with her fingers pointing directly upwards. She lifts the back of the patient's head vertically, elongating the back of his neck while at the same time tipping his chin downwards and inwards (Fig. 5.8a). The movement is particularly useful immediately prior to using grip A for a therapeutic procedure. The therapist keeps the patient's head in the corrected posture and turns carefully to one side until she can place the anterior aspect of her shoulder against his occiput (Fig. 5.8b). She lifts her shoulder and moves it forwards to maintain the elongation of the back of his neck and the flexion of his upper cervical spine as she brings her hand down into position to control his jaw and mouth.

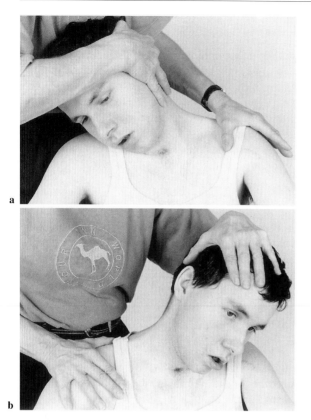

Fig. 5.7a,b. Mobilizing lateral flexion of the neck. **a** Therapist draws patient's head to rest against her chest. **b** Shoulder girdle held in place as head moves sideways

Moving the Face

Normally the face is extremely mobile as it moves so much during the day. The richly innervated muscles are in action for the constant changes and enormous variety of facial expression such as when speaking, smiling or laughing. Their activity is also essential during eating and drinking and for the automatic cleaning of the mouth after partaking of food or swallowing liquids. When the patient is unconscious or unable to move his face actively, its mobility and the extensibility of the muscles need to be maintained by passive movement until voluntary activity has been regained and is being used automatically by the patient.

The muscles of the face are very superficial and their action and the direction in which they shorten can be easily felt. Before commencing treatment, the therapist who is not familiar with the anatomy and actions of the facial muscles can rest her fingertips gently on her own face to feel their activity and direction of pull as she

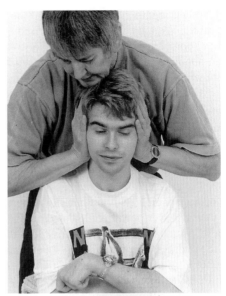

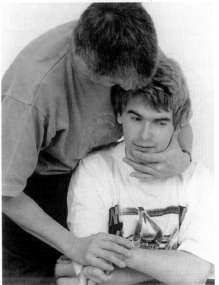

Fig. 5.8a,b. Optimizing the position of the head. **a** Elongating the back of the neck with upper cervical flexion. **b** The therapist's moves round to one side, her shoulder maintaining the head posture as she adopts grip A

moves her own face in different ways. It is also helpful for her to study an illustration of the arrangement of the muscles of the face in an anatomy textbook. Placing her fingers on the patient's face she can then move it in such a way that all the various movements are performed passively through their full range. As the patient's condition improves, he can participate actively in the treatment, with the movements becoming progressively more selective and refined, for example, moving the eyebrows down and towards the midline as when concentrating, looking puzzled or frowning.

When regaining consciousness, it is common for the patient to have his eyebrows constantly raised as if surprised and to have difficulty in relaxing his forehead completely or frowning actively. As a result, the eyes themselves often have an abnormal appearance because they are held very wide open with the whites showing all around the iris.

The therapist places her finger ends on the patient's forehead just above the middle of his eyebrows and moves them downwards and medially. When supporting the patient's head with one of the recommended grips, she performs the passive movement with one hand, using adduction of her fingers to bring the eyebrows towards each other (Fig. 5.9a).

When the patient is sitting out of bed, the therapist stands behind him and uses the fingers of both hands to perform the movement, while keeping his head in the correct position with the anterior aspect of her shoulder (Fig. 5.9b).

Whichever passive or assisted active movement is being carried out, the therapist's fingers should not slide over the skin at all, but instead, with sufficient pressure over the appropriate area of skin, must move the muscles lying beneath it. The amount of pressure applied is crucial because too much is uncomfortable and too little is ineffective or tickles. Practising on a normal subject who can give exact feedback will guide the therapist as to the right amount. As the patient starts to regain consciousness, he can be asked to carry out the movements actively with the help of the therapist who gives only as much assistance or facilitation as is necessary. Most patients find it easier at first to hold a position into which the therapist has moved a part of their face passively. She gives a verbal instruction such as, "Keep it there!" or indicates the aim nonverbally by doing the same movement with her own face as she takes her fingers away.

Treating the Inside of the Mouth

The mouth with its rich nerve supply offers an excellent opportunity for stimulation, not only during therapy sessions but also in association with routine oral hygiene or early attempts at oral feeding. The normal mouth is extremely active and receives a great deal of sensory input during the day through eating, chewing and drinking, as well as through the repeated movements of the tongue, cheeks and lips to clean the teeth and remove any foreign particles from the oral cavity. To collect and swallow saliva automatically at regular intervals both day and night, the muscles of the tongue, soft palate and pharynx are repeatedly activated. When speaking an enormous amount of coordinated activity takes place involving all the movable structures within the area. The patient who is unconscious or whose mouth is significantly paralyzed experiences an almost total sensory deprivation interrupted only by certain nursing or medical procedures, sometimes unpleasant ones. Muscles and joints in the area suffer from the lack of movement. Without the circulatory stimulation provided by active movement, chewing solids or brushing the teeth vigorously, the condition of the gums and the teeth deteriorates. It is, therefore, imperative that the inside of the mouth be treated from the beginning to provide stimulation and movement until the patient is able to eat and talk again.

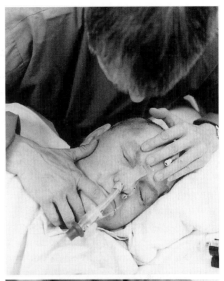

a

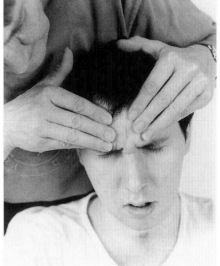

b

Fig. 5.9a,b. Moving the eyebrows downwards and medially. **a** An unconscious patient in intensive care unit. **b** A patient seated in his wheelchair

The Notorious Bite Reflex

Before routine nursing procedures inside the patient's mouth are performed or oral therapy initiated the possibility of an existing bite reflex should be considered in order to ensure the safety of both the patient and the staff.

Although often the subject of intense discussion in professional circles, the bite reflex observed in adults with severe neurological impairment is not clearly understood, and has received scant attention in scientific publications. The suggestion that it could be the reappearance, in an exaggerated form, of the primitive biting seen in normal babies is not generally accepted. Explaining the bite as a spasm in the musculature responsible for jaw closure is contradicted by the fact that muscle relaxants appear to have no effect.

Clinical observation reveals that the hyperactive reflex is bilateral and symmetrical and occurs in association with marked sensory loss or disturbance. When suddenly elicited, it causes the patient's jaws to close forcefully and incredibly swiftly so that his teeth snap together or bite on anything that may be between them and he is unable to open his mouth again voluntarily or let it be opened passively. The power of the bite in severe cases is said to be equal to 90 kg. The patient is in danger of being injured either by biting himself or by breaking an instrument or utensil between his teeth and a part of it remaining within his tightly closed mouth or even being swallowed.

The available literature on orofacial problems of neurogenic origin provides little if any information on how to actually cope with the problem of patients with a pathological and powerful bite reflex. It is, however, a serious problem that not infrequently confronts therapists and nurses working with the severely brain-damaged, and as such cannot be ignored. In fact, the presence of a bite reflex is usually the reason given for no oral therapy having been carried out, and for the poor condition of the patient's teeth and mouth and prolonged tube feeding. Therapists and nurses are understandably afraid of touching the patient's mouth, particularly if one of them has already been severely bitten during therapeutic activities or routine nursing procedures. So strong is the involuntary bite, that finger fractures and wounds requiring stitching have been sustained.

It is, however, imperative for patients who have problems associated with a hyperactive bite reflex to receive intensive orofacial therapy because, without help, a vicious circle effect occurs and the problems are intensified. The area around and within the mouth becomes increasingly sensitive to touch, while gum infection and teeth caries become progressively more painful, causing the bite reflex to be elicited earlier and more frequently, making therapeutic intervention even more difficult than before.

Certainly none of the treatment ideas suggested in the literature can be implemented successfully until the bite reflex has been inhibited sufficiently to allow the patient's mouth to be opened and therapeutic procedures initiated. Through oral feeding and continued treatment, it is often possible to overcome the problem completely.

PROBLEM SOLVING

The first important consideration is that the bite reflex does not appear in isolation but is a part of the problematic whole, sensory deprivation being almost certainly one of the main predisposing causes. It constitutes a problem most commonly in patients who have been left lying in bed for prolonged periods following a brain lesion, with inadequate mobilization and little sensory input. It would be extremely unusual to see a patient who has been turned regularly from the start, sat out of bed in a wheelchair in the early days, stood with support and received orofacial therapy while comatose to have a problematic bite reflex. Prevention is, as always, better than cure, as the old maxim so rightly states, and definitely far easier and less distressing for both patient and staff. Treatment as described in Chaps. 1–4 and in this one will avoid the development of the associated problems in most cases, the secret being to start early before things have started to go wrong.

For the same reasons, when a patient already has a pronounced bite reflex, the first step toward overcoming the problem will be working to regain full mobility of his trunk and limbs, achieving a good sitting posture and upright standing while at the same time striving to improve his level of cognition. The bite reflex cannot be successfully combated if the patient is still being kept in bed in a supine or half-lying position throughout the day in a room on his own without any stimulation, especially in the presence of marked hypertonus and contractures in other parts of his body.

Great care must be taken to avoid eliciting the reflex activity once it is evident that the patient tends to bite involuntarily. Any stimulus which causes biting should be noted and communicated to all members of the team to prevent its being repeated. The patient is afraid of biting himself or someone else, and the fear of doing so increases the risk by raising his muscle tone still further. If he has already had the experience of hurting someone who is helping him, he will be even more nervous of doing so again. The reflex invariably occurs as a reaction to touching some part of the patient's mouth or even his face. Particularly sensitive are the cutting surfaces of his teeth anteriorly, the hard palate and the tongue, but in extreme cases even something coming into contact with the lips or the front of the chin will elicit a bite.

At the start of each daily treatment, before attempting to treat the patient's face and mouth directly, the therapist begins with some activity which is easier for him to tolerate, a movement that establishes contact between them. She chooses one which can be performed without a struggle and with success, however small it may be. She moves the patient's trunk and progresses to his head as he relaxes more, in order to free forward and lateral flexion of his neck and achieves the best sitting posture possible for him at the time. A solid table is placed in front of him close up against his chest, its height being such that it can fit beneath his elbows. If the patient can be brought forward sufficiently, the therapist should help him bring his head down towards the table, turning it to one side so that his cheek rests against the firm surface. Often, with his head fully supported in this way, the bite reflex is inhibited and the patient able to open his mouth far more easily during treatment procedures.

Everything that the therapist will be using for her treatment is placed on the table in front of the patient within his field of vision so that he is not alarmed by an unidentifiable object suddenly touching his face or mouth. The same applies when the patient is being helped to bring food to his mouth during early eating attempts.

It is important that the therapist or nurse should remain calm and confident because any anticipatory nervousness on her part will cause tension which is immediately transmitted to the patient, and the increased tone accentuates the hyperreflexia. The therapist talks to the patient quietly in a soothing, matter-of-fact way, and even if he is unable to understand what she is saying, the sound of her voice will be reassuring and reduce fear. The therapist avoids making any sudden, unexpected movements which might startle the patient when touching or holding him during treatment.

Grip A is recommended, because the close, firm contact of the therapist's arm and hand helps the patient to tolerate the inhibitory and facilitatory handling and also enables her to feel any change in the tone of the muscles of his cheek and lips which will inform her that he is relaxed or give warning of an impending bite. Should the therapist feel tone increasing, she interrupts the activity and moves her finger calmly out of harm's way.

Even if she is feeling somewhat apprehensive, the therapist should apply firm pressure with her fingers when treating the face or mouth because it is easier for the patient to tolerate than any light stroking or shaking which can be irritatingly ticklish or uncomfortable for him and provoke unwanted reactions.

Because the patient has difficulty in tolerating touch, it is helpful if the therapist uses counting when touching his face or mouth, to signify a given duration. For example, she places a finger firmly on his upper lip and says, "one, two" before taking it away again. She shortens or lengthens the period according to which part she is touching and to the patient's tolerance of the tactile stimulus. By counting, she can also note any change in the hypersensitivity. It is advisable for her to start by touching an area which is less sensitive, where she can count up to three or four, and then gradually move nearer to the patient's mouth when he knows what is going to happen. The same system can be used when the therapist is able to treat the inside of the mouth, remembering that a short successful manoeuvre is better than a longer attempt with an unfortunate ending. A count of three seems to be what most people can accept easily and comfortably without having the feeling that they need to swallow, so the therapist need not increase the number when working within the oral cavity itself.

The treatment requires careful progression in consecutive stages, because if the therapist is unable to touch the outside of the patient's face without stimulating unwanted reactions, then in all probability an even stronger reaction will occur if something is placed inside his mouth. For example, only when the therapist can place her hand easily in the grip A position should she attempt to massage his outer gums with her little finger. Certainly she should not place her finger right inside the patient's mouth until she is sure that the bite reflex can be inhibited or adequately controlled. The hierarchical order of progression may not always apply, however, as observation will show and should be adjusted accordingly.

Some patients may have less difficulty in opening their mouth or tolerating its being touched when they are being helped to eat something.

The nature of the bite reflex makes it counterproductive to use force of any sort to hold the patient's mouth open. The strength of the relevant muscles makes it impossible for the therapist to keep the jaws apart with her hands and because tactile stimulation of the teeth can elicit the reflex, any hard, cold instruments placed between them will only cause the bite to increase in strength. The patient then becomes extremely agitated as he cannot release his clenched jaws, clamped with such power on the metal that the result may well be broken teeth.

Coping in an Emergency. Despite every precaution having been taken to avoid eliciting a bite reflex, it may still inadvertently happen. Should the therapist have her finger trapped between the patient's teeth it is important for her to know how to react in the situation. It is equally important if the patient has a spoon, toothbrush or some other object clenched between his teeth and, unable to release it, is in grave danger of being injured. The therapist must be well-rehearsed in the procedure, having studied and practised exactly what she has to do, before she ever finds herself in the rather alarming predicament. She is otherwise liable to react automatically in response to the normal "fight or flight" mechanism, in such a way that the situation becomes even more precarious.

First and foremost, the therapist must resist the very natural impulse to jump back and pull her finger quickly away. The additional stimulus will make the bite even stronger, and either make it impossible for her to remove her finger from the patient's mouth at all or, if she succeeds, her skin may be torn against his teeth. Should some other object be caught between his teeth, the therapist also refrains from withdrawing it rapidly or by force.

Whether it is her finger or the toothbrush or spoon which is trapped, the therapist calmly and quietly reassures the patient, and asks him to try and relax his mouth as she waits for a moment before slowly removing whatever is between his teeth. If the bite still persists, she takes his head back into extension with her free hand and because the bite reflex is associated with flexor spasticity, neck extension will usually facilitate jaw opening enough to enable the therapist to withdraw her finger safely or remove the spoon or brush.

Only as a last resort should a forceful procedure be used to open the tightly clenched mouth, because it is most unpleasant for the patient in an already distressing situation. If the therapist is however unable to release the bite in any other way, she slides her thumb into the space between his cheek and lower teeth and her index finger into the same position on the opposite side. She pushes her thumb suddenly and forcefully down against his mandible on that side, and the asymmetrical pressure mechanically overcomes the power of the contraction of those muscles which are maintaining jaw closure. As she presses downwards, the therapist also tries to draw the patient's jaw forwards with both her thumb and index finger in order to facilitate the opening movement by replicating the normal mechanism of the temporomandibular joint.

After the Event. Whatever method has been used to release the reflex bite, the therapist must make close and friendly contact with the patient immediately afterwards to reassure him that all is well. It is important that she control the normal reaction of feeling anger towards a person who has just caused her sudden, severe pain.

The bite reflex and its consequences must never be misinterpreted as being a wilful or conscious act on the part of the patient, aimed at hurting or punishing the person who is helping him. The bite is a manifestation of his lesion as are all the other symptoms over which he has no control and erroneously interpreting it as an act of aggression will lead to a deterioration in the rapport between the patient and those who care for him. The patient's relatives should also be helped to understand the reflex nature of the problem as they may otherwise be distressed by his apparent "bad behaviour" towards the staff. As the famous Maggie Knott (1970) warned in her inimitable way, "Any therapist stupid and careless enough to get her finger bitten has only herself to blame. She isn't brain-damaged, the patient is!"

Removing Something from the Patient's Mouth. In the event of a piece of some utensil or instrument having been broken off by the unexpected elicitation of a bite reflex and remaining in the patient's oral cavity, the therapist should on no account try to remove it with her fingers immediately, because in the tension of the moment the bite will probably re-occur and cause further problems. Instead, she tips his head forwards to prevent the particle from moving back into his throat and being swallowed and waits to see if the patient relaxes sufficiently to enable her to extricate the piece. If all else fails, it will be necessary for two hard plastic wedges to be inserted between his teeth with the help of an assistant so that the foreign matter can be removed with forceps.

To avoid any such alarming and inherently injurious occurrences, nothing which is breakable should be put into the patient's mouth for treatment purposes or used when he is being helped to eat or drink if there is any risk of a sudden, powerful bite being elicited. Use of a laryngeal mirror for thermal stimulation of the soft palate (Logemann 1986) could for instance be particularly dangerous and is contraindicated in the presence of an active bite reflex.

Assessing and Treating the Mouth

The Gums

The therapist massages the patient's upper and lower gums firmly with her little finger, starting from the middle and continuing right back to the angle between the upper and lower jaw. Sliding her finger underneath his lip, she moves it back and forth along the gums on the outside before turning her hand so that she can move the inside of his cheek with her finger before she withdraws it each time (Fig. 5.10). It is recommended that the therapist establish a routine when moving her finger in the patient's mouth. For example, she moves her finger back and forth only three times before turning it to bring it out again, closing the patient's lips around her finger as she withdraws it. The number of movements becomes familiar to the patient, who will be better able to tolerate the feeling as a result. It also allows

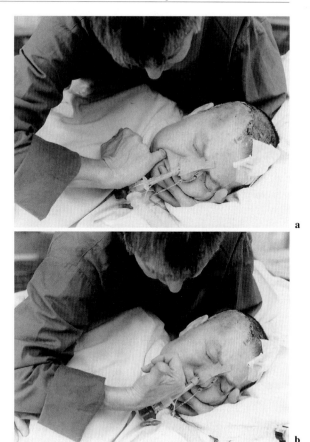

Fig. 5.10. a Massaging the gums. **b** Hand turned so that the little finger can move the inside of the patient's cheek

him time to swallow as he will often do automatically after the movement within his mouth.

Equally important are the gums behind the upper and lower teeth and the roof of the mouth itself, which the therapist massages in the same way. The pressure which she uses will need to be somewhat firmer to avoid unwanted reactions being elicited, because the areas are exquisitely ticklish and the patient may be unable to tolerate a light touch. For example, touching the roof of the mouth immediately behind the upper teeth can easily stimulate a bite reflex.

The Cheeks

The tone in the muscles of the cheeks is often abnormal, being either too high or too low, with the result that active movement is impossible or can only take place in mass synergies. For example when the patient yawns, laughs or cries, his whole face contorts as the activity overflows from one muscle group to another. In the presence of hypertonus the inside of the cheek is often caught between the teeth

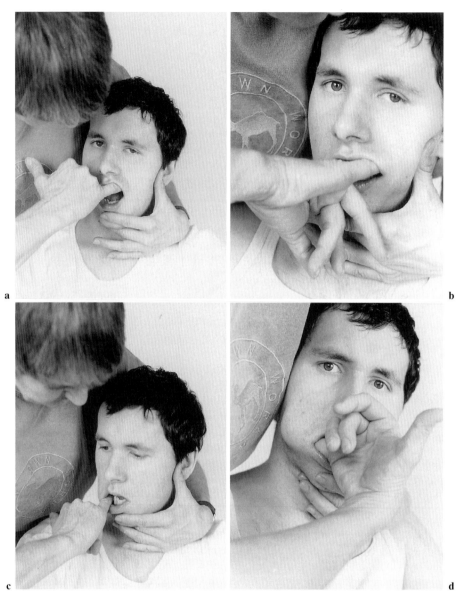

a

b

c

d

Fig. 5.11a–d. Moving the patient's cheek from within. **a** Massaging his gums. **b** Normalizing tone in the cheek muscles. **c** The therapist's little finger rubs along his gums. **d** The tip of her little finger mobilizes his cheek

during chewing movements and on examination reveals small open wounds. If the muscles are hypotonic, not only is it difficult for the patient to close his mouth or chew at all, but the food falls into the space between his teeth and his cheek. The therapist normalizes the tone and stimulates active control by manipulating the inside of the cheek with her finger.

After massaging the patient's gums on the side furthest from her, the therapist pronates her forearm and moves the end of her little finger to the inside of his cheek either from above or from below (Fig. 5.11a,b). Her finger is slightly flexed so that its tip makes contact behind the orbicularis oris muscle to avoid stretching the corner of the patient's mouth as she draws his cheek away from his teeth. The therapist's finger tip presses so firmly against the inside of his cheek that it is clearly visible from without as it moves up and down or eases the part well away from his teeth and then forwards.

To repeat the procedure on the other side, after massaging the patient's gums with her forearm pronated, the therapist turns the palm of her hand towards her; the supination enables her to bring her little finger into position well back inside his cheek (Fig. 5.11c,d).

The therapist moves the cheek passively to maintain its full mobility, to stimulate sensation and to normalize tone. If she feels that the muscles are hypertonic, she performs the movements slowly and in a gradually increasing range. For hypotonicity, she moves her finger more rapidly and vigorously, carefully building up the tone. As soon as the patient is able to participate in some way, she can try to stimulate active control by asking him to suck in his cheek against her finger or try to prevent her from pushing it out sideways. The activity is often easier if done bilaterally. The therapist sits in front of the patient and places both little fingers in his cheeks at the same time by crossing her forearms and he pulls his cheeks in against them (Fig. 5.12).

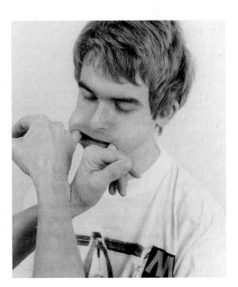

Fig. 5.12. A patient tries to suck his cheeks in actively against the therapist's little fingers

Treating the patient's cheeks from within is also important for assessment purposes because the therapist is able to feel and note any abrasions or lumps on their inner surface. She also discovers if leftover food particles have been left in the pocket of the cheek, which would indicate poor sensation and/or lack of the tongue movement required to remove them.

Treating The Tongue

Due to the extreme complexity of its movements, the tongue is frequently the most affected of all the structures in and around the mouth. The tongue is so important because coping with saliva, eating, drinking and speaking are directly dependent upon its intact functioning. Even the slightest loss of selective movement or sensation can cause considerable difficulties with regard to these activities. Dribbling, which is so upsetting for the patient and his relatives, is not due to the fact that he cannot close his lips adequately, but occurs because his tongue cannot collect the saliva and initiate the repeated swallowing which must take place on an automatic level. It is clear that lip closure cannot be essential to prevent dribbling because when speaking normally, even using long sentences, no saliva escapes from the mouth. The mistaken idea that the patient must learn to keep his lips tightly closed at all times causes self-reinforcing problems. If he is encouraged by the staff and his relatives to press his lips together constantly, then the return of normal movement and changes in facial expression will not be possible. Patients who are unable to eat or have obvious difficulties may be erroneously classified as having "swallowing problems" when in fact the problem exists in the preswallowing phase within the mouth itself. The actual mechanism of swallowing may well be intact, but the affected tongue is unable to transport the prepared food to the back of the mouth.

Passive Mobilization

Before manipulating the tongue directly the therapist normalizes tone in the muscles attached to the floor of the mouth and mobilizes the tongue passively to ensure full mobility and a good starting position.

The therapist stands behind the patient and places her thumbs one on each side of his face with her middle fingers fitting into the space between the bony surfaces of the jawbone underneath his chin (Fig. 5.13a). With the front of her shoulder she steadies the patient's head.

Pressing her finger ends upwards and forwards with rhythmic wave-like movements, she relaxes the muscles of the tongue and then moves it towards the front of the mouth until its tip rests in the midline just behind the patient's lower teeth. (If the patient's tongue is always too far forward at rest, the therapist can correct its position by moving her middle fingers up and then back instead of forwards.)

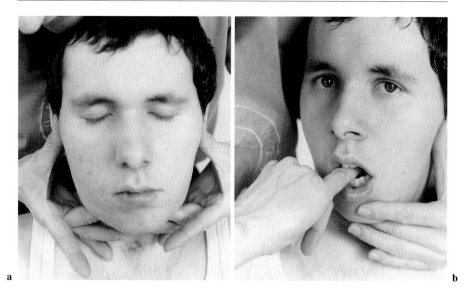

Fig. 5.13a,b. Passive mobilization of the tongue. **a** From the outside moving the tongue upwards and forward. **b** The therapist draws the tongue forwards with her finger

Facilitating Movement Within the Mouth

With a Finger

The therapist can influence the tone of the patient's tongue by direct contact. She places the tip of her little finger on the middle of his tongue and with a firm pressure takes small steps towards the back of his mouth. With her little finger she draws the tongue forwards oscillating it slightly from side to side should she feel some resistance to the passive movement (Fig. 5.13b). With her finger she is also able to guide his tongue to either side or she can ask the patient to push his tongue against her finger actively and follow it as it moves towards the side.

With a Spatula

The spatula, or tongue depressor as it is also known, should always be moistened before being used inside the patient's mouth as the dry wooden or plastic surface is otherwise uncomfortable when brought into contact with sensitive structures.

The therapist places the end of a spatula in a certain position and asks the patient to find it and touch it with his tongue. It may be easier if the spatula is in contact with his tongue and he tries to follow its movement (Fig. 5.14).

If the patient is unable to bring his tongue forward actively the therapist uses the flat side of the spatula to draw it forwards passively (Fig. 5.15a). She can also push his tongue over to the sides, asking the patient to try and move with her help or stay in a position when she removes the spatula.

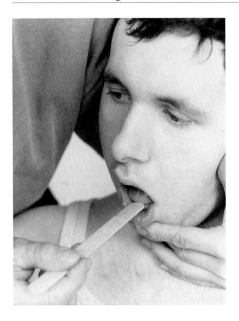

Fig. 5.14. The patient trying to touch the spatula with his tongue

A piece of gauze wrapped firmly round the spatula will provide more hold and enable the therapist to give more assistance should her finger or the spatula alone tend to slip off the tongue (Fig. 5.15b).

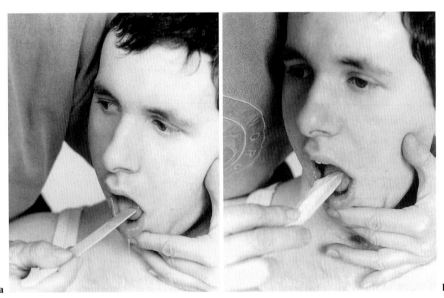

a   b

Fig. 5.15a. Moving the tongue forward with a spatula. **b** Gauze wrapped round the spatula provides more hold

Moving the Tongue Outside the Mouth

Many patients have difficulty in bringing their tongue forwards out of their mouth and in moving it to their upper lip or to one or both sides. The movements are important for licking the lips to remove food particles as well as for cleaning the teeth. When drinking from a cup, the tongue needs to come forward to the inside of the lower teeth so that the liquid can flow along the groove in the middle

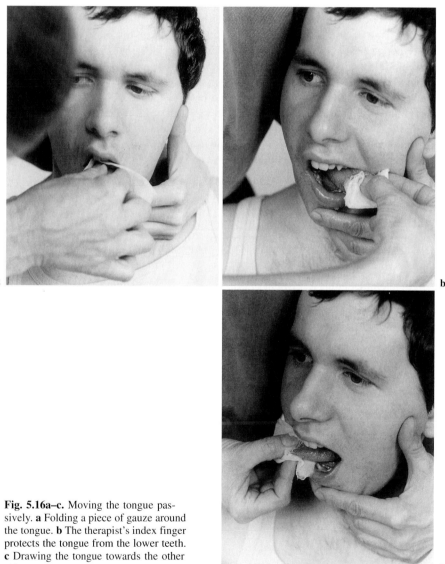

Fig. 5.16a–c. Moving the tongue passively. **a** Folding a piece of gauze around the tongue. **b** The therapist's index finger protects the tongue from the lower teeth. **c** Drawing the tongue towards the other side

to be swallowed. The swallow itself requires an upward movement of the front of the tongue for it to press against the roof of the mouth immediately behind the front teeth. When speaking, the tongue moves behind the upper teeth to form consonants such as those represented by d, t, l, n and s. Moving the tongue passively through as full a range possible outside the mouth paves the way for active movement by normalizing tone and giving the patient the feel of the movement.

When the patient's tongue has been brought as far forwards as possible, the therapist folds a piece of gauze around its anterior third and takes hold of it between her thumb and index finger (Fig. 5.16a). Her thumb is placed on the upper surface while her index finger below prevents the tongue from scraping on the patient's bottom teeth as it is drawn forwards. The therapist lifts the tongue before moving it out of his mouth. Once she feels that there is no resistance to the forward movement, she moves the tongue right over to one side (Fig. 5.16b) and then back to the middle again where she releases it to give the patient time to swallow with his tongue back in its original position and his mouth closed. The procedure is then repeated for the tongue to be taken to the other side (Fig. 5.16c). Once the passive movements can be performed easily, the therapist asks the patient to move his tongue actively in a certain direction or she can place something in a specific position for him to remove with his tongue, for example a blob of yogurt, a smear of chocolate or some mashed banana.

Stimulating Activity with an Orange Segment

When a patient is unable to move his tongue actively (Fig. 5.17a), a strong taste in his mouth may stimulate active movement. Things which taste sour may well be difficult for him to tolerate but can be most effective in helping him to regain lost tongue function.

The therapist holds a segment of orange between the patient's lips and asks him to try and suck it. Using grip A, she helps his lips to make contact with the orange and brings his tongue to the front of his mouth by moving her middle finger underneath his chin (Fig. 5.17b). If necessary she squeezes the orange lightly with her fingers to ensure that a drop or two of juice reaches his tongue.

Directly after the therapist has taken the orange away again, the patient tries to move his tongue forwards as far as he can on his own. Frequently an immediate improvement can be observed (Fig. 5.17c). The same activity can be carried out equally successfully with slices of different fruits such as pears, peaches or melons.

Regaining Selective Movements of the Tongue

For automatic cleaning movements inside the mouth, for eating and drinking and especially so for speaking, the tongue must be able to move selectively and at a considerable speed. Selective movements are those where the tongue moves without the jaw or other parts of the head, face or mouth moving at the same time, for example licking the top lip or repeating the sound "d" rapidly while the lower jaw remains completely still. Once the patient can carry out gross movements in total patterns such as sticking his tongue out on command or licking his bottom lip, more

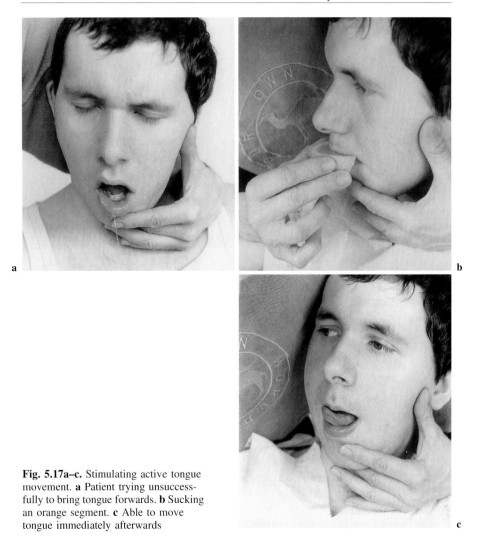

Fig. 5.17a–c. Stimulating active tongue movement. **a** Patient trying unsuccessfully to bring tongue forwards. **b** Sucking an orange segment. **c** Able to move tongue immediately afterwards

selective movements should be practised with the facilitatory help of the therapist and other members of the team including the patient's relatives.

The patient moves the tip of his tongue inside his cheek, trying to reach the spot which the therapist is indicating with her finger touching the outside of his face (Fig. 5.18). He tries to keep the rest of his face still as he moves the tongue to the required position. When he can find the therapist's finger easily, he can try to push the side of his cheek away from his teeth and then move his tongue up and down with increasing rapidity. Because the movement can be observed from without, the therapist is able to assess improvement by counting the number of times the tongue can move in say 5 s without loss of quality.

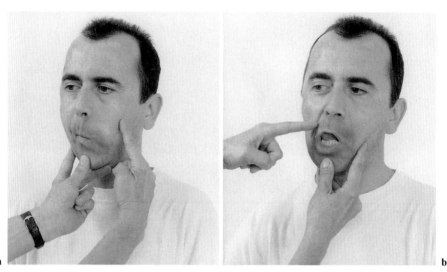

Fig. 5.18a,b. Regaining selective tongue activity. **a** Tongue in cheek to point indicated by therapist. **b** Difficulty in moving to other side.

The therapist touches different places around the patient's mouth and he tries to reach her finger with his tongue, quickly and accurately (Fig. 5.19a). It is often difficult for the patient to bring the tip of his tongue to touch the outside of his top lip, as the lip needs to be tensed and kept in position, and the lower jaw depressed and stabilized while the tongue nevertheless moves selectively and independently (Fig. 5.19b). The movement needs to be practised slowly and carefully at first until it is possible without undue effort and concentration at an appropriate speed. Later, the point of the tongue in the elevated position can also be moved rapidly from side to side while maintaining contact with the top lip.

The patient brings the tip of his tongue to touch the back of his top teeth exactly in the middle. The therapist uses a spatula to facilitate the lifting movement and to guide the tongue into the correct position (Fig. 5.20a). The patient tries to keep his tongue in the same place when the therapist moves the spatula away and then make the sound "d" or "t" (Fig. 5.20b). Each sound can be repeated faster and faster as the tongue becomes more agile, always without associated movements of the chin. The sound "ng" is also practised because the tongue moves in a way very similar to that required for swallowing food or liquid, with the tip flattened and pressing up against the hard palate anteriorly right behind the upper teeth.

Another important movement for the tongue is the elevation of the posterior portion, which takes place when the sound "ga" is made as well as during swallowing in order to transfer the masticated and moistened food back in the mouth to initiate the swallow itself. When drinking, the "humping" movement has to be even more rapid. Practising the sound with facilitation from the therapist will help the

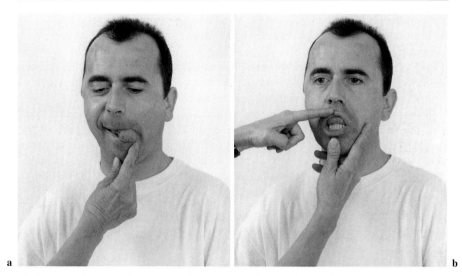

a   b

Fig. 5.19a. Trying to touch the therapist's finger. **b** Difficulty with selective movement when trying to lick the top lip

patient to retrieve the movement which is difficult to perform in isolation and the acoustic feedback he receives will enable him to monitor his performance and then try to improve it. Increased activity at the back of the tongue will also help to activate the soft palate.

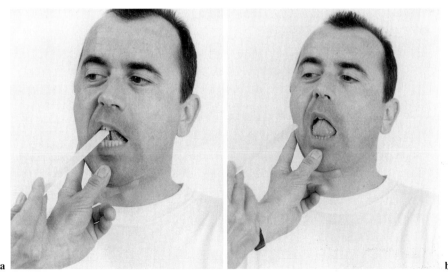

a   b

Fig. 5.20a,b. Facilitating elevation of the tongue tip. **a** Lifting the tongue into position behind the top teeth. **b** Holding the position before saying "d"

With the tip of the patient's tongue remaining in position against the inside of his bottom teeth, the therapist presses firmly down on the middle of its upper surface with a spatula and as she releases the pressure asks the him to say "ga" (Fig. 5.21a). The patient repeats the sound each time the spatula is lifted away and is reminded to keep his tongue forwards touching his teeth, as it will tend to pull back each time in a mass movement pattern.

If the patient if unable to prevent the retraction of his tongue when he says "ga", or if the therapist wishes to increase the amount of activity at the back of the tongue, then she holds it forwards just outside his mouth with a piece of gauze in the way described in Fig. 5.16. At the same time she uses the spatula in her other hand to stimulate the appropriate part of his tongue by pressing down briskly as she asks him to try to produce the "ga" sound (Fig. 5.21b).

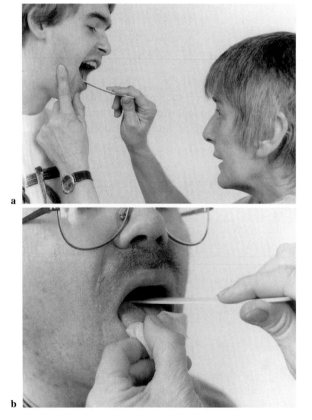

Fig. 5.21a,b. Stimulating elevation of the posterior portion of the tongue. **a** A quick downward pressure before the patient says "ga". **b** Holding the tongue forward while stimulating movement

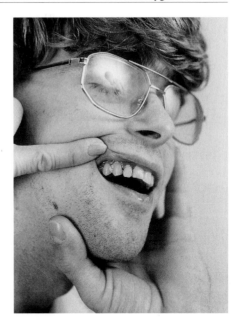

Fig. 5.22. A patient with very inadequate tongue movement has coated teeth and gums which bleed easily

Oral Hygiene

If the patient cannot move his tongue, lips and cheeks selectively, they will not be carrying out the vigorous polishing and cleansing movements inside the mouth that normally occur automatically throughout the day to keep the teeth and gums clean and remove any extraneous matter. As the patient will also not be brushing his teeth and gums vigorously as usual, the condition of both can easily suffer if adequate measures are not taken. The teeth become coated and soon show signs of caries, while the gums develop a characteristic sponginess and bleed easily (Fig. 5.22). Not only would it be a shame for young patients to lose their teeth, but the pain caused by the unhealthy condition of the teeth and the infected gums will also intensify already existing sensorimotor dysfunction.

Care of the Teeth and Gums

In addition to the massaging of the patient's gums which is carried out during therapy to promote circulation and give sensory stimulation, from the very beginning his mouth should be cleaned thoroughly at least three times a day by an assistant, either the therapist, the nurse or an appropriately trained relative.

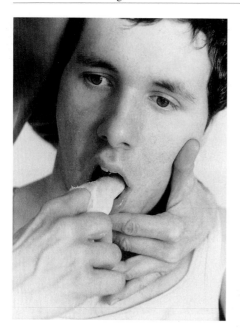

Fig. 5.23. Cleaning the patient's teeth with a piece of moistened gauze wrapped round the assistant's finger

Cleaning the Teeth and the Oral Cavity

In the early days when the patient is still confined to bed and using a toothbrush may be mechanically impracticable, the therapist or nurse can use a piece of gauze wrapped round one of her fingers to clean the patient's teeth and also the inside of his mouth. She moistens the gauze in a pleasant tasting liquid before rubbing the patient's upper and lower gums from the middle towards both sides right along to the back on the outside as well as the inside of his teeth. With a fresh piece of wet gauze she then removes any debris. To clean the patient's teeth adequately, the assistant uses her gauze-covered finger, rubbing it horizontally back and forth along their outer and inner aspects as well as on the cutting surfaces (Fig. 5.23). In order to remove any extraneous matter, she also draws the gauze vertically downwards over the upper gums and inner and outer surfaces of the top teeth or vertically upwards in the case of the bottom teeth.

Finally the assistant inspects the whole of the oral cavity and, with her finger, removes anything that has remained inside his cheeks or is adhering to the roof of his mouth or tongue.

Brushing the Patient's Teeth

As soon as the patient is sitting out of bed in a wheelchair, even if only for short spells, the therapist or nurse can start brushing his teeth with a toothbrush. With a little effort and ingenuity it is possible to brush the patient's teeth while he is lying on his side so that the very therapeutic procedure can be commenced even before

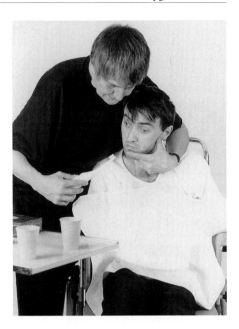

Fig. 5.24. When brushing the patient's teeth the therapist uses grip A and has everything she requires placed ready in front of him.

he is able to sit out of bed. When using a toothbrush instead of a piece of gauze, a far more satisfactory result can be achieved. In addition to the enhanced cleanliness of the teeth themselves, the condition of the gums improves and the stimulation helps to normalize tone and sensation in the mouth. An electric toothbrush is not essential but is strongly recommended because of its many advantages. The small brush is easier to insert under the patient's lip, its intrinsic movements facilitate teeth-cleaning by replacing the complex motions and dexterity normally required, and the vibration in the mouth has a therapeutic effect. The brush can also be turned so that the smooth surface behind can be moved over the patient's lips, cheeks or throat from the outside, which frequently helps to normalize tone and stimulate active movement.

The therapist stands beside the patient using grip A to facilitate the movements of his mouth and control the position of his head (Fig. 5.24). Two beakers of water, toothpaste, paper towel and anything else which she may require are placed on a table in such a way that the patient is able to see them easily. A towel is draped over his chest to protect his clothing from becoming wet.

The therapist slides the brush under his lip, turning it so that the bristles do not scratch him as she brings the brush into his mouth (Fig. 5.25a). If necessary she uses the index finger of her other hand to move his lip out of the way.

Once the brush is in the correct position, the therapist brushes the patient's teeth thoroughly taking care to include all three surfaces of each tooth. Because it is impossible for her to see whether all have been adequately cleaned, it is a help if she mentally divides his mouth into four sections and follows a routine when brushing his teeth. For instance, the therapist starts at the midline of the patient's

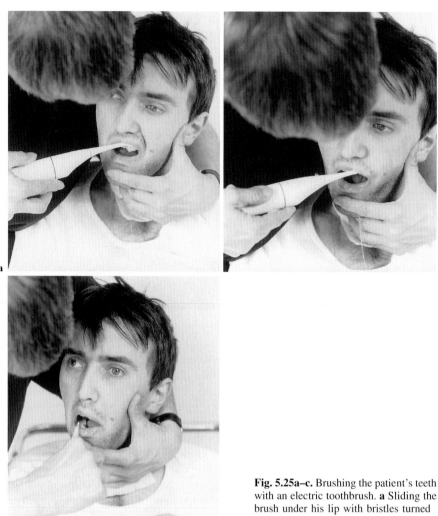

Fig. 5.25a–c. Brushing the patient's teeth with an electric toothbrush. **a** Sliding the brush under his lip with bristles turned away. **b** Brushing along the outside surface. **c** Moving right to the back teeth

upper teeth and brushes the side furthest from her right to the back as far as she can go (Fig. 5.25b) and then withdraws the brush from his mouth. Moving the brush on to his lower teeth, she once again proceeds from the midline to the back. She then repeats the procedure on the side nearest to her, cleaning first the upper section, removing the brush and allowing a pause before continuing with the lower teeth on that side (Fig. 5.25c). Having brushed the outside of the patient's teeth, the therapist follows the same sequence to clean the inner surfaces and then the cutting edges of the teeth in all four sections. When brushing the inside of the teeth, the therapist holds the toothbrush vertically instead of horizontally and draws the brush down from the gums to the distal end of the upper teeth or upwards

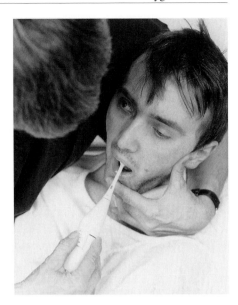

Fig. 5.26. Drawing the brush vertically
downwards behind the front teeth

from the gums to the edges of the lower teeth as if she were scraping away food
particles from between his teeth (Fig. 5.26).

If the patient's mouth is particularly sensitive to touch or vibration and unwanted reactions are elicited, then the electric toothbrush should be used in the
same way but without current at first until he can tolerate the sensation. Usually
the therapist will be able to brush the outside of his teeth with the brush switched on
long before it is possible for her to take the vibrating brush inside his mouth and
clean their inner surfaces. The patient's tolerance is slowly increased until the
therapist can clean all aspects of his teeth without switching the current off.

A patient who has not had his teeth brushed nor his face and mouth treated with
direct contact for a considerable time will often be extremely hypersensitive, and
the same careful progression will be necessary.

Rinsing the Mouth

Rinsing out the patient's mouth after his teeth have been brushed is often the most
difficult part of the procedure, as he is unable to perform the swift, coordinated
movements normally required to rinse the mouth, collect the fluid and spit it out.
For the same reason it is usually not feasible to solve the problem by using any type
of water-jet instrument or spray.

In clinical practice the following ideas have proved helpful:

- If the rinsing procedure is particularly difficult, no toothpaste is used because if
  any remains in the mouth it tends to have an abrasive effect after a time. The
  brush is moistened with a gentle disinfecting fluid instead.

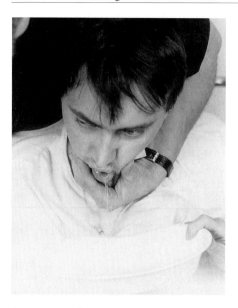

Fig. 5.27. Rinsing the mouth — the assistant facilitates spitting out the water

- The therapist carefully places a small amount of water in the patient's mouth in the way shown in Fig. 5.3c, tilting his head back slightly or to one side, but not allowing any fluid to run back into his throat. As soon as the water is in his mouth, the therapist quickly tips his head forwards with her shoulder, moving her hand simultaneously from its grip A position to facilitate spitting the liquid into a container positioned directly in front of the patient. Her index finger, which previously rested on the anterior aspect of his chin, slides round to draw his cheek and the corner of his mouth forwards and pout his lips, while her thumb moves down to do the same on the other side. The therapist's flexed middle finger beneath his chin pushes firmly upwards and forwards against the floor of his mouth to move his tongue and the water to the front (Fig. 5.27). If she needs to use her middle finger to assist the index finger for the manipulation of the patient's cheek and the corner of his mouth, then her ring finger can be used beneath his chin instead.
- A piece of moistened gauze can be used to clean the mouth if the rinsing has not been adequate or if it is impossible to facilitate.

PROBLEM SOLVING

For Bleeding Gums. Infected or unhealthy gums will tend to bleed when oral hygiene is being carried out, and the therapist or nurse may think that her treatment has been too vigorous or too prolonged. Quite the opposite is in fact the case and intensive measures must be undertaken to overcome the problem until the teeth and gums can be brushed with impunity with no signs of bleeding even when the electric toothbrush is switched on for brushing.

While the gums are still extremely sensitive and in a very poor condition, they should be massaged gently with gauze dipped in a suitable medication to counteract the infection as the brush, even with the current switched off, may be impossible to tolerate. Not only the gums outside the teeth where the bleeding is more obvious should be massaged with a slowly increasing amount of pressure, but the area behind the front incisors often requires particular attention. Once vigorous massage can be tolerated, a toothbrush is introduced to clean the teeth and surrounding gums in less affected areas with the current on or off as is appropriate and gradually spreading out to include all the teeth as the condition of the gums improves. If the patient is tolerating the brushing without showing signs of pain or over-reaction to the stimulus, then some slight bleeding should not deter the therapist from continuing as the circulatory improvement will speed up the healing process. The massage with the therapist's finger wrapped in gauze should be continued until the patient is able to eat solids and have his teeth brushed all over with the electric toothbrush.

Using Dental Floss. Without using a toothbrush, it is extremely difficult to clean the spaces between the patient's teeth adequately and the same difficulty arises when he starts to clean his own teeth and has insufficient manual dexterity for the finely coordinated movements that are normally made. Dental floss can be a great help and the mechanical difficulties confronting either the therapist or the patient himself when manipulating the thin thread with both hands can be overcome by using a device to hold the floss (Fig. 5.28).

Inability to Open the Mouth. If the patient is unable to open his mouth voluntarily and keep it open, then cleaning his teeth adequately can be a difficult task. Brushing his teeth from the outside is not the problem as his lips can be moved away to gain access, but reaching their interior or cutting surfaces becomes almost impossible and both the teeth and gums suffer if the problem is not solved. Whether the patient is holding his mouth tightly closed because he does not understand what is expected of him, or because his mouth is suddenly tightly closed because of a hyperactive bite reflex which he is unable to inhibit, the first line of approach is to treat the outside of his face until he is able to tolerate touch in less sensitive areas. Because the treatment to restore sufficient control of the patient's mouth may take a considerable time, the therapist will need to hold his jaws open mechanically as an emergency measure, in order to be able to clean the oral cavity and maintain the condition of his teeth and gums.

Warning: Metal instruments should never be used to force the patient's teeth apart and hold his mouth open.

In the presence of a forceful bite, his teeth may easily be damaged and the patient's anxiety will increase the problem of opening his mouth the next day. Any broken tooth presents an enormous problem because it is impossible for dental repairs to be carried out at such a stage without a full anaesthetic.

A hard yet slightly yielding material should be used to construct two strong wedges just thick enough so that when placed between the patient's teeth, one

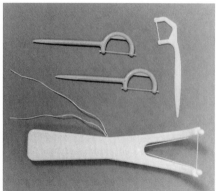

a

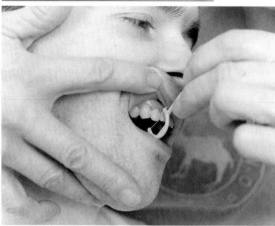

b

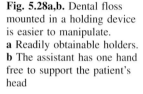

Fig. 5.28a,b. Dental floss mounted in a holding device is easier to manipulate.
a Readily obtainable holders.
b The assistant has one hand free to support the patient's head

on either side of his mouth, the therapist's finger is able to enter the oral cavity easily and safely. A wooden spatula with a bandage wrapped around it and fixed in place with strapping plaster has the right consistency, and two of these could be sufficient, but if the bite is very strong the material may be torn off and pieces be left in the mouth with little possibility of retrieving them again. The therapist waits until the patient's mouth opens during spontaneous oral movement or when she is working on his gums outside the teeth before she or an assistant slips first one of the wedges and then the other as well in between his teeth. Because the experience may well be alarming and uncomfortable for the patient, the therapist talks quietly and calmly to him and as little force as possible is used when inserting the plastic wedges. If necessary, the therapist uses a disinfectant on the gauze to treat any signs of infection inside the mouth. She controls the patient's head and jaw with grip A both while cleaning and massaging his mouth on the inside or when she is brushing his teeth on the outside. The close contact provided by grip A is often comforting for the patient.

Starting to Eat and Drink Again

Although primarily we eat and drink to survive by fulfilling the nutritional requirements of our bodies, eating and drinking are also very much concerned with enjoyment and social interaction. The patient who is unable to partake of food by
mouth suffers a great loss of life quality, particularly as so many other pleasurable
activities are also impossible for him. As well as the pleasure he would gain from
eating and drinking, he is deprived of the regular stimulation they provide within
the mouth for circulation, sensation and movement. In the absence of oral intake,
the condition of the mouth deteriorates and without the motor activity of chewing
and swallowing the muscles and joints suffer in the same way as do those of the
limbs.

From all points of view, the sooner oral feeding is commenced, the better it is for
the patient. All forms of nutritional support have their disadvantages and should
therefore be regarded as transitional or supplementary feeding measures. Only
after determined and prolonged therapy along the lines described should enteral
feeding be accepted as a permanent solution because nearly all patients will eventually be able to eat again even if some are restricted to pureed food. In a retrospective study of 55 with swallowing problems as a result of head injury, 45 of
whom were not able to partake of food by mouth at all on admission to a rehabilitation centre, Winstein (1983) describes the positive outcome following implementation of therapeutic, management programmes for the neurogenic dysphagia.
"Ninety-four percent of those with dysphagia became functional oral feeders.
Thus, the prognosis is very good." In addition, the study revealed that "a concomitant improvement in cognition and disappearance of primitive oral motor
reflexes also appears to take place", a finding which could be attributed to the
increased tactile/kinaesthetic stimulation within the mouth.

Even after prolonged periods of nonoral feeding, patients can with help regain
the ability to eat, which Heimlich (1983), after successfully treating seven stroke
patients with total dysphagia, emphasizes: "Prior to swallowing rehabilitation,
their nutrition had been maintained by tube-feedings for periods of 5 months to
3.9 years." Secondary benefits were also noted in that "there was generally some
improvement in speech soon after regaining the ability to swallow. Gratifying
reports of enhanced social reintegration became routine."

Even if the patient is not able to regain the ability to eat normally again and
requires supplementary nutrition on a permanent basis, his condition should be
reviewed from time to time to ascertain whether there has been any improvement
and intensive periods of therapy repeated if there is the slightest chance of his being
able to eat or drink anything at all.

Even being able to manage small amounts of a favourite dish or beverage can
be an enormous bonus for the patient. After weeks, months or sometimes years
of having nothing in his mouth except disinfection fluid, a morsel of food tastes
wonderful.

A Case in Point

G.B. aged 50 had been unable to eat or drink anything for more than 2 years following bilateral cerebrovascular accidents and received pureed food carefully prepared by her husband through a gastrotomy tube. Despite good return of voluntary function in her arms and legs, her face and mouth remained paralyzed to the extent that she could not even swallow her own saliva, close her eyes or mouth on command, or change her automatic breathing rhythm in any way. When walking in public places, G.B. held a towel to her mouth with her left hand at all times to collect the constant stream of saliva, a towel carefully chosen to match the colour of her clothing perfectly. Within the confines of her home G.B. wore a padded surgical mask to prevent dribbling so that her hands were both free for household tasks. She was unable to speak at all, but when she laughed or was excited a moaning sound was produced. After intensive orofacial therapy and considerable effort on her part, G.B. learned to place titbits way back in her mouth with a teaspoon and swallow them. She was also able to manage sips of coffee in the same way, much to her delight. One day, some 4 years after commencing orofacial therapy, she arrived for treatment, obviously extremely excited about something. Not only was she laughing joyously but in addition making frantic gestures with her hands and moaning repeatedly as she tried to tell the therapist what had happened but all to no avail. Only after the arrival of G.B.'s husband did the picture become clear when he explained that, it being the asparagus season, he had put fresh asparagus in the blender and his wife had been able to eat the delicious puree with melted butter using a teaspoon. To taste asparagus in her mouth again after 6 years was the most wonderful experience for G.B., and it inspired her to keep on trying even harder.

When to Start Oral Feeding

Evaluating Dysphagia

The question as to when oral feeding may safely be attempted is difficult to answer because there are no definite criteria which can be used with absolute certainty for each and every patient. Nurses and therapists feel justifiably anxious about starting too soon, with the possibility of the patient choking or even aspirating, and often the doctor in charge is hesitant about giving permission for the same reasons. Various authors have stressed the importance of evaluating dysphagia by radiography, dynamic imaging with video or cineradiography before the re-education of swallowing is attempted (Bass 1990, 1988; Donner 1986, Siebens and Linden 1985). Videofluoroscopic evaluation of the patient's oral–pharyngeal swallow using a "modified barium swallow" (Logemann 1988; Lazzara et al. 1986) is recommended whenever a pharyngeal swallow disorder or aspiration is a possibility, while Espinola (1986) describes radionuclide evaluation with continuous monitoring to detect aspiration during swallowing. Such procedures can be extremely valuable, not only for assessment purposes but for treatment planning and evaluating the results as well. Their importance is clearly stated by Siebens and Linden (1985) "treating disordered swallowing rationally often requires a therapeutically orientated radiologic examination. Whether a given treatment approach is likely to succeed frequently can be established only by visualizing its consequences. Making the distinction between what is likely to succeed and what is not is significant because re-education in swallowing is time-consuming, complex, taxing, and not without hazard."

> However useful and interesting such dynamic recording techniques may be, they should not be considered as an essential prerequisite before oral feeding is attempted because many patients would thus be deprived of the chance of learning to eat again.

The costly and complex procedures are simply not available or possible for all patients at the present time and as Donner (1986) so rightly points out, "It can safely be said that many physicians, including radiologists, are not sufficiently experienced in the radiologic evaluation of the pharynx and oesophagus to contribute fully to the multidisciplinary evaluation of dysphagic persons."

In most instances, the necessary information and adequate safety measures will need to be provided by careful observation, therapeutic evaluation and proper management. Those who treat the patient on a daily basis will have the advantage of seeing him in familiar surroundings, and he will also feel more at ease in the therapeutic situation to which he is accustomed. The attempted swallow will not need to be performed on command without preparation, but will be an integrated part of the therapy after his mouth has been "warmed up", so to speak. Because swallowing is partly automatic and yet has a voluntary component, it is most complex and can be much influenced by external factors. Trying to swallow at a specific time on command is difficult, as anyone can experience by chewing a mouthful of food and then having another person give verbal instructions like "Wait, keep it there!" and "Now swallow!" Any form of tension alters the pattern of normal swallowing to some degree, and the same will apply during the diagnostic application of dynamic imaging which for the patient is like a test of his ability. The mere fact that other people are scrutinizing him closely and waiting for him to swallow what is in his mouth will make a difference to the activity. As Donner (1986) points out "moreover, one should be aware that a patient evaluation represents a controlled situation, and no matter how carefully performed, it may not accurately reflect the status of the patient at other times".

Eating patterns are also influenced by what the food looks, feels and tastes like and individual habits and preferences. The radiopacification of solids and liquids required for imaging can make them very unappetizing, a problem which could cause conflicting results if not taken into account. For example, the patient may be coping well and safely with food which he enjoys when assisted by the nursing staff or his relatives, but abnormalities are recorded when he attempts to swallow the prepared bolus. To help to overcome the difficulty, Siebens and Linden (1985) thoughtfully suggest "if barium is used, the product is usually unsightly and less savory than its nonopaque counterpart. Having the hospital's kitchen prepare barium-impregnated puddings, gels, purees, mashed potatoes, and hamburgers to be used at the time of the study is very helpful in making decisions bearing on swallowing re-education." In addition, a secondary benefit is rightly pointed out, "fluoroscopic observation of radiopaque boluses with varying physical characteristics can help establish what kinds of food can be ingested safely." Whenever dynamic imaging is being used such factors should be considered, and the advice given by Siebens and Linden followed.

Swallowing Difficulties

Swallowing or deglutition can be defined as "the semiautomatic action of the muscles of the respiratory and gastrointestinal tracts to propel food from the oral cavity to the stomach. This action not only transports the food but also removes secretion and particles from the upper respiratory tract, thereby protecting the respiratory tract from ingesting particles" (Miller 1986). Swallowing involves three separate but interacting phases commonly described as the oral or oral preparatory stage, the pharyngeal stage and the oesophageal stage (Buchholz 1987; Donner et al. 1985; Logemann 1983; Bass and Morrell 1984).

The oral stage divides the food into sufficiently small pieces for transport into the pharynx and hence the oesophagus, and while the material is in the mouth, it is moistened with saliva to facilitate its passage in the pharynx and formed into a comfortable shape preparatory to the swallow. The prepared material in its ready-to-swallow state is described as the bolus. The preparation of solids involves rotatory chewing, with the cheek muscles holding the piece in position between the molar teeth laterally and selective action of the tongue keeping it in place from within, as well as moving it automatically from one side to the other. During mastication, the agile tongue also sorts out pieces of food which are ready for swallowing and forms them into a bolus. While the remaining material is held temporarily in the oral cavity awaiting further preparation, the partial bolus is swallowed. A mouthful of food therefore need not be swallowed all at the same time. The oral phase of swallowing begins with the lips closing and the tongue and facial muscles capturing the bolus. The bolus is propelled posteriorly by a swift, wave-like movement of the tongue, with the tip elevating behind the front teeth and then the blade pressing against the hard palate to squeeze the appropriately prepared food into the posterior oral cavity. At this point the involuntary pharyngeal phase of the swallow is initiated. Although the oral stage can be defined as voluntary, in that any of the movements involved may be stopped or started at will, the chewing and the multiple activities performed by the tongue take place on an automatic basis. The number of times food is chewed prior to being swallowed varies from person to person: it is an acquired or learned preference and is not only dependent upon the consistency and size of the piece. Observation of normal eating can reveal a surprising range of between 7 and 40 chewing movements to prepare a similar solid before swallowing occurs.

The pharyngeal stage commences when the swallowing reflex is elicited as the bolus passes the anterior faucial arches, modified by sensory feedback. The pharynx develops a propelling force as the constricting muscles of the throat contract, while at the same time respiration is inhibited. The soft palate elevates to close the nasal cavity from below, the epiglottis is tipped downwards, and the larynx constricts as it elevates, all of which serve to protect the airway and the respiratory tract as a whole. Once the bolus has passed through the valve at the upper end of the oesophagus the next stage begins. However, the contraction of the pharyngeal phase continues, so that a positive force is developed to continue the movement of the bolus (Miller 1986). The pharynx is cleared of any remaining particles by a few subsequent swallowing movements, the repeated swallows being elicited by continuous feedback from the soft palate, the base of the tongue and the walls of the pharynx itself.

The oesophageal stage allows the bolus to be moved by peristaltic contractions to the stomach and, as quoted by Miller (1986), "begins 600–800 ms after the start of the pharyngeal phase and lasts much longer, extending from 3 to 9 s." Continuing peristaltic activity is stimulated by the bolus, which not only modifies primary but also elicits secondary peristalsis by its presence.

Eating difficulties may be due to problems in any of the three stages of swallowing, but in the patient with head injury they are more commonly located in the oral preparatory phase or pharyngeal stage. The patient diagnosed as having "swallowing problems" may be unable to chew, control the food with his tongue, or transport it back to the pharynx. Loss of sensation may prevent the triggering of the swallowing reflex and, without elevation of the soft palate, fluid or food particles may enter the nasal cavity. Choking or even aspiration may occur if pharyngeal constriction is inadequate or if the larynx does not elevate and constrict to guard the airway. Food particles are often left clinging to the pharyngeal wall and, due to sensory loss, repeated swallows are not triggered to clear them away. Some time later, when the patient is not being so closely supervised, these particles can easily be dislodged and inhaled, particularly if he is lying down.

Although such problems may be observed in isolation, any difficulty during one phase will affect the efficiency and normal smooth functioning not only of that phase, but that of the others as well. As Bass (1988) so wisely points out, "it should be emphasized that the feeding process must be viewed as a totally integrated and interdependent series of behaviours in which an abnormality at any stage will result in abnormal adaptation involving the entire process".

When making the decision to commence oral feeding, the potential for adequate function in all three stages will already have been estimated through assessment, but only when food is actually placed in the patient's mouth can a realistic evaluation of his eating performance be made.

Guiding Factors and Safety Precautions

In the absence of absolute criteria as to when eating can first be attempted, considering the following points in conjunction with certain safety precautions can be helpful.

The Presence of a Cough Reflex. The patient should be able to cough in order to protect the airway. It is not essential that he be able to cough voluntarily on command or clear his throat when requested, as long as he coughs spontaneously in other situations. For example, the patient coughs vigorously during mechanical suctioning of his tracheostomy tube, posterior oral cavity and pharynx or coughing has been observed when secretions have gathered in these prior to suctioning. If the cough is not sufficiently forceful, the therapist can use her hands on his lower ribs or sternum to increase its strength and ensure adequate expulsion. Important is that the cough reflex can be elicited by tactile stimulation. As the patient progresses, he can be encouraged and helped to cough on command to clear his respiratory tract regularly even before the stimulus has been perceived.

The Gag Reflex. The presence of an active gag reflex is in no way a prerequisite for eating as is sometimes mistakenly assumed. The reflex plays no part in normal adult eating performance and, in fact, can cause additional difficulties for the patient if it is hyperactive. No attempts should be made to stimulate the gag reflex during therapy as it is most unpleasant for the patient, serves no useful purpose, and can cause unwanted reactions. Testing for the reflex will provide only some information as to the sensation in the back of the patient's mouth and throat which could be of diagnostic interest but little practical value. "The presence of a reflex indicates sensitivity elicitation in the pharynx but provides little information about competence in feeding. Since this reflex is sometimes absent under normal conditions, unilateral absence is of greater clinical significance than a lack of response to bilateral stimulation" (Bass 1988).

Vocal Sounds. The production of vocal sounds, whether voluntary or occurring spontaneously when the patient laughs or cries, indicates that his vocal cords can be brought together, affording a certain degree of protection for the airway during swallowing. The protection thus provided is enhanced by elevation of the larynx, which should be kept freely mobile to allow the quick, upward movement observed during normal swallowing. The tone in the muscles surrounding the larynx should be normalized before oral intake, and the position of the head should be optimized, as neck extension places the anterior musculature under tension, creating a resistance to laryngeal elevation. The increased difficulty in swallowing caused by such a resistance is readily demonstrable, even in an unimpaired person, if the neck is extended.

Every effort should be made to encourage phonation on a voluntary basis during early treatment to initiate and increase activity in the vocal cords and, whenever possible, pitch changes should be practised so that the larynx moves actively up and down.

Correct Sitting Posture. A correct, upright sitting posture facilitates swallowing considerably, so that it is inadvisable to attempt oral feeding if the patient has not yet been brought out of bed, and is still lying or, at best, half-lying in a slumped position, with the head of the bed raised. When he is seated correctly in a wheelchair with a table in front of him to support the weight of his arms, there is less tendency for his thoracic spine to be flexed and his neck extended. Neck extension not only prevents laryngeal elevation, but also hampers jaw closure. The position of the mandible is an important factor as swallowing is extremely difficult with the jaw lowered. For the same reason, using grip A will facilitate swallowing, because the neck is elongated posteriorly and jaw closure assisted from below.

Swallowing Saliva. The ability to swallow saliva is a good indication that the patient will probably be able to swallow other things as well. Because saliva has no taste or temperature difference and flows relatively quickly with gravity, it can be difficult for the patient to cope with. If the patient is able to lie supine for any length of time without choking or showing signs of distress, then obviously he is swallowing his saliva automatically. Under these circumstances, the problems will usually involve the preparation of the food in the oral stage or the transportation of the bolus back into the pharynx in order for it to be to be swallowed, a supposition that can be verified by placing a small portion of ice cream or yogurt on the back of the patient's tongue where it can easily be swallowed.

Active Tongue Movements. For chewing solids and for transporting liquids or solids into the pharynx, active tongue movements are essential. If at any other time the patient has been observed moving his tongue spontaneously, for example to lick his lips or to pronounce an occasional word clearly, then activity must be present although he may not be able to move it on command. Activity in the tongue is particularly important with regard to eating, not only in the oral stage but also because "the lingual action to initiate the voluntary swallow appears to be a major component of the stimulus for triggering the swallowing reflex" (Logemann 1985).

The fact that the patient is unable to move his tongue should not, however, deter the therapist from attempting oral feeding altogether. Activity may well be regained through the stimulation provided by food in the mouth and assisted chewing as long as adequate safety precautions are observed. In such cases, the therapist will need to find ways to compensate for the absent tongue movements or to facilitate them from without.

Condition of Teeth and Gums. The patient's teeth and gums should be in good condition and, if they have been allowed to deteriorate, any problems which are causing pain must be overcome before eating can be successfully attempted. Pain from infected gums or damaged teeth may be causing the apparent "swallowing" difficulties rather than the actual swallow itself.

Placement of Suction Machine. A suction machine should not be placed ostentatiously near the patient as if a life-threatening choke were expected. Its foreboding presence will only tend to create tension in an already somewhat tense situation and, moreover, suction with a small pliable catheter would serve little purpose in the event of solids being aspirated. Even when cleaning the patient's mouth after he has finished eating, it is preferable to do so with his participation and manual assistance rather than using a machine.

Warning: No piece of food large and hard enough to cause a serious choke should be placed in the patient's mouth until he is able to chew and swallow adequately.

Choking. If the patient chokes during oral feeding or some time afterwards or even on his own saliva, it is important for all members of the team to know how to assist him, calmly and confidently.

Every effort should be made to ensure that the patient does not choke at all, by careful choice of the type of food, a good starting position in sitting, adequate preparation before eating and a relaxed atmosphere. Choking is a very unpleasant experience for anyone, and in the case of the patient, will tend to have a self-reinforcing effect. With each choke he becomes progressively more afraid of it happening again, and the anticipatory fear in turn causes hypertonus, which does indeed increase the likelihood of a recurrence. Should the patient, however, unfortunately choke or show signs of distress prior to choking, as will inevitably happen at some time despite the appropriate measures having been taken, the therapist must help him to clear his airway without any sign of alarm.

She starts by talking to him normally, in a quiet, matter-of-fact way as she places the spoon or fork back on the plate or helps him to do so if he has been holding it himself. She flexes his neck and pats him gently and rhythmically over his upper thoracic spine, while waiting a moment or two to see if the airway clears as he relaxes and swallows. The gentle patting on the back, similar to that of a mother helping her baby to break wind after a bottle feed, seems to relax bronchospasm and free something which has been inadvertently inhaled. It is important to keep the patient's head and trunk flexed, because if he pushes them back into extension, inspiration is accentuated and the piece of food or the liquid is taken in still further. If the patient does not succeed in coughing out or swallowing whatever is causing the trouble, the therapist uses the palm of her hand to give a firm tap over his upper back, the tap timed to synchronize with his next expiratory breath, which usually results in the offending substance being dislodged and expelled. The Heimlich manoeuvre has been advocated to overcome choking, but for minor chokes of this nature it would seem too extreme and carries the risk of the patient sustaining rib fractures unnecessarily (Heimlich 1978). The therapist can instead assist the patient's cough if it is too weak by placing her arm around his lower ribcage and pressing his ribs together and downwards when he attempts to cough. Only in the unlikely event of a patient ever being unable to breathe in at all should emergency procedures be implemented, such as bending him right forwards with his head between his knees or lying him face down with his head over the side of the bed and pushing down suddenly on his thorax or inserting an airway to allow suctioning with a hard, large-bore catheter. Such a situation should never occur if the type of food has been carefully selected, the patient's eating supervised, and appropriate assistance given. The measures are described only to ensure that adequate steps are taken in an emergency, one which is far more likely to arise at a later stage in rehabilitation when the patient is eating on his own.

Residual Food Particles in the Mouth and Throat. The patient's mouth and throat must be completely clear of any food particles after he has eaten before he is left unsupervised or lies flat in bed. Any pieces of food which have adhered to the roof of his mouth or the pharyngeal wall could be dislodged later and aspirated when he is alone with serious or even fatal results. To eliminate the danger, routinely after every meal or eating attempt the nurse or therapist uses a pocket torch to make a quick inspection of the oral cavity and pharynx and, if she sees that particles have remained, ensures their removal. It will often be sufficient for the patient to drink something, with help as required, and then to make repeated swallows, which he is encouraged to do. The therapist may need to rinse out his mouth, either with facilitation or with her finger covered with moistened gauze. Larger morsels can be removed with a spatula or toothbrush. As a further safety precaution, the patient should remain in an upright position for 1 h after eating and should not partake of food for 1–2 h before going to sleep (Bass 1990).

Facilitating Eating

Once the decision to commence oral feeding has been made, the patient should be assisted in every way possible to ensure that the eating attempts are successful and pleasurable for him and that the transition from tube-feeding proceeds smoothly without undue stress. The following suggestions have proved helpful for patients in the transition phase.

Removal of Nasogastric Tube

The presence of a nasogastric tube influences swallowing adversely even in the absence of neurological deficits, so that if the patient is receiving supplementary feeds the tube should be removed before he tries to eat. At first he may be unable to take sufficient fluid by mouth and the tube will need to be replaced each evening to ensure an adequate fluid intake. Because of the loss of sensation in the pharynx, which is almost always a predisposing factor, replacing the tube is usually not difficult and so much is gained that the additional effort is well worthwhile.

It must also be remembered that if the patient has just had a nasogastric feed he will not be hungry at all, a fact which could easily affect his eating successfully. Early oral feeding attempts should be timed to coincide with periods when the patient has a feeling of hunger, before the next tube-feed would normally be due.

Correct Posture

The patient should be helped to sit up as straight as possible in a chair, with a table of the correct height in front of him on which his arms can be supported if necessary. It is extremely difficult for him to eat if he has slid down in his chair into a half-lying position or if his trunk is too flexed. For a patient who has problems with eating, it would be counterproductive to attempt oral feeding while he is lying in bed, a position which in itself hampers normal swallowing.

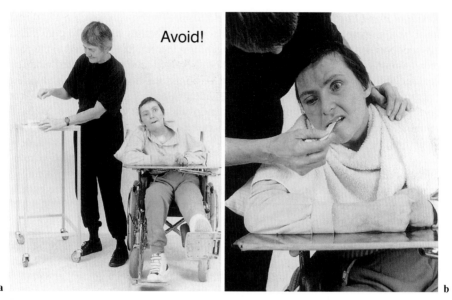

Avoid!

a   b

Fig. 5.29a,b. Before eating attempts the patient's posture must be corrected. **a** Incorrect position of helper and patient. **b** Bite reflex elicited by unexpected arrival of implement

The plate of food should be placed on the table within the patient's field of vision so that he can see what he is being helped to eat in order to make the situation as normal as possible. From earliest childhood onwards, people are accustomed to having food presented to the centre of their lips from a position directly in front of them. It can be very disconcerting for the patient if a mouthful of food is brought from one side by the person feeding him so that it arrives without warning and suddenly touches his mouth. The unexpected contact may cause a reflex withdrawal of his head with neck extension or even elicit a bite reflex (Fig. 5.29).

Manual Facilitation of Eating

If the patient is unable to eat on his own, eating is facilitated manually by a member of the team or one of his relatives who has been carefully instructed.

The helper stands beside the patient and will usually need to use grip A to ensure an optimal eating pattern. With her other hand, she brings the food to the his mouth with a spoon or fork (Fig. 5.30a).

She places the underneath surface of the spoon or fork on his tongue before bringing his lips together with her index finger to initiate the swallowing cycle (Fig. 5.30b). During normal eating, the portion is removed from either implement by an active movement of the closed lips as it is withdrawn from the mouth. If the patient however is unable to move his lips actively, a fork is the implement of

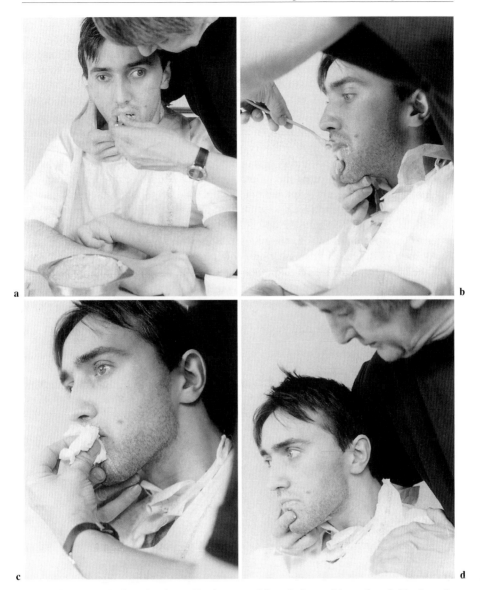

Fig. 5.30a–d. Facilitation of eating. **a** Food presented from in front of the patient. **b** Lips brought together to remove food from fork. **c** Firm pressure with napkin stimulates lip closure. **d** Therapist's middle finger facilitating tongue movement

choice, because its shape makes it easier for the helper to facilitate the required lip action passively. When using a spoon, much of the food remains in the hollow, and the helper may be tempted to scrape it off against the patient's teeth, so causing an abnormal pattern right at the beginning of the swallowing programme, i.e. by-passing lip closure which will affect the swallow itself.

After replacing the fork on the plate, the helper removes any food which has remained on the outside of the patient's mouth with a soft, absorbent paper napkin. She first compresses the napkin into a manageable form and then presses it firmly against his lips with a small rotatory movement, which stimulates lip closure (Fig. 5.30c). The helper should not clean the patient's lips by rubbing them repeatedly because the skin around the mouth can easily become chafed and painful.

Once the food is safely in the patient's mouth, the helper waits for a moment to see what the patient can do on his own before using her middle finger beneath the floor of his mouth to facilitate the upward and backward movement of his tongue in order to transport the bolus to the pharynx for swallowing (Fig. 5.30d).

As soon as the patient can swallow more easily and requires less manual help with the oral phase, the helper can guide his hands to enable him to bring the food into his mouth himself, following the principles described in Chap. 1 (Fig. 5.31). Not only does using his own hands facilitate eating, but hand function is often improved as well.

Assistance from Relatives

The patient's relatives will be more than willing to help him with eating at mealtimes which not only lightens the load on the hospital staff but can also be a positive experience for the patient and those helping him. In the beginning, eating may be a

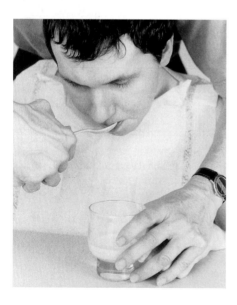

Fig. 5.31. Guiding the patient's hands during eating

slow process, which makes it very time-consuming for busy members of staff, so that a more relaxed atmosphere may prevail if a caring relative is assisting. When the patient first starts to eat again, whoever is assisting him must be relaxed and have sufficient time at his or her disposal. With a helper who is tense, constantly looking at her watch and consciously or subconsciously trying to chivvy him along so that he finishes his meal more quickly, the patient will be more likely to choke or have other difficulties with eating. As soon as it has been ascertained that the patient is able to swallow relatively safely, the therapist should practise the correct manual facilitation with his relatives because, left to their own devices, they might otherwise unwittingly feed him in a way that reinforces abnormal postures and patterns (Fig. 5.32).

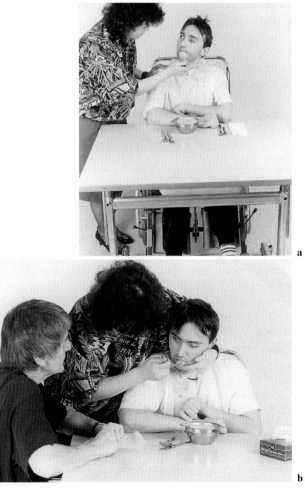

a

b

Fig. 5.32a,b. Relatives helping the patient to eat. **a** A mother unwittingly reinforces an abnormal pattern. **b** With careful instruction she assists therapeutically

Quality of Food

It is important that the food should look appetizing and be something that the patient enjoyed before. A number of psychological factors are involved in the process of eating, many of which, such as individual preferences, are learned in early life. Patients who can still only manage a soft diet are often faced with a most unattractive looking, brown puree in which all the ingredients have been mashed up together. With care, the same ingredients prepared and arranged separately can be presented in an attractive way, so that the patient is not put off eating them but stimulated to taste them instead.

The patient's likes and dislikes will also need to be considered and the relevant information should be obtained from his family or friends if he is unable communicate in any way. For example, yogurt has an easy-to-swallow consistency and is, therefore, often chosen for early eating attempts. If, however, the patient previously disliked yogurt intensely, he is hardly likely to gulp it down willingly when he is learning to swallow again, merely because he has sustained a brain injury! On the other hand, it is inadvisable for the patient to eat only sweet things, as many will tend to do, finding jellies, chocolates and cream cakes easier to manage and more enjoyable. On such a diet, he will inevitably gain too much weight, which could impede his physical rehabilitation, and the sweet foods will cause his teeth and skin to deteriorate. Sugary substances also tend to stimulate primitive, stereotyped movements in the mouth. Once the patient is able to swallow some specific edibles again he must be helped and encouraged to progress to other types of food in order to improve the activity required both for eating a normal diet and for speaking.

Appropriate Type of Food

Certain types of food are easier than others to manipulate within the mouth and to swallow, so that what is chosen will also facilitate early eating attempts. It is difficult to state exactly which type of food will be right for which patient as there will be individual variations, but certainly substances that are intrinsically moist and glide slowly and smoothly toward the pharynx are usually the easiest in the beginning, for example, yogurt, custard, ice cream, mashed banana, or vegetable puree.

When the patient is not yet able to chew, then obviously hard solids which require mastication cannot be offered to him unless they can be held and removed from his mouth again (see "*Problem solving*" below). If he can make some chewing movements, these should be encouraged and strengthened by his being offered "easy-to-chew" solids such as lightly cooked vegetables or fruit, or biscuits which do not crumble and are quickly reduced to pulp.

The sorts of food to be avoided when swallowing is in any way difficult for the patient, are those which incorporate a mixture of different consistencies, for example, stews, minced meat in gravy, minestrone soup or fruit salad.

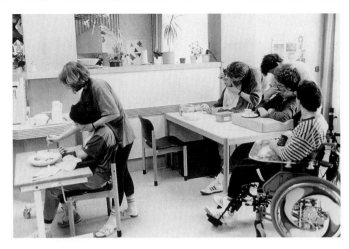

Fig. 5.33. Eating at table with others creates a more normal atmosphere

Eating with Others

Whenever possible, the patient should take his meals together with others and not alone in his room (Fig. 5.33). Eating at table with others creates a more normal atmosphere, and the familiar ritual may help him to retrieve temporarily lost functions. Sitting and eating a plateful of food while someone else who is not eating anything watches every move intently is a stressful situation for anyone.

The problem posed by the patients eating in a group is that the nursing staff would be unable to help all those requiring assistance at the same time. It is a problem which is easily solved, however, if all members of the team have learned the manual facilitation and are prepared to join in and assist. Such mealtimes can be a most rewarding experience as well as providing invaluable, additional assessment information for the different professionals. Each patient can then be helped according to his specific needs (Fig. 5.34).

PROBLEM SOLVING

For the Patient Who Is Unable to Chew. Many patients are unable to chew at first, or only inadequately, and as a result begin their swallowing re-education with a soft or pureed diet. It must be remembered, however, that because chewing is an automatic action albeit under voluntary control, if a patient has nothing in his mouth hard enough to require chewing, then chewing will not be initiated. Mastication cannot be practised in isolation without solid food in the mouth, nor can the complex rotatory grinding action be manually facilitated despite some claims to the contrary. At most, a primitive up-and-down motion of the jaw can be achieved passively if muscle tone is sufficiently low, a fact that can easily be verified by attempting to replicate the components of chewing manually on a normal subject

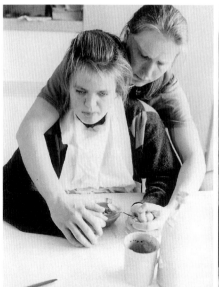

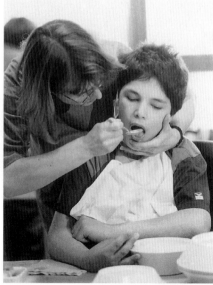

a

b

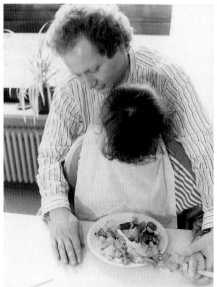

c

Fig. 5.34a–c. Eating in a group is possible with all members of the team able to give individual help. **a** An occupational therapist guiding. **b** A physiotherapist assisting. **c** A psychologist guiding well too.

in the absence of oral content. A vicious circle effect can, therefore, arise in that a patient who is unable to chew never has anything which would stimulate chewing placed in his mouth, and he may well remain on a soft diet for a very long time, if not forever.

In order to interrupt and change the self-reinforcing situation, solid food must be placed and held between the patient's teeth without his being in danger of swal-

Fig. 5.35a–c. Re-educating chewing.
a Wrapping a piece of apple in gauze.
b Placing the piece between the molars.
c Keeping the piece in place for chewing

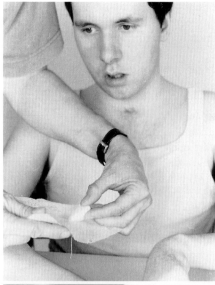

a

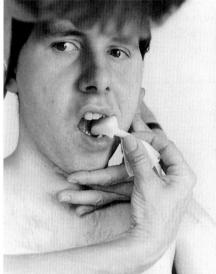

b

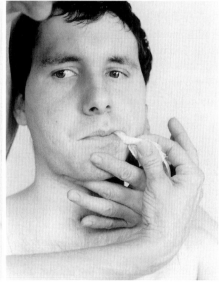

c

lowing and choking on an inadequately masticated bolus. Safe chewing practice using a variety of edibles can be carried out as follows:

The therapist wraps a piece of food with a firm, crisp consistency in a piece of gauze, the patient watching her as she does so (Fig. 5.35a). Particularly suitable for the purpose are apples, pears, dry toast, rusks or raw carrots which have been cut into cubes, because they all have the property of stimulating chewing and providing some taste in the mouth when compressed.

Using grip A and facilitating jaw opening, the therapist places the piece of wrapped food between the patient's molars on one side, keeping it carefully in place by holding the wound end of the gauze (Fig. 5.35b).

After helping the patient to close his mouth and keep his lips together, the therapist encourages him to chew the piece of food (Fig. 5.35c). If chewing is not initiated, it may help if she facilitates an up and down "chomping" motion to start the action by compressing the solid morsel. Frequently, the reason why a patient is unable to chew successfully is that he is unable to keep the piece of food in position between his back teeth. Without skilled tongue movement, after one bite the morsel is pushed back into the oral cavity, and, if there is too little tone or activity in his cheek, the piece falls down into the space on the outside of his teeth. With the therapist maintaining the position of the solid, not only is he able to perform repeated chews, but the muscles of the cheek, lips and tongue are activated by the movement within his mouth.

The therapist removes the gauze containing the chewed piece of food from the patient's mouth and, after a pause to give him time to swallow saliva which has gathered, repeats the procedure on the contralateral side with a freshly prepared bite-sized portion (Fig. 5.36).

For the Patient Who Is Too Afraid to Attempt Eating. The patient who has had an unpleasant and alarming experience through choking when trying to eat may be too afraid and refuse to try again. Other patients may be afraid simply because they feel that they are not in a position to clear their airway should something "go down the wrong way". Any patient whose teeth and gums are in a poor condition may be

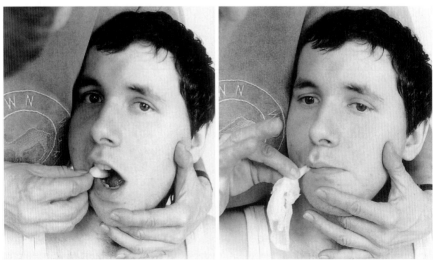

a   b

Fig. 5.36a. Placing a fresh piece of apple for chewing on the other side. **b** Lip closure with chewing initiated

unwilling to attempt eating because of the pain which is elicited when anything is placed in their mouth and touches their teeth or gums. To solve the last problem, as has already been explained in the section on oral hygiene, the gums must be treated to clear any infection or painful condition and the patient must be seen by a dentist in order to have his teeth restored to their preaccident state. Only when he is pain-free can he be expected to take food by mouth and the re-education of swallowing proceed successfully.

The patient who is afraid of swallowing presents a very different problem. He should on no account be exhorted or forced to eat, because the already tense situation will only tend to worsen. Instead, eating attempts should be temporarily suspended and intensive orofacial treatment continued but without his being required to swallow anything. Once the stress has been alleviated, it can be helpful if he is assisted to dip his own finger in yogurt, custard or ice cream and bring it to his lips or tongue. Renewed attempts with small successes in this way can have a positive effect. The same applies to letting him chew on solids wrapped in gauze which he knows he does not have to swallow. Often when he is chewing the piece of food he will automatically swallow his saliva which has mixed with the juice of the apple or pear for instance. Improvement in eating ability will usually occur in conjunction with improvement of the patient's general condition, but if an inordinate fear of swallowing persists despite significant return of sensorimotor function, then much time and patience will be necessary to help him to overcome the problem.

Drinking

Nearly all patients with dysphagia of neurogenic origin will have more difficulty in managing fluid intake than they do with eating, the reason perhaps being that fluids travel faster into the pharynx and unlike a formed bolus are more dispersed if not adequately controlled by the active tongue. They also provide less solid tactile information for the patient with diminished sensation and, unless very cold, their temperature makes them difficult to distinguish from saliva. It is not uncommon for a patient to be eating enough not to require supplementary nutrition but still need additional fluid to be administered via nasogastric or gastrostomy tube in order for the recommended requirement of 2 l per day to be met. Once the patient has begun to swallow soft foods, he can be helped to start drinking with careful facilitation.

Manual Facilitation of Drinking

With a Spoon

Controlling the patient's head position and jaw with grip A, the therapist brings a spoonful of some thick liquid such as yogurt to his mouth, which he should open only as the spoon is almost touching his lips and only just enough to allow it to pass unimpeded between them (Fig. 5.37a). Many patients tend to open their mouths excessively wide even before the fluid has left its container and by so doing can

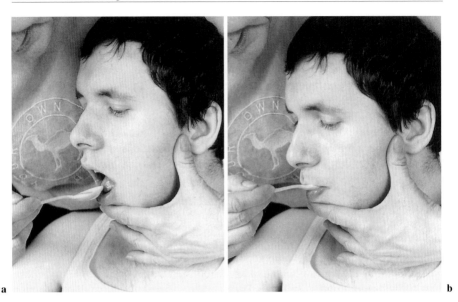

a   b

Fig. 5.37a,b. Facilitation of drinking using a spoon. **a** Preventing excessive mouth opening.
b Facilitating lip closure to remove liquid from the spoon

develop a habit which is not only unaesthetic but also disturbs the oral phase of
drinking. Subluxation of the temporomandibular joint can often be observed when
the jaw is opened through an extreme range of movement before each mouthful. If
such wide opening of the mouth is allowed to continue, the joint and its surrounding tissues can be damaged.

The therapist places the spoon on the patient's tongue, which should be as far
forward as possible, and facilitates lip closure with her index finger from below.
The liquid is taken from the spoon by the patient's lips as the therapist draws it from
his mouth (Fig. 5.37b).

From a Cup

When the patient can manage fluids that have been presented on a spoon, he should
be helped to drink from a cup so that he can progress to taking repeated swallows
instead of only one spoonful at a time. The viscosity of the liquid will have to be
adjusted accordingly to allow it to flow into the patient's mouth as he takes a sip.

With one hand again in the grip A position, the therapist lifts the cup to the
patient's mouth and rests it on his lower lip, which she has brought forward with
her index finger to receive it (Fig. 5.38a).

During normal drinking, the same movement is made after which the fluid is
drawn actively into the mouth, not running in passively with the help of gravity as
is sometimes thought. The patient is, therefore, asked to take an active sip once the
cup is in place. On no account should his head be tipped back by the helper in order
to pour the liquid into his mouth, because it would then flow too quickly to his

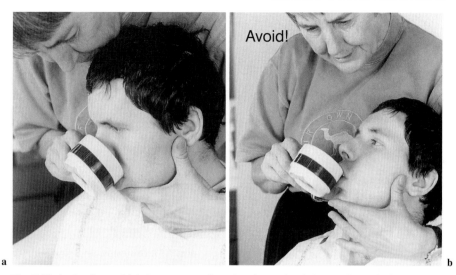

Avoid!

Fig. 5.38a,b. Starting to drink from a cup. **a** Cup placed on patient's bottom lip ready for an active sip. **b** The liquid should not be tipped into his mouth

pharynx and in all probability cause him to choke (Fig. 5.38b). Normally when drinking, the head is only tipped back when the cup or glass is nearly empty, so that to have the patient's head in an optimal position for swallowing it is advisable for the cup to be relatively full.

From a Glass

When helping the patient to drink from a glass, which as an adult he usually enjoys doing and feels is a sign of progress, the therapist uses the same facilitation as she did before (Fig. 5.39).

Using a glass when facilitating drinking has the advantage that the therapist is able to see exactly how much fluid is actually going into the patient's mouth, something that can be difficult to judge with a cup or mug. In the past it was advocated that a cardboard or plastic container be used so that the uppermost side could be partially cut away to allow such visual control. However, the result was that less fluid could be held in the beaker and the patient's neck needed to be extended in order for the contents to reach his mouth, which made the subsequent swallow difficult. In any event, a nonpliable container is easier for the therapist to handle in the situation, particularly when she starts guiding the patient's hands so that he can hold the cup and bring it to his lips himself.

If the patient has an active bite reflex, a beaker of unbreakable material should be used as a safety measure.

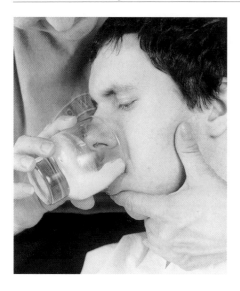

Fig. 5.39. Drinking from a glass with the lower lip brought forward into position

PROBLEM SOLVING

If the Liquid Flows Too Fast for the Patient. The patient who can still only move his tongue slowly, clumsily and with effort will not be able to control fast-flowing fluids in his mouth. In order to offer him a greater variety of choice than yogurt or custard, the therapist can thicken and so slow down the flow rate of any drink that the patient enjoys by adding one of the available thickening agents. Winstein (1983) describes the successful use of clear gelatine for that purpose in a progressive eating programme. "Adding clear gelatine thickens the liquid and thus slows its progression through the oral pharynx to the oesophagus, which allows time for the often delayed swallow".

As the patient's tongue movements and swallow improve, the amount of thickening can be reduced accordingly.

When the Patient Is Unable to Use His Tongue to Move the Fluid or Puree Back into the Pharynx for Swallowing. Some patients will have too little active tongue movement to guide the liquid back towards the pharynx, while an uncontrolled thrust of their tongue may cause others to push it forwards involuntarily. In both instances, drinking or attempting to swallow puree will be unsuccessful and the patient unable to experience the feeling of swallowing with the result that any progression towards oral intake is considerably delayed. Placing a small amount of thick liquid far back on the patient's tongue may overcome the problem mechanically and, when a swallow is elicited, lingual activity may be stimulated. The therapist uses an instrument which allows her to control both the amount and exact location of the fluid. An ordinary roasting baster, such as is normally used to moisten a roasting joint with melted fat or gravy, can be obtained in stores

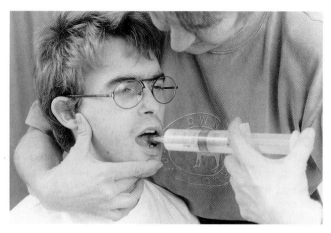

Fig. 5.40. Placing a small amount of thickened fluid well back on the patient's tongue

supplying kitchen utensils and serves the purpose extremely well. Made of a hard plastic material, the cylinder is of a comfortable size to insert in the patient's mouth. A rubber air-filled bulb at one end is manually compressed and then released to draw fluid into the cylinder. Equally efficient is a large 60 ml syringe of the disposable type used for pleural punctures.

The therapist fills the syringe with a slow-flowing liquid and, while supporting the patient's head and jaw with grip A, allows a small amount to run on to the posterior third of his tongue (Fig. 5.40).

Withdrawing the syringe, she helps the patient to close his mouth and facilitates the required movement of his tongue from below with an upward and backward movement of her middle finger. The patient can swallow more easily with his neck in slight flexion, a position which the therapist makes possible by using her arm against his occiput to tip his head forwards and tuck his chin in.

The therapist repeats the procedure several times, and usually with every successive swallow the movements become more and more active until the liquid can be presented on a spoon. The patient gains confidence through realizing that he can swallow safely and enjoys the experience of being able to drink something by mouth again.

When the Patient's Problems Are Less Obvious. Patients who are not able to eat or drink at all clearly require and will usually receive orofacial treatment, but care must be taken that many others with less obvious difficulties are not overlooked. "Adaptive neuroplasticity may mask clinical signs and symptoms of neurogenic dysphagia" (Bass 1988), and the resultant compensatory mechanisms could be the reason for the erroneous assumption that, following head injury or stroke, "most patients will be able to eat and drink normally" (Lynch and Grisogno 1991). In fact, it would be unlikely for patients with sensorimotor disturbances involving the extremities and trunk sufficient to require therapeutic intervention, not to reveal some change in feeding performance as well and hence the need for treatment. The patients themselves, are often unaware of any difficulties and, when questioned, state that they have no problems at all. Careful assessment is required, an assessment which must include both observing the patient managing a whole meal unaided in a normal eating situation with others at table with him, and questioning his relatives and the nursing staff with regard to any problems they may have noticed. Normal, mature eating and drinking involve a series of complex, sensory-cued, interdependent behaviours, so that even a comparatively slight disorder can have distressing consequences. Although the patient may appear to be getting enough to eat, the risk of his choking and possibly aspirating is increased and his choice of food limited to the extent that eating is less pleasurable for him. Weight loss is common and draws immediate attention to eating difficulties. If, however, a patient is eating large amounts of high-calorie food such as ice cream, jelly, custard, chocolates and cream slices, which are easy for him to swallow, he will inevitably put on weight. The increase in weight can be deceptive and may lead to the conclusion that he has no problems with eating.

Finally, in a comprehensive assessment it should not be overlooked that unaesthetic social eating will detract from the patient's enjoyment and family life, because the problem upsets him and those at table with him. He may even choose to eat alone.

Prolonged Postacute Tube Feeding

Patients whose swallowing difficulties persist after the acute phase will require supplementary nutritional support which may have to be continued for a considerable time. It is important that the method chosen should be effective, safe, not cause delay in the relearning of normal eating, or interfere with and impede progress in the total rehabilitation of the patient.

The procedure of choice is percutaneous endoscopic gastrostomy (PEG), which fulfils these criteria better than any other. As soon as it becomes evident that a patient will need to be tube-fed for a prolonged period, be it for his total nutritional requirements or only for fluid intake, medication and additional alimentary support, the method should be implemented without delay to avoid the problems associated with nasogastric intubation.

The conventional nasogastric tube, used almost exclusively for this purpose in the past, is no longer recommended for the nutritional support of patients with neurogenic dysphagia on a long-term basis because of its undesirable side effects:

- The position of the tube makes swallowing even more difficult for the patient and thus interferes with the re-education of eating. Any irritation of the nasopharyngeal area adds still further to the problem (Nehen 1988; Schlee et al. 1987).

- The tube does not permit nasopharyngeal closure, and the constant pressure it exerts on the soft palate over a long period would appear to have an adverse effect on later return of efficient functional activity. When patients continue to have significant problems with soft palate closure despite remarkable return of function in other related spheres, it could well be that localized peripheral damage rather than the original central lesion is responsible.
- The nasogastric tube is frequently pulled out by the confused patient, and as a result he is subjected to having his hands tied to the bed. He pulls desperately against the restraining bandages which increases his restlessness, causes skin abrasions and can impede circulation. Furthermore, if active movements of his hands are restricted, the patient will be deprived of valuable sensory input. The tube is also easily dislodged when the staff are moving the patient and, in both cases, the frequent reinsertions can lead to mucosal irritation (Winstein 1983).
- Cosmetically, the presence of the tube stuck to the patient's face with pieces of adhesive plaster is a disaster and does little to help restore his self-image, particularly when he is able to leave the confines of his room, either in a wheelchair or even on foot.

The Merits of PEG

Personal observations of many patients in the clinical setting and the positive experiences of several authors reveal that PEG has distinct advantages over other means of administering nutritional support. However, a recent review, quoted by Moran et al. (1992) suggests "that PEG is an underused technique", a finding borne out by the large number of neurologically disabled patients still seen today with nasogastric tubes despite the following positive statements:

"Percutaneous endoscopic gastrostomy is a safe and effective method for long-term enteral feeding avoiding complications of surgical gastrostomy and side effects of nasoenteral tubes (Burghart et al. 1989)"

"PEG enables adequate enteral nutrition of patients with neurological impairment. The advantages of PEG over parenteral nutrition are fewer complications, lower costs and above all, its superiority in meeting physiological requirements (Peschl et al. 1988)"

"Percutaneous endoscopic gastrostomy should be performed in all patients referred for a gastrostomy and should be considered in all patients requiring long-term tube feeding"

"Many patients currently maintained or supplemented by nasogastric tube feeding, often in the community, would benefit from this relatively simple procedure. Long-term follow-up confirms the safety and efficacy of the technique (Moran and Frost 1992)"

Specific Advantages

The first obvious advantage is that the gastrostomy tube is discreetly tucked away beneath the patient's clothes and not hanging in front of his face all the time like the nasogastric tube, which immediately makes him look better and feel more normal (Fig. 5.41).

With the tube not always dangling within his field of vision, he is far less likely to pull at it and dislodge it. Perhaps because the abdominal area is not as sensitive as the richly innervated face, the patient is less aware of the small tube beneath its simple gauze dressing, and it is therefore extremely rare for a patient to pull out the gastrostomy tube. His hands, therefore, do not have to be tied down as is often the case with a nasal tube. Larson et al. (1987), in a study which included 235 patients with neurological involvement, found that using an abdominal binder decreased the incidence of the tube being dislodged accidentally as it was in six of their cases, but such measures are seldom necessary. Tube dislodgement, should it occur, can in any event be easily remedied "The gastrostomy catheter can be conveniently replaced if accidentally dislodged" (Foutch et al. 1986).

PEG is a relatively simple procedure with very few insertion complications (Moran et al. 1990; Ponsky and Gauderer 1989) and can be performed under local anaesthesia, thus avoiding the risks of a general anaesthetic. In the Larson study, in fact, 23 out of the 314 patients were out-patients when the procedure was carried

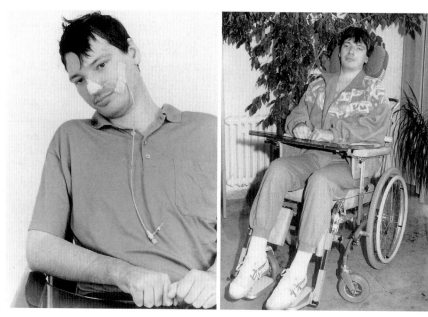

Fig. 5.41a. Nasogastric tube with adhesive plaster fixation looks unsightly. **b** The same patient with gastrostomy tube invisible beneath clothes

out. Only a very short operating time is required, usually within 15–30 min according to Foutch et al. (1986) and less than 10 min according to Larson et al. (1987).

Kirby et al. (1986), reporting on 51 successfully performed PEGs, states that "there were no deaths directly related to the procedure" and that "no patient required laparotomy or developed fistulae from the procedure." Burghart et al. (1989) and Foutch et al. (1986) also report that no procedure-related deaths occurred. Any peritubal or wound infections were successfully treated with antibiotics or avoided by their use prophylactically.

An advantage of PEG which must be stressed is that it appears to enable patients to learn to swallow again and be able to manage without supplementary feeding sooner than those being fed via nasogastric tube. Possibly the fact that there is not a foreign body in the nasopharynx to irritate the mucosa or hamper elevation of the soft palate facilitates the whole process. Certainly without the anaesthetic effect caused by accommodation to the pressure of the tube over a long period, sensory feedback will be less disturbed. With reference to clinical outcome following PEG, Moran and Frost (1992) write, "patient tolerance and carer satisfaction have been excellent and early results suggest that recovery of speech and swallowing in acute neurological disorders may be enhanced." It is interesting to note that the authors add, "we were surprised with the number who recovered allowing tube removal" when 11 of their patients resumed swallowing at a mean of 122 days (range 20–390 days) post insertion. Winstein (1983), although stating that a "G tube [gastrostomy tube] would not usually be indicated within the first five months after injury" admits in contrast that her clinical experience has been that "patients with persistent neurogenic dysphagia often improve more quickly after a gastrostomy and removal of the NG [nasogastric] tube".

Because the patient can receive nutrition through the PEG tube while he is resting (Fig. 5.42), more time is available for providing the different forms of therapy which he so urgently needs. The gastrostomy tube can be left in place without jeopardy for as long as is necessary, even for years, should the patient still require additional nutritional support, perhaps solely to ensure an adequate fluid intake. A patient may in fact be able to eat and drink enough for his nutritional requirements, but only with so much time and effort required that the strain placed on him and those caring for him can become unacceptable. Because it is so safe, even on a long-term basis, PEG provides a preferable alternative which relieves stress and leaves time not only for continued therapy but also for enjoyment. The patient can eat and drink then for pleasure, and let the tube take care of the rest of his daily intake requirements.

And lastly, when the patient is able to eat and drink again, the gastrostomy tube can be easily removed and the stoma closes spontaneously, usually within 48 h and without the need for surgical intervention.

With so many advantages to offer, it is understandable that Larson and co-authors "concluded that endoscopically placed gastrostomy is the procedure of choice to achieve long-term enteral nutrition in patients who cannot swallow but have an intact gut". These criteria would apply to patients with traumatic brain injury almost without exception.

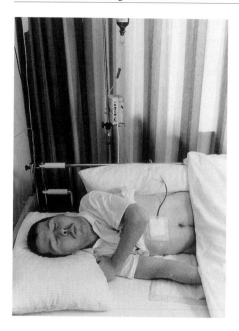

Fig. 5.42. Receiving nutrition while asleep saves treatment time

Explaining PEG to Staff and Relatives

All concerned with the patient should be well-informed about PEG, particularly about placement, functioning and removal, so that any worries or fears which they may have can be allayed. Especially his family need to understand the whole procedure because it will be someone close to him who will be required to sign consent. Certain unfortunate misconceptions with regard to PEG exist and, if the patient's relatives have heard these, they will naturally be unwilling to take responsibility for something that could be detrimental for him. Another important aspect is that if they have had adequate explanation from the beginning and are encouraged to become familiar with the routine tube feeding, they will feel confident enough for the patient to be able to spend periods at home far sooner, despite his not being able to take food by mouth.

Easily understandable, illustrated information sheets should be available to familiarize carers with details of PEG, and placed so that they can be studied at leisure before the event. Kirby et al. (1986) also report positive results after developing a special information sheet for nursing and house staff whom they felt "did not know enough about PEGs (or even standard gastrostomies)". It can also be helpful if the tube itself is displayed, handled and attention drawn to its small size and unthreatening appearance (Fig. 5.43).

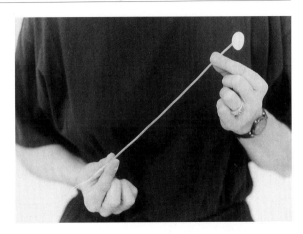

Fig. 5.43. The small tube can be held comfortably in position after insertion

Placement of the Gastrostomy Tube

The patient lies supine and is awake. Topical anaesthetic spray in the back of the mouth and the throat makes the passing of the gastroscope less uncomfortable and suppresses the gag reflex if one is present. For a patient who is very restless and uncontrolled, intravenous sedation can be administered as a premedication.

The outside of the abdominal wall is carefully disinfected and, once the inside of the stomach has been reached by endoscopy and is clearly visible, a local anaesthetic is injected into the area through which the gastrostomy tube will be passed via a small incision. (Fig. 5.44a). Prior to anaesthetising the abdominal wall, the assistant locates the optimal site by pressing his fingers over the anatomical position of the stomach, guided by feedback from the doctor manipulating the gastroscope and the image it provides on the monitor screen. (Fig. 5.44b,c). A percutaneous cannula is then advanced into the stomach through the anaesthetized abdominal wall at the chosen location. A thread is introduced through the cannula so that one end can be grasped with an endoscopic snare or biopsy forceps and pulled out of the patient's mouth together with the endoscope, while the other end remains protruding from the abdominal wall. The thread is then tied to the tapered end of the gastrostomy tube and, by traction being applied to its abdominal end, the tube is pulled down the upper digestive tract into the stomach and out through the abdominal wall until its flange is seated against the gastric mucosa and so held in place. A face plate is applied at the exit site to maintain the position of the tube from the outside (Fig. 5.45a). A small gauze dressing covers the site and is held in place with a nonirritating, adhesive plaster (Fig. 5.45b).

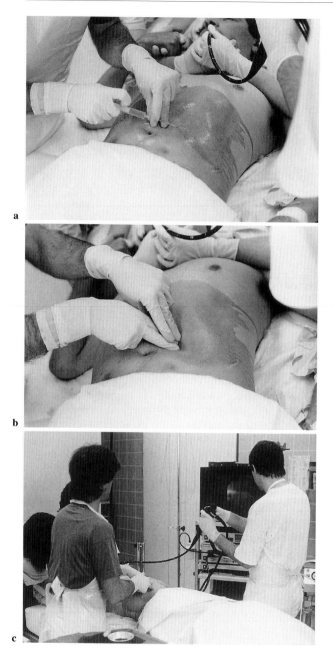

Fig. 5.44a–c. Placing the gastrostomy tube. **a** Only a local anaesthetic is required. **b** Assistant first locates the exact site. **c** Viewing the inside wall of the stomach with a gastroscope to find the optimal position.

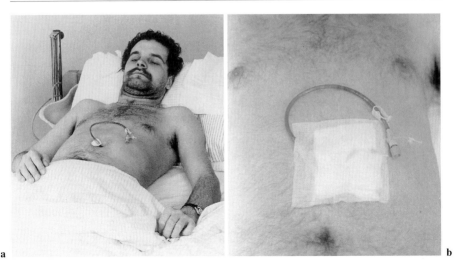

a   b

Fig. 5.45a. Patient comfortable immediately after tube placement. **b** A small dressing covers the site

Removal of the Tube

Once the patient has regained the ability to eat and drink again, and can do so in a reasonable time, the tube is removed, once again without the need for anaesthesia.

The patient lies supine, and the endoscope is passed into his stomach so that the end of the gastrostomy tube can be grasped with the forceps under endoscopic control (Fig. 5.46a). The tube is withdrawn together with the endoscope (Fig. 5.46b,c) and a dressing applied to the stoma, although very little seepage occurs, even directly following tube removal.

Within a few days the stoma has usually healed completely, and the dressing is no longer required (Fig. 5.47). During the period when supplementary feeding by means of the gastrostomy tube is required, it is possible for the patient to participate fully in an active and comprehensive rehabilitation programme, enabling him to make progress in many different areas.

Learning to Speak Again

Many of the activities already described will help to improve the tongue and facial movements required for articulating, and the same applies to regaining more normal eating patterns. Particularly the tongue and soft palate will have to move far more quickly than they do during swallowing, although basically the movements

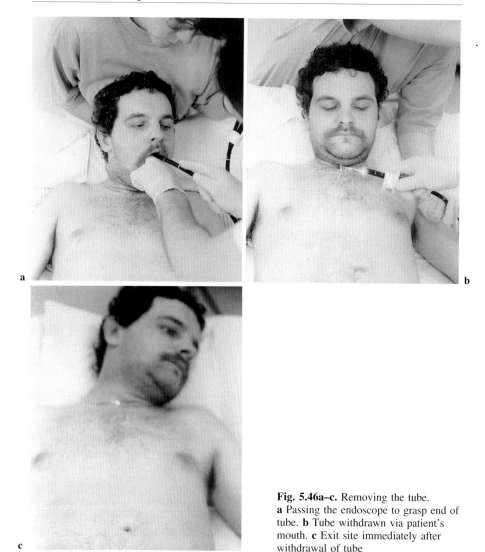

a

b

c

Fig. 5.46a–c. Removing the tube.
a Passing the endoscope to grasp end of
tube. **b** Tube withdrawn via patient's
mouth. **c** Exit site immediately after
withdrawal of tube

for both are similar. An adequate volume of air and the ability to control its flow are
essential for producing voice and making speech sounds.

It is of prime importance for the patient to be able to communicate with others
again, because only then can he make his wishes known and enable others to know
what he is thinking. If his voice is too soft or if he cannot speak clearly, it can be
most frustrating for him because he will constantly have to repeat what he is saying, as the listener will not be able to understand him and will often misunderstand
what he has said. For those communicating with the patient, it can be very frus-

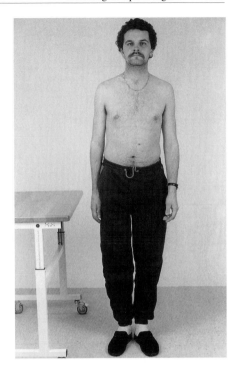

Fig. 5.47. Four days after removal of gastrostomy tube, the dressing is no longer required, and the patient's progress has not been delayed by 3-month period of intubation

trating, too, as they cannot grasp what he is trying to say. In addition to the measures described in the previous chapters, specific activities aimed at improving each patient's ability to produce voice, make speech sounds and enhance the quality of both should also be included in the treatment. Even the aphasic patient will benefit from the activities, because producing sounds will make his eating safer through activating his vocal cords, and his respiratory function will also improve. The fact that the patient can make sounds when other people are talking to him is also a great help towards his being integrated in the group.

Mobilizing the Larynx

It is difficult for the patient to produce sounds if the larynx is not free to move, either through tension in the muscles which surround it or because his neck is constantly in an abnormal, stiff position, e.g. when sitting the patient's neck is extended with his chin poked forwards. The larynx is also required to move swiftly up and down during swallowing to provide a safety mechanism to protect the airway so that the mobilization can also be performed before eating is attempted. The posture of the whole body should be corrected and sufficient support

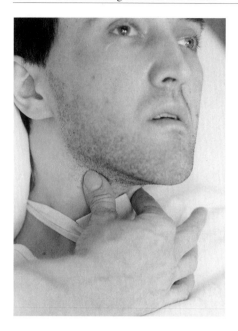

Fig. 5.48. Mobilizing the larynx directly with head in corrected position

given before the therapist moves the larynx itself. It may be necessary at first for the patient to be totally supported in a half-lying position in bed so that he does not have to hold his head against gravity.

Standing beside the patient the therapist holds the patients larynx gently between her finger(s) and thumb, taking care not to exert any pressure which can be very uncomfortable (Fig. 5.48). She moves the larynx from one side to the other and diagonally upwards and downwards, increasing the range and speed of movement as she feels the resistance lessening.

Assisting Deep Expiration

Right from the start, when the patient is still in intensive care, the therapist mobilizes his ribcage, using her hands to simulate the movement which occurs during expiration.

With the patient in side lying, the therapist stands behind him and places her hands over his ribs, one hand on top of the other (Fig. 5.49). She waits until the patient has inspired naturally or with the assistance of the respirator before pressing firmly downwards and medially towards his umbilicus during the expiratory phase, moving the ribs through their full range of motion in that direction. Not only is expiration increased through the facilitation, but the flexibility of the ribs retained passively. When the patient is able to cooperate, he can be asked to lengthen the outward breath with the help of the therapist, which he will need to do in order to

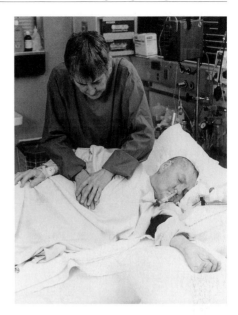

Fig. 5.49. The therapist maintains the expiratory excursion of an unconscious patient's ribcage

speak. During normal quiet breathing, inspiration and expiration are of almost equal length, but during normal speaking the latter is about ten times longer and the inspiratory phase shortened to allow a quick intake of air.

Later, when the patient is sitting or standing during treatment, the therapist can assist expiration with overpressure, placing one hand on either side of his chest wall and pressing downwards and inwards as he breathes out.

Facilitating Phonation

Many patients will require help to produce vocal sounds at first, and even if they are not yet able to speak will be delighted to hear their own voice again. Producing a sound entails the vocal cords approximating actively, an activity which also serves to protect the airway during eating and is, therefore, most important.

With the patient seated in a good position with his arms supported on a table in front of him, the therapist places her hands over his sternum and assists expiration by pressing his chest wall firmly downwards. The patient tries to make a sound, but if he tries too hard he may not succeed due to increased muscle tone (Fig. 5.50a). Moving one of her hands to a modified grip B position, the therapist helps him to open his mouth at exactly the right moment, just as he starts to breathe out, while at the same time keeping his tongue forwards with her middle finger beneath his chin (Fig. 5.50b). Very often, immediately after the patient has produced a tone with the therapist's hand timing the movement of his mouth he will be able to do so again when both her hands are being used to increase expiration as they did before

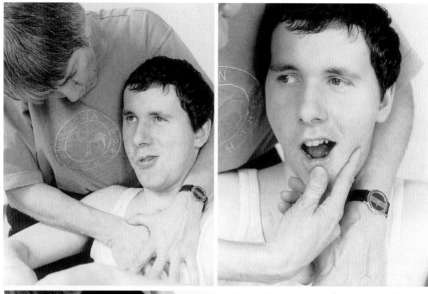

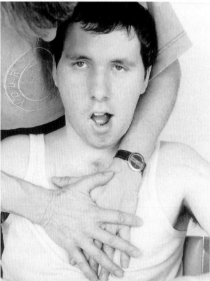

Fig. 5.50a–c. Initiating voice production. **a** Patient using too much effort is unable to make a sound. **b** Therapist facilitates mouth opening and expiration. **c** Voice produced with assisted breathing afterwards

(Fig. 5.50c). The same facilitation can also be used with the patient who requires more support in a half-lying position in bed or on a plinth (see Fig. 5.4b).

The patient should be encouraged to produce sounds frequently during the day, but only with sufficient help to ensure that he does so in the normal way while breathing out. If the patient phonates on inspiration, as many with severe problems will tend to do, for example when laughing or crying, a habit can develop that is hard to break and which is detrimental to his learning to speak again. The tendency should be actively discouraged by all concerned with the patient, and not deliberately provoked as can happen inadvertently if the danger is not appreciated. A member of staff may say or do something that makes the patient laugh and produce a tone as he does so, while breathing in. The staff are so pleased to hear the patient uttering a sound after his long silence that the phrase or action is repeated often to elicit the response again, and the habit is reinforced. Instead, as soon as the therapist or someone else in his vicinity hears the patient begin to phonate in this way, they should change the situation, placing their hands on his chest wall to assist expiration and so help him to produce the sound as he breathes out.

Facilitating Different Vowel Sounds

Once the patient can produce a sound and maintain it for a few seconds, the therapist asks him to try to form the different vowels. Not only will the muscles of his lips and cheeks be activated automatically as the vowel changes, but he will also be learning to sustain a longer sound. Through loss of the necessary sensory information, the patient often has difficulty in grading the movements of his jaw, always opening his mouth very wide when he says "ah" for example, when he laughs or when he takes a mouthful of food. As has been explained in Chap. 1, he moves the joints and muscles into extreme range to gain some information as to their position, with the motion frequently ending only when a total, mechanical resistance is encountered. By forming the different vowel sounds, he receives acoustic feedback which can enable him to experience a greater variety of jaw positions. Although the sound "ah" may be easier for him at first, it is one which encourages the wide-open mouth together with neck extension. If he needs to start with "ah" in order to produce a voice at all, then after commencing he can change to "ooh", for example, which will bring his lips forward and his jaw into a more closed position.

The therapist sits in front of the patient so that he can watch the shape of her mouth and uses grip B to facilitate his jaw and lips. When the patient is saying a long "aah" she helps him to limit the movement of his jaw with her middle finger and thumb (Fig. 5.51a).

To facilitate the "ooh" the therapist changes the position of her thumb and index finger so that she can use them to draw his lips forward from both sides while at the same time lifting his jaw with her middle finger from below to close his mouth slightly for the correct aperture (Fig. 5.51b).

When the patient attempts the sound "ee", the therapist's thumb on one side and her index finger on the other help him to draw his lips outwards, while at the same time her middle finger elevates the lower mandible until his teeth are almost together (Fig. 5.51c).

As the patient's ability improves, the therapist can alter the order in which the vowel sounds are produced, starting with different ones and changing the consecutive sequences. It is also important for the patient to learn to change the pitch of his voice because it will give it variety and melody once he is able to speak

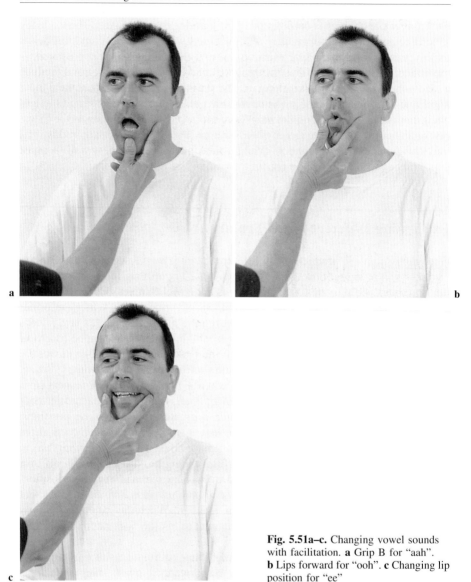

Fig. 5.51a–c. Changing vowel sounds with facilitation. **a** Grip B for "aah". **b** Lips forward for "ooh". **c** Changing lip position for "ee"

again, avoiding the typical monotone which otherwise sounds abnormal. Furthermore, when changing pitch, the larynx moves up or down accordingly and practising high and low sounds will also help to reduce the risk of choking during eating and drinking, because the elevated larynx is part of the normal safety mechanism to protect the airway. It is easier for the patient if there is a big difference in pitch at first and also if he uses sounds which facilitate pitch for example, using the vowel "ee" can make a high note easier to attain and "ooh" a low one.

Activating the Soft Palate

Either due to the neurological lesion itself or as a result of long-term nasogastric intubation, the soft palate often fails to function adequately and causes difficulties with both eating and speaking. If the nasopharyngeal closure is incomplete or absent, then fluids or particles of food may be pushed up into the nasal cavity when the patient swallows. His voice is very much affected by the loss of the quick, selective activity required of the soft palate during normal speaking. His voice will have an unattractive nasal quality or sound strange as air escapes through the nose, and both problems can make the patient's speech difficult to understand.

Even before the patient is able to speak, activity in the soft palate should be stimulated both actively and mechanically, and such stimulation should be continued later to improve the quality of his regained voice.

To stimulate activity mechanically, the therapist can use ice in direct contact with the soft palate, provided that the patient does not have a pronounced bite reflex and is able to open his mouth voluntarily. A wet cotton bud is placed in the freezer some hours before the treatment and taken out again only just before it is required, because the ice melts very quickly.

With the patient's mouth well-illuminated, the therapist holds his tongue down with a spatula to allow her to see the soft palate clearly and brings the iced cotton bud into position. It may be possible for the therapist to stand beside the patient and use her chest and shoulder to keep his head in the correct position, with her hands free to hold both the spatula and the cotton bud (Fig. 5.52a). If, however, the patient cannot hold his head in position actively himself, it is probably easier for him to be in a well-supported half-lying position to enable the therapist to look into his mouth from the front.

With the patient's head supported in bed or held actively the therapist sits in front of him and stimulates his soft palate with the iced tip of the cotton bud (Fig. 5.52b). She can apply the stimulation either to the centre of the palate immediately above the uvula or laterally to the arch on one or other side, in each case pressing the bud quickly and firmly against the anterior aspect. Another possibility is to press upwards and outwards along the length of the arch from below which has the additional effect of stretching the elevators of the palate. Whichever location is the most effective will be determined by the result, so that it is important for the therapist to have some means of comparing activity before and after the stimulus. She chooses a sound, a word or combination of words which demonstrate the problem caused by the malfunctioning soft palate clearly and then after applying the ice asks the patient to repeat the task. Effectiveness can also be evaluated by comparing the patient's subsequent swallows, as suggested by Logemann (1986), after applying thermal stimulation with a laryngeal mirror. Although the ice makes it more tolerable for the patient, direct stimulation of the soft palate can be quite uncomfortable and should, therefore, only be used if it is effective and improves a specific function.

Immediately following mechanical stimulation, activities which elevate the soft palate and affect nasopharyngeal closure are practised such as the patient being

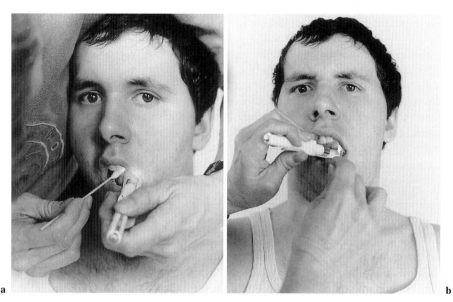

Fig. 5.52a,b. Stimulating the soft palate with an iced cotton bud. **a** With patient's head supported by therapist's chest and shoulder. **b** Illuminating the mouth from in front while touching the palate with the iced cotton bud

asked to make explosive oral sounds with the therapist assisting quick expiration. A simple yet effective exercise, which the patient usually enjoys doing and will practise on his own as well, is to blow air into both cheeks and hold it there. The therapist may need to help the patient to hold his lips together at first and, once he succeeds, she can press her fingers against the outside of his cheeks while he tries to prevent any air from escaping, either through his nose or from between his compressed lips (Fig. 5.53a).

Progressing further, the patient transfers all the air into one of his cheeks which requires the cheek and lip muscles on the contralateral side to work actively as well as those of the soft palate (Fig. 5.53b). The patient moves the air into the other cheek, and continues to transfer it from one side to the other at increasing speed. The faster he changes the sides, the more difficult it becomes to maintain complete nasopharyngeal closure.

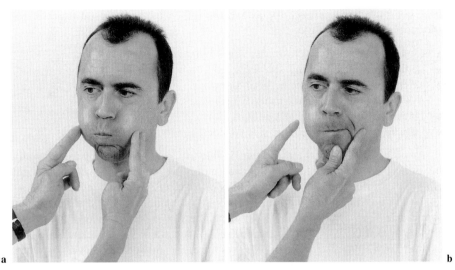

Fig. 5.53a,b. Active elevation of the soft palate. **a** Blowing air into both cheeks and keeping it there. **b** Transferring air from one cheek to the other

Providing an Alternative Means of Communicating

From the start, every effort must be made to find a way by which the patient can communicate with those caring for him and later those with whom he mixes socially. As soon as any signs are observed which indicate that he is regaining consciousness, the staff and his relatives should begin trying out different possibilities and, as the patient's ability progresses, more comprehensive and satisfying means should be sought. Because regaining the ability to speak may take a considerable time for some patients, and others may have on-going difficulties even after their rehabilitation, the best solution should be found for each patient. Modern technology is developing so rapidly that more sophisticated, lightweight, alternative communication devices are constantly being designed and becoming available.

Movements to Signal "Yes" and "No"

In the beginning, when the patient is still very helpless, the simplest form of communication is for him to move some part of his body to answer questions which are put to him in such a way that they only require an affirmative or negative response, one movement signalling "yes" and another "no". The part that he is best able to move reliably is chosen, and a system evolved. Some common examples which have been used successfully are as follows (given in the list as affirmative response/negative response):

- Closing the eyes once/closing the eyes twice.
- Looking upwards/looking sideways.
- Chin up as if to nod/turning head sideways.
- A squeeze with the better hand/two squeezes.
- Thumb or finger up/thumb or finger down.
- Foot up and down/foot from side to side.

Any other movement that the patient is able to execute more easily can naturally be used in a similar way. The helper must only be sure that the question is put correctly and does not offer alternatives. For example, if the patient appears restless and is asked, "Would you like to turn on to your side or would you rather sit up for a while?" he will be unable to say which he would prefer. Instead, the person helping him asks, "Are you uncomfortable?" and waits for his response before asking, "Would you like to lie on your side?". If the answer indicates no or seems doubtful, then the patient can be offered an alternative, "Would you prefer to sit up for a while?"

Using an Alphabet Board

In order to spell out words, the patient has to be able to move his eyes or one of his hands actively in order to indicate the relevant letters on the board. If he can move his head but not his hands, it may be possible for him to hold the pointer in his mouth. A pointing board comprised of organized lists of frequently used words can also be constructed (Horner 1984). Pictures illustrating everyday requirements can be used instead of letters to speed up the communication, and also for those patients who are unable to spell because of a concomitant aphasia, but the alphabet board allows the patient to communicate a wider range of ideas.

The advantage of a board is that it is light, easily transportable, and virtually cost-free, but it is also slow and can be tedious for both the patient and the person with whom he is communicating.

The ZYGO augmentative communication system (ZYGO Industries, Inc., Portland, Oregon; Horner 1984) has a 16-item display that can be readily individualized, either with words or pictures. A patient with very little active movement possibility can use it because the scanning light is stopped at the desired item by means of a remote control switch which can be adapted to suit his needs.

Complex Computer-Based Communication Augmentation Systems

Intermediate stage systems will enable the patient to type sentences on a keyboard of some description and the typewritten material will either appear on a monitor or be printed on paper. All such systems are, of course, dependent upon the patient having the necessary language ability as well as being able to move a limb in a sufficiently controlled way. The Canon Communicator is one of the best known, and its small, compact size is a great advantage because it fits easily onto a wheelchair table or can be attached to the arm of the chair or even held on the patient's lap. Another advantage is that the message is printed on a strip of paper which can be kept until required or maintained for assessment purposes. For patients who have difficulty with the fine coordination required for the small keyboard, an larger overlay is available. Any electric typewriter can be used for the patient to type out thoughts and messages, using an appliance if he cannot use his fingers or a finger selectively. One severely disabled patient was able to type with a plastic extension fitted to her right foot, which was the only part she could move selectively. Using a computer has the advantage that what the patient has typed he can store away, avoiding the embarrassment of someone reading something that was not intended for their eyes.

If very little movement is possible for the patient, with time and effort almost anything becomes possible including "discrete eye position recording for alternative communication" (ten Kate et al. 1985), an "eye operated keyboard" (Ignazzi and Ramsden 1984) or an "eye gaze communicator" which enables the user to achieve faster communication speeds, incorporating a multipage dictionary derived from word frequency lists which eliminates the need to choose each letter separately (Downing 1985). Communication systems can even be adapted for patients with severe visual impairment in addition to their sensorimotor handicaps (Beukelmann et al. 1984).

Unfortunately, however, most systems when adapted for severely disabled patients have a common disadvantage which can lead to frustration and possibly resignation in some cases. Normally, most people can converse at speeds of about 150 words per minute, but when using a communication aid many patients will often only be able to manage 3–5 words per minute,depending upon their level of purposeful, controlled movement and whether a scanning, encoding or direct selection method is employed (Downing 1985). For many, the immense concentration and effort required for a short message may well make using the computer a theoretical possibility rather than a practical reality.

Using a Voice Output Communication Aid (VOCA)

What the patient really longs for is to be able to speak again, using his voice, and not having someone peering over his shoulder trying to read what he is spelling out or waiting patiently while he slowly types a message. He wants to be able to speak "in a world where speech is an integral part of life" (Creech 1980). Creech, using a Phonic Mirror 120 Handi-Voice because he himself is unable to speak without an aid, goes on to explain, "speech is the most important human faculty. We are social beings. Our psychological development and well-being is dependent upon interaction with others — without communication there is no interaction with others. When there is little or no interaction with others, it has a detrimental effect upon a persons psychological development and sociological development." He confirms what many other patients have experienced, the prevalence of the idea that if a person cannot speak, there must be something wrong with his mind as well, that he is in fact mentally retarded. Like the other patients he wants to be treated as the adult that he is.

Perhaps the biggest advance in alternative communication has been the development of the artificial voice systems activated by touch-sensitive panels, all of which share the special feature that messages can be conveyed by way of a synthesized (electronic) voice or be stored for later use. Being able to actually "talk" to someone makes a world of difference to the patient. Such battery-operated devices are now available in sizes which make it possible for them to be constantly with the patient in his wheelchair (Fig. 5.54). The modus operandi can be adapted so that even the most severely paralyzed can manage to operate the device as long as he is able to move some part of his body voluntarily, learn the complex system and, of course, can spell.

Using whichever system most suits him, the patient should be encouraged by all to communicate as much as possible because it is his only possibility for doing so until such time as he has regained his voice. Intensive therapy must, however, be continued to give him the chance of learning to speak again. On no account should it ever be thought that by giving the patient a communication aid return of speech will be delayed or even prevented or that he will no longer be motivated to learn to speak, erroneous ideas that unfortunately continue to prevail in certain groups. In fact, quite the opposite is true. Speaking is one of the ways in which human beings communicate with one another, a part of the whole complex process which makes communication and acquiring the ability to communicate possible. Because it is not a separate entity, a skill learned in isolation, stimulating, practising and improving any part of that whole will help to improve the other parts as well, just as reading and listening help someone who is trying to learn to speak a foreign language.

Conclusion

For every human being, the ability to communicate with others is of the utmost importance not only for survival but in order to share with others and be a part of the group. Eating and drinking play a significant role in enjoying life and being together with others and even more so for the patient who is unable to participate in other pleasurable pastimes such as sport, dancing, or gardening, to name but a few.

Fig. 5.54a,b. An artificial voice system. **a** Battery-operated device small enough for wheelchair use. **b** Severely paralyzed patient uses touch sensitive panel to "talk" or store messages for later use

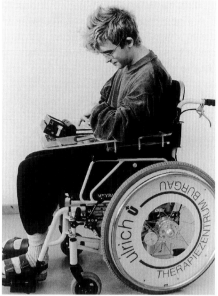

a

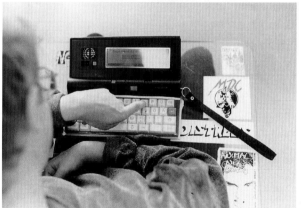

b

For these reasons alone, it becomes obvious that orofacial treatment is an essential part of any rehabilitation programme and cannot be neglected because of lack of time or knowledge, no more than can the retraining of walking or the activities of daily living which are automatically given such a high priority in every form of treatment or evaluation.

In addition to the role the face and mouth play in the enhancement of life quality, however, there is another important reason for intensive treatment for both areas. Their rich innervation provides an ideal area for stimulation which can affect the whole patient and through the input influence his general condition considerably.

The information in Chap. 5 is based on lectures and demonstrations given by Kay Coombes during courses on the rehabilitation of the face and oral tract held in the Post-graduate Study Centre Hermitage, Bad Ragaz (1977–1990). Additional reading will be found in Coombes' own book which is nearing completion (Coombes 1995).

6 Overcoming Limitation of Movement, Contracture and Deformity

To all intents and purposes, the development of contractures in muscles and joints can be prevented if the therapeutic procedures and activities that have been described in the previous chapters are carried out diligently right from the start. Adverse mechanical tension in the nervous system can also be minimized and that which has arisen as a result of the initial lesion can be mobilized to allow full range of movement. The devastating physical and psychological consequences of contractures make their avoidance imperative. Prevention becomes particularly important because experience has shown that although gross muscle and joint contractures can be overcome, some permanent disabilities may remain such as in the fine motor function of the hand and fingers.

Much has been published with regard to predicting outcome for patients following traumatic brain injury (Lewin and Roberts 1979; Jennet et al. 1979, 1981; Teasdale et al. 1979) but seldom, if ever, has any mention been made that the development of contractures could be a significant factor in preventing the attainment of more positive results. Such painful and significant limitation of movement must surely influence the individual patient's potential adversely and not merely the factors "chance", "the extent and location of the lesion" or "destiny", as has been suggested. There would be no way in which a patient in a condition similar to that of T.B. (see Fig. 2.40a) or E.S. (see Fig. 4.25a) could show improvement in his or her functional ability and thus attain a higher score on any type of assessment chart. Such a patient would be virtually "locked in" by the contractures and the ensuing vicious circle of pain, depression, failure and eventual resignation would render him incapable of benefiting from any spontaneous recovery of sensorimotor activity or intellectual ability which may take place. Cope and Hall (1982) emphasize the enormity of the problem by citing a review of 127 patients with head injuries whose average length of coma was 3 weeks and whose entry into rehabilitation had been delayed. On admission to a rehabilitation centre, examination of these patients reveals 30 "frozen shoulders" and 200 other major joint deformities.

The development of contractures should never be accepted as inevitable because they are not a symptom of the brain damage itself but of its management. Whenever extensive correction of contractures is necessary in any centre, the therapeutic approach must be urgently revised. Prevention of contractures by appropriate treatment and handling is equally important in acute care hospitals, because for many patients there will be long delays before admittance to specialised rehabilitation centres, either due to the severity of the lesion or to the limited number of available places. It is easier to prevent contractures, or overcome those which already exist, if the reasons for their development are understood.

Reasons for the Development of Contractures

Sitting or Lying in Stereotyped Positions. If the patient always lies or sits in one stereotyped position, muscles shorten adaptively as a result. He may be pulled into the position by spasticity, for example with his elbows constantly flexed, or he may hold his limbs actively in a certain position and resist any attempts to adjust his posture. If he is unable to move actively at all, he remains in the position in which he is left lying or sitting by the staff, and, unless the position is changed regularly, muscle shortening will likewise occur.

Disturbed or Confusing Sensation. The patient with disturbed or confusing sensation will tend to search for more reliable information in some other way, one of which is to hold his limbs in extreme positions. When the joints are at the end of their mechanical range, no further movement is possible and an absolute resistance is encountered. The limbs may be pulled into total flexion, total extension or a combination of the two where some joints are fully extended while others are flexed.

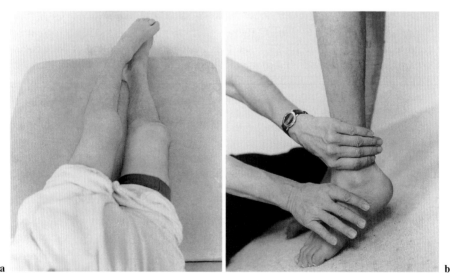

a   b

Fig. 6.1a,b. The classical pattern of extensor spasticity. **a** Legs extended and adducted with plantarflexion of feet. **b** Shortened Achilles tendon

The patient whose legs extend and adduct at both hips and knees with the feet in plantarflexion (Fig. 6.1a) fits the classical pattern of extensor spasticity as described by B. Bobath (1968, 1971, 1978) and K. Bobath (1966). Any resultant shortening of the Achilles tendon makes standing on a plantigrade foot impossible before corrective measures have been carried out (Fig. 6.1b). The stereotyped nature of the spastic patterns both in the upper and lower limbs was stressed to the extent that Karel Bobath (1988) claimed that, "if the therapist can imitate the exact posture and movement synergy of her patient then it is spasticity because it is always the same. If she cannot copy the position of his arm or leg and says that it varies, then it cannot be spasticity."

It is, therefore, possible, that when variations in posture or combinations of extreme positions are seen in the limbs of individual patients, they are caused not by spasticity as such, but by the patient's efforts to obtain additional information. More intense information is provided by increased tension in muscles, joints forced into end of range positions or by touching one part of the body with another. For example, a patient may hold his legs in a flexed position, but with his hips adducted and his feet plantarflexed (Fig. 6.2). Another patient may have his hips and knees extended but his feet dorsiflexed and supinated so that they touch each other (Fig. 6.3). In the case of the hands, it may be observed that some fingers remain extended while the others are strongly flexed.

What causes the variation of flexion and extension between patients or even the difference between the positions of the same patient's limbs is not clear, nor is it fully understood why some patients lift their hands or feet off any supporting surface while others press down hard against the bed, the floor or a table. Perhaps different types and degrees of tactile/kinaesthetic disturbance are responsible, or possibly some other seemingly insignificant factor or occurrence leads to the predominance of one position rather than another.

A normal baby, if left lying on the floor on its own, without any contact to other persons or objects in its vicinity will demonstrate a similar phenomenon by either extending its limbs strongly or flexing them tightly as it cries in distress

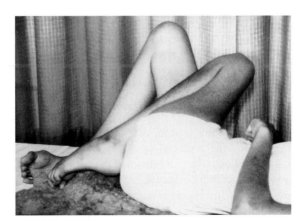

Fig. 6.2. Legs in flexion but with hips adducted and feet plantarflexed

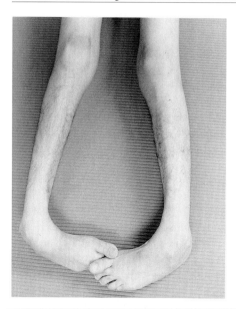

Fig. 6.3. Feet dorsiflexed and supinated despite extended, inwardly rotated legs

(Fig. 6.4a,b). The moment it has close contact to its father or mother again and reaches out for an interesting object, the extreme positions disappear and are replaced by normal postures and movement (Fig. 6.4c,d).

Pronounced Adverse Tension in the Nervous System. Pronounced adverse tension in the nervous system will tie or fix the patient in positions with progressive loss of range of movement and eventually contractures. The degree of abnormal tension in the nervous system itself is not only dependent upon the severity or location of the lesion, but also on individual predisposing factors. It has been noted that certain people tend to exhibit excessive tension following even slight trauma to neural structures. It is possible that such individuals would be those patients more prone to contracture development following a lesion of the central nervous system. Certainly every patient who does develop contractures will also reveal significantly increased adverse tension.

Incidents Which Cause Pain. Any incident which results in the patient experiencing pain can start the process of a contracture developing. A muscle may be overstretched during therapy or nursing procedures, the patient may fall out of bed and injure a limb, or a burn may result from a hot-water bottle that has been inadvisably placed to warm up a cold limb. Whatever the initial injury may have been, the part hurts and the patient holds the limb tightly in a protective position to prevent either active or passive movement of the painful part. Even an intravenous drip leaking fluid into the tissues at the elbow can lead to a serious loss of extension.

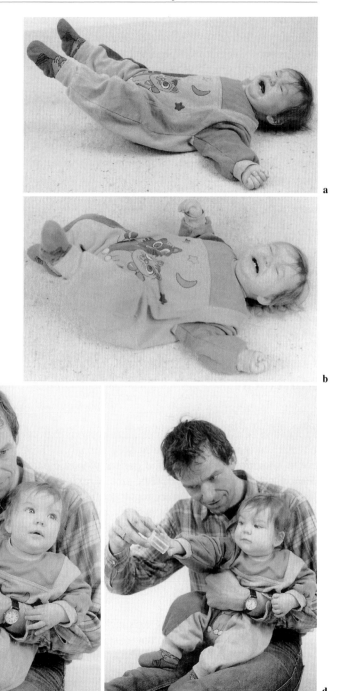

Fig. 6.4a–d. A normal baby . **a** Left alone without contact legs extend strongly with feet plantarflexing. **b** Legs and arms flex as if spastic. **c** Immediate normalization of posture when held close by father. **d** Reaching for an object with no sign of abnormal tone

Delay in Commencing Mobilization. Pain can also be the result of delay in commencing mobilization after onset of coma. The patient will later hold the part constantly in such a position that the shortened muscles or soft tissue structures are prevented from moving into a painful range, either with gravity or when his limbs are being exercised passively. The situation is a self-reinforcing one, because with any painful loss of range causing the patient to hold the joint in a protective position the tissues will tend to shorten still further.

Fractures. Fractures which have occurred at the time of the original accident or due to a fall while in hospital may prevent adequate mobilization, particularly if they are not stabilized and fail to unite for prolonged periods. Even without a fracture, other traumatic injuries such as sprains or bruising can lead to contractures if they are not carefully treated.

Heterotopic Bone Formation. Heterotopic ossification (HO) at one or more major joints can cause grave limitation of movement by forming a mechanical impedance which, according to its size and location, prevents or blocks motion in certain directions. A relatively high incidence of this disabling complication has been reported in patients with spinal cord lesions or following traumatic brain injury.

Overcoming Contractures and Restoring Functional Movement

Prevention is, as always, better and less arduous than cure but, should contractures have arisen through any of the reasons described above, then they must be overcome immediately to allow the patient to participate fully in a comprehensive rehabilitation programme, and be free to experience normal movement so that he can learn from the correct input and is able to move without the inhibitory effects of pain. Pain inhibits activity in muscles and because the contractures are painful, motor function can only be improved or regained once full painfree range of motion has been restored.

Theoretical Principles

The principles for overcoming existing contractures and preventing further deterioration are closely related to the reasons which have been given for their development in the first place and can be summarized as follows:

1. Move the patient, change his position regularly and start standing him with support.
2. Provide reliable tactile information through guiding and active movement in the performance of actual problem-solving tasks.

3. Mobilize the nervous system and reduce adverse tension.
4. Avoid causing pain so that the patient does not have to prevent movement by actively holding his limbs in fixed postures.
5. Stabilize any fractures in the best possible way, as for individuals without brain injuries, and stand and move the patient despite fixation measures. Treat any soft tissue injuries with the same up-to-date treatment that other young individuals would receive.
6. If HO has developed, mobilize all surrounding areas to enable the patient to compensate for any loss of range of motion at one or more involved joints. Assess carefully whether the ossification is really the reason why the patient is unable to perform a certain function so that appropriate treatment can be introduced and fruitless surgery avoided.

Putting the Principles into Action

Moving the Patient and Changing His Position Regularly

Before any other form of intervention is considered, range of motion can often be regained purely by mobilizing and activating the patient if the contractures are not too long-standing and too extreme. Even if other measures should prove to be necessary at a later stage, general mobilization should always be carried out first.

The patient must be brought out of bed and must sit in a wheelchair for increasing periods each day. The wheelchair will usually need to be of a type that can be adjusted in many different ways to make sitting possible for him despite his contracted limbs and trunk (Fig. 6.5a,b). As joint ranges increase, the chair can be altered to attain a progressively improved sitting posture. Ways must be found to support him as comfortably as possible, with additional pillows when necessary to accommodate severely contracted limbs or to avoid pressure on existing decubitus (Fig. 6.5c).

Once the patient can sit in a supported position, teaching him to propel his wheelchair can help to reduce contractures. If possible, the patient pushes his chair with his hands on the wheels, and the goal-orientated activity required of his arms encourages elbow extension. He can also be helped to push the wheelchair with his feet on the ground, the active movement increasing the mobility of his knees.

When the patient is lying in bed, he is turned regularly to prevent static postures from being reinforced, and the supine position is avoided whenever possible.

Prone lying is commenced, using supporting foam-rubber packs, wedges and pillows to accommodate the flexion contractures of the hips and knees and to relieve pressure from the stiff painful shoulders (Fig. 6.6).

The benefits to be gained from lying prone cannot be emphasized enough. The hips and knees slowly relax and extend with each attempt at prone lying; there is no pressure on the vulnerable sites of sacrum, buttocks and heels and spasticity is also reduced in the supported position. With care and determination, the therapist and nurse working in unison will find a way to achieve the position, even if only for short periods at first, and they can then gradually increase the time as the patient's

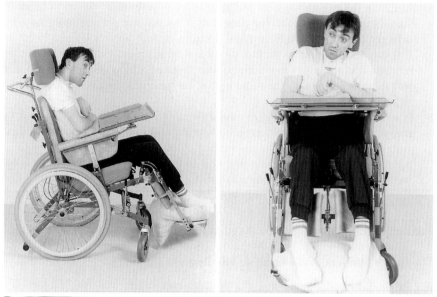

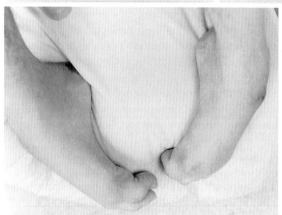

Fig. 6.5a–c. Bringing the patient with contractures out of bed. **a,b** An adjustable wheelchair to make sitting possible. **c** Extra pillows to accommodate severely contracted feet

tolerance and mobility increase. At no time should he be left too long in prone. The nurse or therapist must return at the specified time and turn him again as promised into a more comfortable side lying position or sit him up out of bed. Unable to move himself, if he is left alone and becomes uncomfortable and distressed then he will be unwilling to lie prone again.

Walking with help can be attempted if the patient has active movement in his legs, despite any slight contractures of his hips or knees. The therapist assists the patient in whichever way is necessary. He may be able to manage more successfully if he walks behind his wheelchair and pushes it along in front of him.

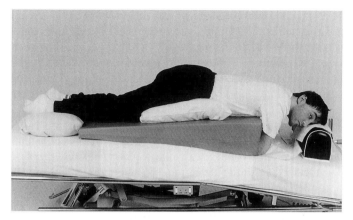

Fig. 6.6. Prone lying commenced despite contractures

Standing the patient daily will almost always overcome any slight contractures of the hips, knees or shortening of the Achilles tendon if his knees are supported in extension by means of back slabs in the way described in Chap. 4 (see Figs. 4.6 and 4.15).

Knee-Extension Splints

A knee-extension splint is used for all patients who cannot actively maintain selective knee extension without compensatory movements and excessive effort when standing upright. A firm splint is required for activities in standing if any of the following problems are observed:

- Plantarflexion of the foot occurs when the patient tries to extend his knee and it is difficult to bring his heel down to the floor.
- Ankle clonus interferes with weight-bearing.
- The patient extends his trunk strongly and/or pushes his head back when trying to keep his knee straight.
- The patient is unable to extend his knee if his hip is extended and can only maintain the extension mechanically by pushing his hip backwards in flexion with his trunk inclined forwards.
- The patient habitually stands with his knees flexed to some degree. If there is no actual structural shortening of the tissues, using the splint for standing will prevent the development of contractures and at the same time give him the feeling of standing in a normal position. Should some loss of extension already have occurred, it can be regained by standing in the splint with the amount of extension being gradually increased.
- After serial plastering to overcome a long-standing knee-flexion contracture, the patient may at first not be able to maintain knee extension actively. Standing with the posterior slab will help him to regain active control.

Using the splint for standing activities will improve active knee extension and not as is sometimes thought decrease muscle strength through reduced demand. It should, therefore, not be regarded as a retrograde step for patients who are able to stand in some way without such support. On the contrary, immediately after the patient has stood with the back slab, it can be removed and he will be better able to stand and control his knee actively without the use of compensatory movements.

Type of Splint
In order to support the patient's knees adequately, the splint must be of an inflexible material which is bandaged firmly in place with slightly elastic crepe bandages. The therapist eases the knee gradually into more extension with each consecutive turn of the bandage.

Various types of ready-made splints are available in "fit-all" sizes, and can be used as long as they are completely stable and do not allow the patient's knees to sag into flexion when he is standing (see Fig. 4.1). A back slab can be made for the individual patient, using a suitably hard material. Plaster of Paris is readily available, relatively inexpensive and quick and easy for the therapist to use.

Making a Plaster Back Slab
When plaster of Paris is used, the knee splint can be made either on the ward with the patient in bed or in the physiotherapy department while he is lying on a plinth. The exposed surfaces of the bed or plinth and the floor can be protected by plastic sheeting or old newspapers.

Before positioning the patient, the therapist prepares the three sections of plaster which will be required for the slab. She measures the distance which will allow the splint to reach from about 7 cm beneath his ischial tuberosity to 3 cm above the

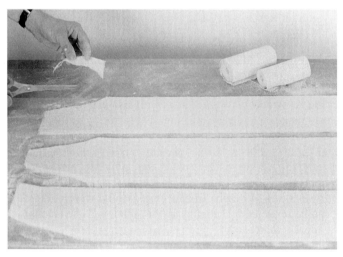

Fig. 6.7. Plaster of Paris strips for making a knee-extension splint, each seven layers thick and shaped to fit the ankle

lateral malleolus of the ankle. She then cuts to the required length three strips of plaster, each of them seven layers thick. One is used as a central strip and the others are for the medial and lateral aspect of the leg, respectively. Depending upon the size of the patient's legs, either 10, 12 or 15 cm plaster bandages will be the correct width. The therapist narrows one end of the plaster strips by cutting off diagonal pieces appropriately in such a way that the splint will fit the shape of the patient's ankle neatly. The central strip is trimmed on both sides and the medial and lateral strips are trimmed only on their outside edges (Fig. 6.7).

While the patient is still lying supine, a gauze stockinet is placed on his leg, to extend beyond the extremities of the plaster of Paris when it hardens (Fig. 6.8). The patient is turned over onto his belly with his legs fully extended. An assistant holds one of his legs in position with one of her hands over his buttock and the other pressing down on his heel to prevent any sudden flexion of his knee from occurring before the plaster has set solid.

The therapist dips the central strip in warm water, holding both its ends firmly between her index fingers and thumbs with the rest of the bandage folded concertina-like between her other fingers (Fig. 6.9a). The plaster is judged to be sufficiently moist when air bubbles cease to escape from it into the water. The therapist squeezes the excess water from the bandage and smoothes it into place down the back of the patient's leg (Fig. 6.9b). The medial strip is moistened in the same way and positioned on the inside of the patient's leg so that it overlaps the central strip, but also extends half-way up the inner aspect of his knee to provide support when he is standing. The lateral strip is placed on the other side of the central strip, and the plaster slab allowed to harden (Fig. 6.9c).

Once the splint has set firmly, the patient's leg is rotated either medially or laterally, whichever offers the least resistance, to enable the therapist to cut through the gauze down one side (Fig. 6.10a). The therapist lifts the patient's leg to allow the gauze to be withdrawn as the assistant removes the plaster slab

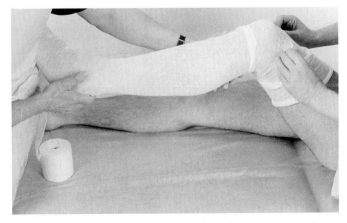

Fig. 6.8. Gauze stockinet covering the patient's leg prior to plastering

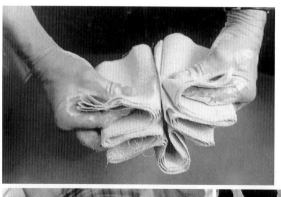

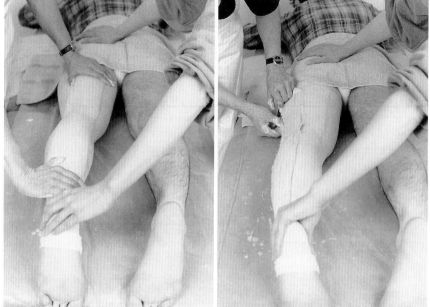

Fig. 6.9a–c. Making the plaster back slab. **a** Holding the folded plaster strip securely to immerse in warm water. **b** Smoothing the central slip into place. **c** Arranging the lateral strip

(Fig. 6.10b). Finally the gauze is trimmed along the edges of the back slab and fixed neatly in place with a single narrow plaster strip, moistened and then smoothed along over the line of the cut gauze on the outside of the splint. No padding material is required because the patient will only wear the splint for relatively short periods while he is standing during therapy sessions. The back slab should not be left on for positioning purposes after therapy or when the patient is in bed.

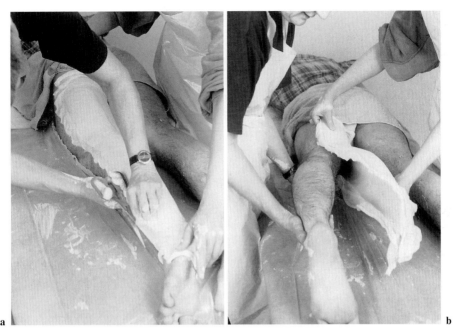

a   b

Fig. 6.10a,b. Removing the back slab. **a** Leg laterally rotated while cutting the gauze. **b** Leg lifted to allow removal of plaster shell

PROBLEM SOLVING

If for some specific reason a patient cannot be turned to lie prone, the back slab can be made with him in a supine position, his foot resting on a block of some description to allow the therapist to place the wet plaster strips on the underneath side of his leg (Fig. 6.11). The plastering is rendered more difficult because the strips will tend to fall off and need to be held in place by the assistant while they are being moulded. Once the plaster has set it will adhere to the gauze stocking.

Providing Additional Information from the Environment

Merely through changing the patient's position regularly, already different parts of his body will have made contact with his surroundings so lessening the tendency for his limbs and trunk to be held constantly in one stereotyped posture. By sitting out of bed in a wheelchair which supports him adequately, the patient will have received yet another beneficial input, particularly when a firm table is placed in front of him, touching his chest and supporting his arms. The mere fact that he is not being left lying on his back in bed, alone in a room, will change the tendency for him to flex or extend his limbs in a way similar to that of a normal baby in the same circumstances (see Fig. 6.4a,b). In addition, guiding his hands and his body as a whole during purposeful tasks will provide him with more meaningful input. The information he perceives through contact with actual objects will reduce the need

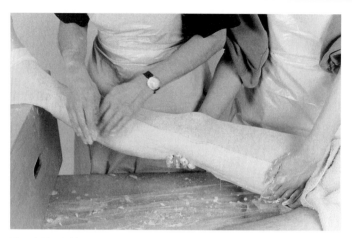

Fig. 6.11. Making the splint with the patient in supine

for him to pull his limbs into end of range positions or increase tone in muscles as has been explained in Chap. 1.

Before serial plastering or any other form of intervention is deemed necessary or repeated, the patient should be guided in many and varied real-life situations. Not only will his mobility improve, but also his ability to cooperate, should some form of intervention prove necessary at a later stage.

If the patient's limbs are extremely contracted, the therapist chooses an appropriate task for guiding, one which does not require a greater range of movement than is attainable at the present time. For instance, if a patient's elbows have less than 90 extension and his wrist and fingers gross flexion contractures, reaching out to grasp a large object some distance away would not be feasible (Fig. 6.12a).

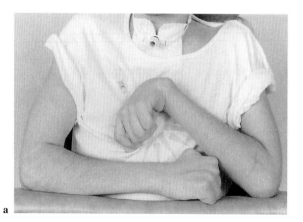

Fig. 6.12a–e. Guiding to overcome upper limb contractures. **a** Patient with marked contractures. **b** Testing the soil in a pot plant. **c** The pot held close to the patient. **d** Bringing the watering can to the plant. **e** Watering the plant after changing hands

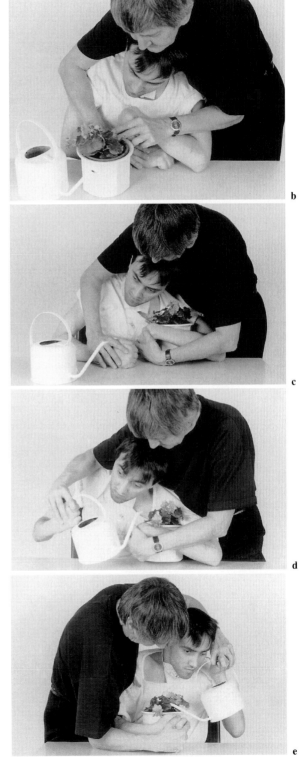

Fig. 6.12a–e

By preparing a more suitable task the therapist can ensure that it will be possible to complete successfully, e.g. watering a pot plant with a small watering can which has a handle (Fig. 6.12b–e). Many of the activities of daily living lend themselves very well to guiding and, if suitably selected and organized, will increase the range of movement in the desired area.

The patient's family can be a great help if they too guide activities frequently during the day. The patient may in fact be more relaxed with someone whom he knows well, trusts implicitly and does not associate with any form of painful or uncomfortable therapy. Certainly he will often be able to let the contracted limb move more easily when guided by a close relative than he can during attempts on the part of the therapist to perform passive stretching in isolation (Fig. 6.13).

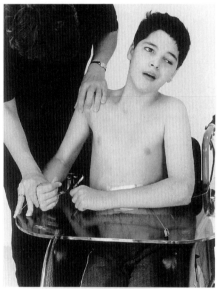

Fig. 6.13a. Patient resisting painful passive extension of his contracted elbow. **b** Goal-orientated activity with the help of his father

a

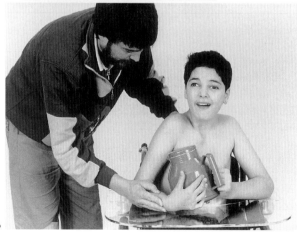

b

Mobilizing Adverse Mechanical Tension in the Nervous System

It should be remembered that it is not only the elasticity of muscles and soft tissues or the mobility of joints which allow full range of motion, but also the adaptive lengthening of the nervous system as well. Any contracture will certainly have an abnormal neural tension component in addition so that mobilization of the nervous system will help considerably to overcome contractures wherever they may be.

The therapist, by moving some part of the patient's body which is not painful, such as his neck, trunk or a less involved extremity, can influence the more affected areas. It is amazing, for instance, how lateral flexion of the neck will increase the range of movement in a contracted elbow, without the patient's arm having been handled directly. All the mobilization procedures described in Chap. 3 should be gradually introduced and performed daily, the emphasis being on moving to mobilize and not stretching to lengthen.

Eliminating Painful Stretching of Contracted Structures While Increasing Range of Motion

Because the patient with brain damage is unable to tolerate pain, any therapeutic measures involving active or passive stretching will not be successful in overcoming contractures. The patient actively resists any attempt to move the contracted part beyond the point where pain is elicited. It is contraindicated to anaesthetize the part locally or sedate the patient heavily before passive stretching is carried out, because pain is the protective response which prevents structures from being traumatized.

Where gravity would cause the shortened muscles to lengthen the patient also holds his limb actively in such a way that the painful lengthening does not occur. For example, where there is a loss of extension at the elbow, the elbow flexors are in a state of constant activity, and with a knee flexion contracture, the patient dare not relax the flexors when he is lying supine because his knee would move into more extension if he did as a result of the pull of gravity.

Once a contracture has developed, pain is the key factor which perpetuates it. The pain causes the constant protective postures and the resistance to movement and a vicious circle ensues. The patient moves less because it hurts, which in turn will result in more pain occurring on movement, and he will, therefore, resist movement even earlier in an ever-decreasing range.

Severe contractures are, therefore, more likely to present problems for patients with head injury, hemiplegia or multiple sclerosis than for those who have suffered a complete spinal cord lesion and have no pain sensation. Should a patient with a complete transection of the spinal cord develop contractures below the level of the lesion, these are far easier to overcome through positioning, passive stretching and supported standing because no pain is experienced. The spinal tetraplegic, on the other hand, with a lesion at C5/6 has absent elbow extensors and is at risk of developing elbow flexion contractures because he can feel pain in that area and has active flexors with which he can prevent movement into a painful range.

If a brain-damaged patient has a contracture so marked that it prevents standing or functional activities and an intensive treatment period with positioning, active therapy and guiding has failed to overcome the difficulty, then other procedures will need to be considered. The three possibilities are:

- Serial casting
- Surgical intervention
- Nerve blocks

Serial Casting

Serial plastering, whereby the contracted limb is held in a progressively corrected position by a cast of plaster of Paris, is the method of choice and should always be considered in preference to any other procedures. It is amazingly effective in correcting even the most severe contractures, including those which have been present for some years.

Serial plastering with circular casts can be used successfully to overcome the following contractures:

- Knee flexion. Any concomitant hip flexion contractures will be reduced simultaneously because the patient's whole leg will no longer pull up into a flexed position. The knee cast, used in conjunction with prone lying and assisted standing will regain lost hip extension at the same time as correcting the flexion contracture at the knee.
- Plantarflexion of the ankle with shortening of the Achilles tendon and possibly the toe flexors as well.
- Elbow flexion.
- Wrist flexion, usually with shortening of the finger flexors.

Advantages of Serial Plastering over Other Methods

There are several reasons as to why serial casts should be used in preference to other procedures. First and foremost, all muscles remain intact for later use, retaining their original length, coordination and function. Once the contracture has been overcome and the limb is being used again, adequate power is quickly and easily restored.

Every muscle in the body plays a significant role in the execution of normal movement, whether performing an obvious action by contracting to move a certain part or by subtle changes in tension to enable other muscles to work more efficiently. It is sometimes overlooked that such changes in tension provide invaluable sensory information for the maintenance of balance in upright positions as well as the control of movement, since muscles are also an essential part of the body's sensory system. Another important function is the breaking action provided by eccentric contraction to regulate the speed of movement in the direction of gravity, while isometric contractions make static postures possible. Unfortunately it is all too common to hear statements like "just cut the hamstrings" when a knee flexion contracture is causing problems. But, these important muscles are essential for normal gait, for stabilizing the knee and extending the hip and for taking steps backwards. It would be a pity to cut them or interfere with their length when knee extension can be successfully regained with no loss of function by employing circular plastering techniques.

Because it is never certain how far the patient will recover, it is advisable to keep every door open so that in the event of return of functional activity there will be no retrospective regrets. The potential for normal movement remains.

No anaesthetic is required and the risks however slight, inherent in any surgical undertaking are avoided. Physical and other forms of therapy can be continued without interruption immediately the plaster has dried. Guiding the patient during the performance of goal-orientated tasks can be continued despite the cast, because the changing resistances can still be perceived through the plaster, and the information provided by the contact with actual objects will further reduce the tension in the patient's contracted limbs.

Very little pain is experienced by the patient, neither when the plaster is being applied nor during the subsequent period of casting required to correct the contracture. With the limb securely encased, the relevant muscles can relax because the patient no longer has to guard against any increased range of motion which might occur as a result of passive or active movements. For this reason, circular plastering is used with the cast left intact, because if it is bivalved or even if some portion is removed, then the patient will once again need to guard against any painful lengthening of the structures which might occur during therapeutic or nursing procedures. Without surgical intervention, there is also not the pain of an incision.

The development of a contracture can be prevented by applying a circular cast prophylactically, even in the early days if the therapist has the feeling that she is in danger of losing range of motion at some joint.

Requirements for Serial Plastering

General

The plaster cast can be applied when the patient is in the intensive care unit, on the ward in bed or in the physiotherapy department, if no special plaster room is readily available. Plastic sheeting is used to protect the patient's bed or the plinth as well as the surrounding floor area. In addition, newspapers can be spread out and are an inexpensive and time-saving way of keeping the surfaces clean.

Sufficient time for applying the plaster cast is necessary and usually requires about 30 min, but if the preparation of the materials and the patient are taken into consideration then an hour is a more realistic estimate. An assistant must hold the patient's limb in the correct position during the plastering, a task which can be very taxing physically. Another person should always be present to talk to and entertain a restless patient, and to hold him in place on the bed should he tend to wriggle or slide out of position. One of his relatives may be ideal for the role.

Materials

The following items are required for serial plastering:

- Sufficient rolls of plaster of Paris of an appropriate width, namely 12 cm for the knee cast, 10 and 12 cm for the ankle, 10 cm for an elbow and 8 and 10 cm for the wrist.
- Six to eight bandages may be sufficient for the cast itself, but it is advisable to have a few extra rolls near at hand.
- A portable basin or a bucket of warm water in which to immerse the plaster bandages.
- Rolls of smooth, soft padding material to bandage on to the patient's limb before applying the plaster of Paris. The material should not be too bulky and the rolls should be of the same width as the plaster bandages or, if they are slightly narrower, it will be easier to prevent their wrinkling.

Some therapists and orthopaedic nurses favour the use of a crepe tissue paper bandage applied over the padding to hold it smoothly in place and to absorb some of the moisture. It is not generally necessary, but may be useful, for example, for the final cast for the wrist when the contracture has been almost completely corrected to ensure a close fit.

Instruments

To facilitate removing and changing the cast and to eliminate stress, four instruments are strongly recommended (Fig. 6.14).

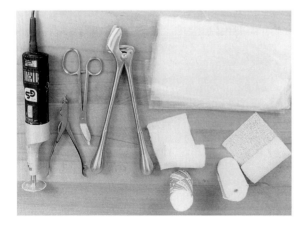

Fig. 6.14. Instruments and materials for serial plastering

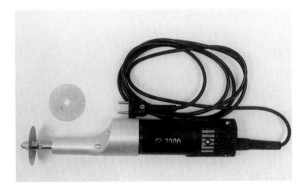

Fig. 6.15. An electric plaster saw for easy removal of plaster cast

- *A plaster saw* (Fig. 6.15). An electric plaster saw with an oscillating blade which will not cut through the padding material and cannot cut the patient's skin is essential. Various models are available and those which make the least noise and have adjustable speeds are advocated.
- *A plaster spreader* (Fig. 6.16). Once the cast has been cut through with the saw, it is difficult to pull the two edges apart as the plaster is relatively thick. The tips of the spreader are eased into the opening and, when the handles are pressed towards each other, the cut is prized open without effort. Using a spreader to open the gap allows the padding to be divided easily so that the cast can be removed. When the contracture has been overcome, the spreader is most useful for making the hinged plaster which requires that the edges remain undamaged and the shape of the cast unchanged.

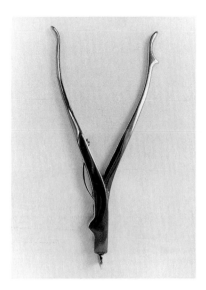

Fig. 6.16. A plaster spreader to part the cut edges of the cast

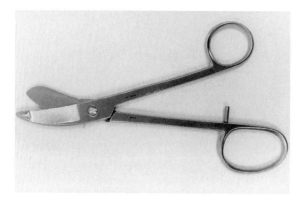

Fig. 6.17. Blunt-tipped scissors to cut through the padding material

- *Blunt-tipped plaster scissors* (Fig. 6.17). A pair of sharp scissors is needed to cut through the padding before the plaster can be removed. Because the padding is pulled tightly against the patient's skin after the cast has been prized open, the tips of the scissors should be smoothly rounded to avoid possible injuries. It is important that the scissors be sharpened regularly, because it is most frustrating if the padding proves difficult to cut, and newly gained range of motion may be lost.
- *Plaster shears* (Fig. 6.18). To cut through the thinner plaster at the extremities of the cast, plaster shears can be used instead of the saw, particularly if the patient becomes agitated. The shears can also be used to trim the cast should any hard pieces be pressing against the patient's skin. In the event of a power failure or if a child is very nervous of the electric saw, the whole cast can be removed with shears.

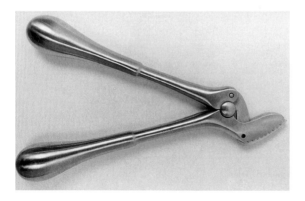

Fig. 6.18. Plaster shears to open or trim the extremities of the cast

General Principles for Serial Casting

Once the decision has been made to correct a contracture by means of serial plastering, the following principles should be followed to ensure maximum safety and success:

- If the patient has been receiving treatment on an out-patient basis, he should be admitted to hospital or to a rehabilitation centre for the duration of the procedure whenever possible. Observations, total management and intensive therapy are far easier for all concerned if the patient is an in-patient.
- A plaster cast should only include one joint in order to avoid complications, although it may be tempting to plaster the knee and foot or the elbow and the wrist simultaneously, as indeed experienced staff may decide to do in individual cases.
- If both lower limbs have knee-flexion contractures, it is advisable to plaster both legs at the same time, because when only one leg is plastered the skin of the other may be damaged by rubbing against the cast.
- Force must never be used to gain an increased range of extension, either before or during the application of a cast, and no anaesthetic should be used in an attempt to achieve a better correction. For an extremely anxious or restless patient, slight sedation may be given but is seldom necessary. The best possible position of the limb at the time which does not cause the patient undue pain or fear is accepted and the plaster applied. Thus any injury to joints or tearing of muscles is avoided and, if the patient's bones have become osteoporotic, any danger of a fracture is eliminated.
- Care must be taken that the padding material is not too thick, as more movement within the cast would be possible as a result, leading to an increased risk of pressure sores developing. No extra pieces of padding should be placed over bony prominences or other vulnerable areas, because instead of being a protection they will only serve to increase the amount of pressure over that part.
- The cast is changed only once a week because it has been found that nothing is gained by more frequent changing and valuable treatment time is lost. In the course of the 7 days, the limb has time to adapt to the new position, and a considerable increase in the range of extension can be achieved when the next cast is applied.
- When changing the cast, the new plaster must be applied immediately after the old one has been removed. While the old cast is being taken off, the assistant should already have her hands in position to draw the limb into an improved range and hold it there. After a quick inspection of the patient's skin, the therapist starts to roll the padding material into place, and commences plastering. On no account should the limb be moved passively into flexion before the new cast is applied, because by so doing the newly won accommodation to stretch and the increased range of extension can easily be lost again.
- Every effort must be made to avoid pressure areas, but should a small open area or blister have developed, it should be quickly cleaned, a zinc cream dressing placed over the area beneath the padding, and plastering commenced. With the

new cast in place, there will no longer be pressure over the same area and, in all probability, the skin will have healed by the time the next change is due.

- Only in the unlikely event of a significant pressure sore having been caused should the casting be interrupted prematurely, because the regained range of motion will certainly be lost otherwise. Many centres are unwilling to use serial casting because of the fear of decubitus formation, but it should be realized that a pressure sore will cause infinitely less suffering for the patient than a permanent contracture and no chance of being able to use his limb again. Once the contracture has been overcome, the decubitus will heal swiftly with appropriate treatment.

- After the cast has been applied, the patient may experience some discomfort as he is not accustomed to his limb being held in a more extended position. It is not unusual for him to complain that the plaster is causing "pain", and care must be taken to differentiate between the two feelings. If routine observations of colour and temperature indicate that the circulation is adequate, changing the patient's position may help to alleviate the problem. A window should not be cut in the cast in order to check the area because its edges will cause more pressure. The decision whether to remove the plaster completely or not is a most difficult one, particularly during the first night after it has been applied. Bivalving the cast is not recommended as it is very difficult to hold the two halves in position afterwards, and the danger of pressure areas is in fact increased. The patient may untie the bandage or a night nurse release the cast to afford him some relief for a short while. In both instances valuable ground is lost, as the limb will have flexed again and there will be renewed resistance to correction the next day.

- Most patients will require some sedation during the first night or two until they have become accustomed to their flexed limbs being held in increased extension. Once the muscles have relaxed, the discomfort disappears and no further medication is required.

- Intensive physiotherapy must be continued throughout the period of serial plastering because the casts alone will not achieve the desired results. Mobilizing the nervous system is particularly important and the therapist emphasizes mobilization of the cervical spine, the shoulder girdle and the trunk in all starting positions. When the knee or elbow is in plaster, the foot and hand require considerable attention to prevent the transfer of tension or "spasticity" to distal muscle groups with the risk of muscle shortening in these areas.

- Localized passive movements are performed as well, whenever applicable, by moving the patient proximally, especially in weight-bearing positions. As soon as the knee is sufficiently extended to allow standing, the therapist supports him while he flexes his trunk and returns to an upright position again (see Fig. 4.22), shifts weight from one leg to the other with a rolled bandage placed beneath his toes to increase the extensibility of his calf and intrinsic foot muscles.

- Usually about 6 weeks will be required to overcome a contracture completely. After the final cast has been removed, the previously immobilized part will tend to become oedematous for a short time. Such oedema is to be expected, however, and should not cause alarm. The therapist treats the swelling with ice, elevation and active movements, and it soon resolves. The swollen limb should be replaced in a hinged cast at night and for unsupervised periods during the day. The therapist may fear that the patient may not be able to regain flexion of the joint again, but her fears are unfounded. Passive flexion should be omitted until all signs of oedema have disappeared as it would only aggravate the condition while inflammation is still present. Flexion soon returns when the patient is moving or being moved during the activities of his daily life, to the extent that care will have to be taken to avoid the flexors from shortening again.

Serial Plastering of the Knee

Correcting a knee-flexion contracture by means of repeated casting presents fewer problems than do any of the other joints, even if the knee is flexed beyond 90 and has been contracted for a considerable time. Much is gained by correcting the deformity, because standing becomes possible and walking can be attempted, leading to an overall improvement in the patient's condition and compliance.

Applying the Initial Cast

With the patient lying supine, a layer of padding is applied to his leg with an extra layer at the two extremities where more pressure is exerted by the cast. Particular care is taken to ensure that the padding at the thigh end extends far enough up to be beyond the edge of the completed plaster (Fig. 6.19). With the assistants already holding the patient's limb in the corrected position, one preventing hip flexion and the other applying traction from the ankle, the therapist rolls the padding material smoothly around the leg from proximal to distal. The padding extends right down over the malleoli with each layer of the bandage partially covering the previous one to avoid any gaps (Fig. 6.20).

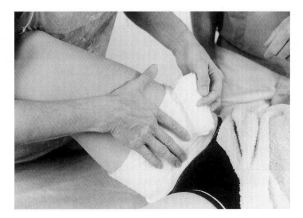

Fig. 6.19. Padding material around the top of the thigh

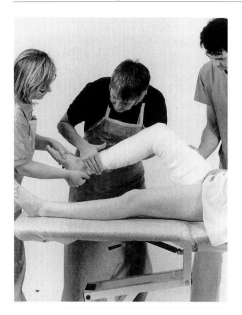

Fig. 6.20. Patient's leg held in corrected position by two assistants while padding is applied

Successive plaster of Paris bandages are placed in the container of warm water and, when the bubbles cease to escape, the therapist starts bandaging them round the patient's leg, starting at the upper thigh and moving on down to the knee. The assistant who holds the patient's ankle extends the knee by applying traction and lifting the tibia in an upward direction, as she will do throughout the procedure. The other assistant provides counterpressure to prevent the whole leg from being lifted by pushing down firmly on the patient's thigh in the small exposed space available (Fig. 6.21).

Once the plaster on the patient's thigh has set somewhat, the assistant can place the palm of her hand over it and by applying gentle pressure can maintain the

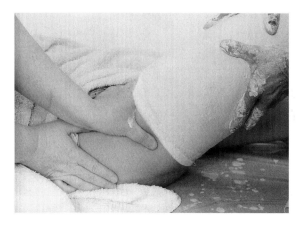

Fig. 6.21. One assistant holds the femur down while the plaster is being applied around the thigh

Fig. 6.22a,b. Completing the plastering.
a Assistants achieving maximum correction of contracture before plaster
hardens. **b** Padding material extending
beyond the ends of the cast

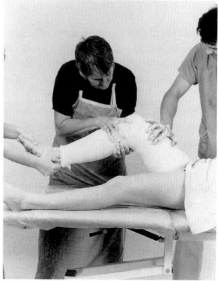

a

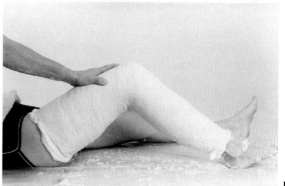

b

maximum amount of knee extension while the therapist continues plastering the
lower leg (Fig. 6.22a). Care must be taken that no indentation in the plaster is
caused.

When the last plaster bandage has been applied, the padding material is folded
back over the edges of the cast, and the patient is kept lying down until the plaster
has set hard (Fig. 6.22b).

Changing the Cast

The same procedure is carried out each week when the cast is changed, with the
assistants holding the patient's leg in position even before the old cast is removed.
Firm pressure and additional traction applied immediately after each successive
cast has been taken off usually achieves a marked increase in knee extension,
which then needs to be maintained until the new cast has been completed.

Preventing a Downward Sliding of the Cast

When the patient's knee is more extended, the plaster will tend to slide down his leg particularly during standing activities but also as he moves in and out of bed. A suspension mechanism is incorporated in the subsequent casts to prevent the downward shift and resultant damage to the skin over the knee, Achilles tendon or malleoli.

The patient's leg is shaved in two strips, one on the medial and one on the lateral side below his knee. A length of 4 cm wide Elastoplast or adhesive extension plaster is stuck along each of the shaved areas and cut off so that they extend approximately 30 cm beyond his foot (Fig. 6.23).

The cast is applied as before, with the padding material being bandaged on over the strips of extension plaster. Before using the last plaster of Paris bandage, when the cast has almost hardened the therapist pulls the strips of adhesive plaster firmly up on each side for the assistant to hold tightly in place (Fig. 6.24a). With the last roll of plaster, the therapist covers the two strips which will thus be fixed in position when the plaster dries and will act as a suspender for the whole cast (Fig. 6.24b,c).

Avoiding Pressure on the Patient's Heel

With the patient's knee more extended, the weight of the cast together with that of the straightened leg will place considerable pressure on his heel, as can be seen in Fig. 6.24c. The skin over the heel will have become very soft and tender as it will not have been in contact with any surface for some time, due to the flexed knee. A pressure sore could easily develop if the heel were left constantly in contact with the supporting surface.

In order to prevent the weight of the cast from being taken through the patient's heel, the therapist places a dry plaster bandage underneath the distal end of the newly applied cast and plasters it firmly in position, while the assistant lifts the leg (Fig. 6.25a). The roll beneath the cast ensures that the patient's heel is

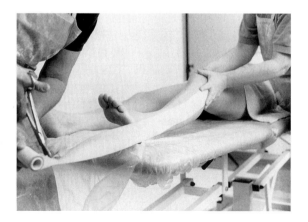

Fig. 6.23. Adhesive plaster strips applied to each side of the leg and cut off well beyond the foot

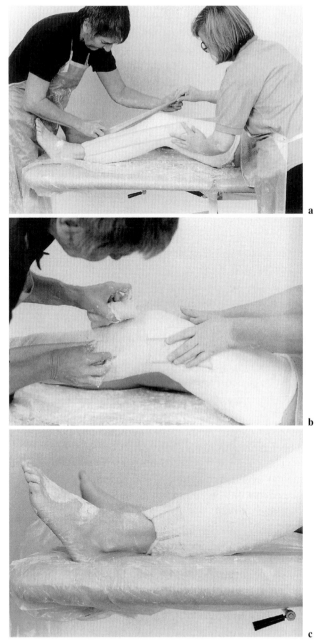

Fig. 6.24a–c. Suspending the plaster cast. **a** The strips of adhesive plaster pulled up firmly on each side of the cast. **b** Fixing the strips in place with the last roll of plaster. **c** No downward sliding possible

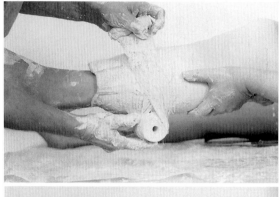

a

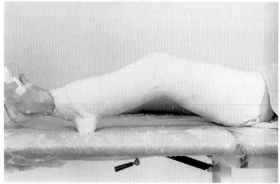

b

Fig. 6.25a,b. Relieving pressure over the heel. **a** Roll of dry plaster being plastered into position. **b** Patient's heel no longer in contact with the supporting surface

never in contact with a hard surface, whether he is lying in bed or sitting in a wheelchair with his leg supported straight out in front of him (Fig. 6.25b).

The plaster roll beneath the cast can also serve another purpose by preventing medial or lateral rotation of the patient's leg. A 12 cm wide bandage can be so placed that one end protrudes further on that side to which the leg would otherwise constantly rotate.

Duration of Serial Casting

Serial plastering is continued until full knee extension has been regained, because if there is any residual shortening the knee flexion contracture will in all probability develop again. Before cessation of casting the patient should, therefore, have no pain on full knee extension even when overpressure is applied by the therapist and she should not feel any tension or resistance when performing the passive movement (Fig. 6.26).

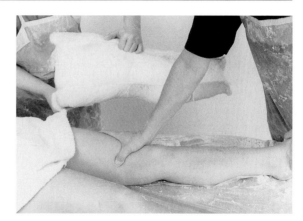

Fig. 6.26. Full painfree knee
extension without resistance

Maintaining Full Range of Knee Extension with a Hinged Cast

Immediately following the weeks of serial casting, it is usually necessary to support the patient's knee in the corrected position until active control has been regained or daily standing with splints or braces has become a routine. A removable cast with a hinge mechanism is made which can be bandaged on for certain periods during the day to prevent prolonged knee flexion when the patient is sitting in his wheelchair. For therapy sessions, the cast is removed so that activity can be stimulated and normal movement facilitated. It is important that the cast be left on for the night because the patient is likely to curl up when asleep and may lie for some hours with his knees flexed, with the result that the regained extension could easily be lost.

Making the Hinged Cast

When full painfree knee extension has been achieved the therapist applies a final light plaster with the patient's leg in the corrected position (Fig. 6.27a). Using the pointed ends of a pair of scissors, the therapist bores a row of small holes on the outside of the cast along its entire length (Fig. 6.27b). With the plaster saw she cuts open the medial side of the cast neatly, marking the plaster first with a pencil to ensure a straight line (Fig. 6.27c). Using the spreader the edges of the cut are gently prized apart (Fig. 6.28a) and the underlying padding divided with the blunt-tipped scissors (Fig. 6.28b).

The therapist and her assistant carefully open the cast, pressing their thumbs against the row of holes to ensure that these are the fulcrum of movement or hinge when the top section of the plaster is rotated upwards and outwards (Fig. 6.28c). When the opening is sufficiently wide the patient's leg is lifted and the cast removed (Fig. 6.28d). The edges and the padding at the opening are trimmed with a single layer of plaster or adhesive strapping.

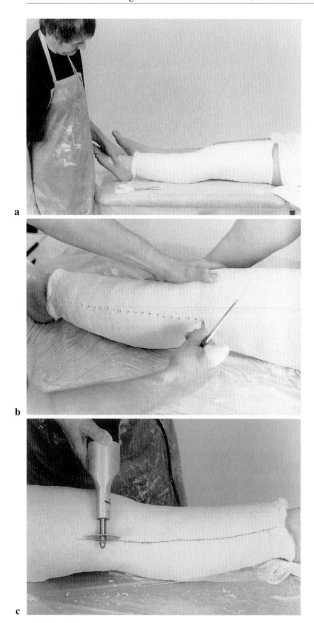

Fig. 6.27a–c. Making a hinged cast. **a** Lightweight cast with knee fully extended. **b** Boring a row of holes with a pair of pointed scissors. **c** Cutting open the medial side of the cast

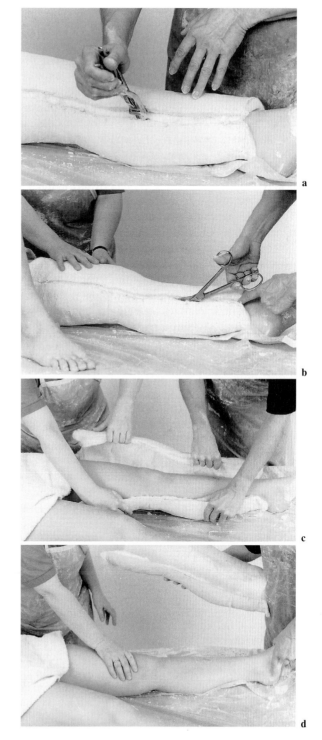

Fig. 6.28a–d. Removing the cast. **a** Parting the cut edges. **b** Cutting through the padding. **c** Prizing the cast open. **d** Lifting the cast away

Putting on the Hinged Cast

The patient's leg is placed in the lower shell of the plaster and the opening on the medial side is closed with care to avoid the skin from being pinched between the two edges (Fig. 6.29a). If it is particularly difficult to close the cast without trapping the patient's skin, either because of some oedema or because the knee is flexing somewhat, the assistant uses the edge of a wooden spatula to press the flesh away from the opening as the therapist draws it closed with an elastic crepe bandage (Fig. 6.29b). The therapist bandages the cast firmly into place, starting at the knee but continuing right from the top down to the distal end to ensure a secure fit (Fig. 6.29c).

A patient who is still extremely restless and not able to understand why the cast is necessary, may remove it at night by unwinding the bandage on his own. In such cases, a narrow plaster bandage can be moistened and used to fix the cast in place. The single layer of plaster is easy to cut with a pair scissors on the following day when the cast needs to be removed.

The hinged cast is left off for increasingly long periods during the day and eventually the night as well, and need only be replaced if any loss of range of extension reappears or seems imminent. Should any loss of range be observed, perhaps after a holiday weekend without therapy, the hinged cast can be plastered on with a single plaster-bandage and left in place for a few days without being removed at all. Within a short time the muscles will once again relax and full range be regained.

Serial Plastering for a Plantarflexed Foot

The patient who has lost range of dorsiflexion of his ankle will have difficulty in standing with his heel on the floor. Because weight is taken through the ball of his foot which presses against the floor, activity in the plantar flexors will be stimulated and the Achilles tendon will tend to shorten. The patient's weight will be always behind the line of gravity and his hips flexed as a result. Whether there is actual shortening of the calf muscles or whether marked spasticity is causing the plantarflexion, the problem can be overcome by serial casting.

Applying the Cast

The patient lies supine and the assistant stands beside him to hold his leg in position. She flexes and abducts his hip, flexes his knee against her body and, with both her hands, keeps his foot in as much dorsal flexion as possible (Fig. 6.30a). With the leg thus in the total pattern of flexion, more dorsiflexion is possible and is easier to maintain. The therapist rolls on the padding material, moulding it carefully to cover the bony points around the ankle, and continues down to below the metatarsal heads (Fig. 6.30b).

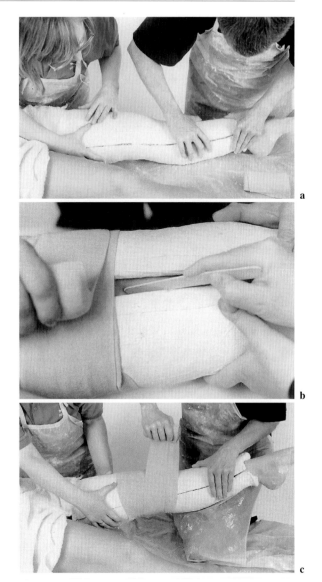

Fig. 6.29a–c. Replacing the patient's leg in the hinged cast. **a** Carefully closing the gap. **b** Pressing the skin away with the edge of a spatula. **c** Bandaging the cast firmly in place

Pieces of foam rubber are placed in the spaces between the patient's toes to ensure that there will be enough space for them when the cast has been completed (Fig. 6.31a). The resultant abduction of the toes will also help to reduce the hypertonus in the plantar flexors and facilitate dorsiflexion of the foot. Before starting the actual plastering the therapist measures and cuts several layers of plaster and padding material a little wider than the patient's forefoot, which will be applied beneath his toes at a later stage in the procedure (Fig. 6.31b).

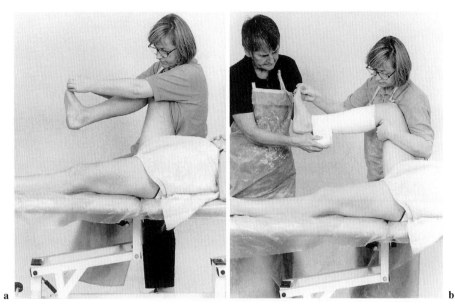

Fig. 6.30a,b. Preparing to plaster a plantarflexed foot. **a** Holding the leg in total flexion. **b** applying the padding material

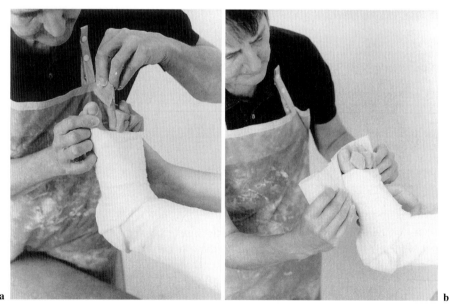

Fig. 6.31a. Placing pieces of foam rubber between the toes. **b** Preparing layers of plaster for beneath the toes

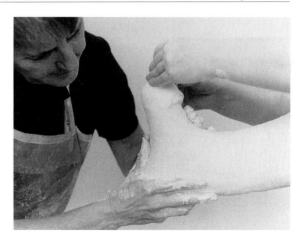

Fig. 6.32. Moulding the plaster to fit snugly around the ankle

The therapist starts plastering the lower leg and continues down over the ankle as far as the ball of the foot, carefully moulding the wet plaster to achieve a snug fit around the heel and ankle (Fig. 6.32). The assistant continues to hold the patient's toes and maintain the position of his foot until the plaster which has been applied as far as the metatarsal heads has dried.

Once the plaster has set, the assistant can take her hands away from the toes to enable the therapist to place the prepared padding in position (Fig. 6.33a). After moistening the precut layers of plaster, the therapist lays them beneath the toes so that they overlap the already hardened plaster below the ball of the foot, but still extend beyond the tips of the toes and winds the rest of the roll around over the top of the foot (Fig. 6.33b). The layers are plastered firmly in place by bandaging on an additional plaster roll which passes underneath them and round over the dorsum of the foot. The therapist presses the wet plaster up beneath the patient's toes using her thumbs to hold them in an extended position, while her fingers against the top of his foot give counterpressure (Fig. 6.33c). At the same time, the assistant pulls the edges away from the proximal ends of the toes taking particular care that the extensor tendon of the great toe is completely free and will not rub against the edge of the cast above it (Fig. 6.33d).

The assistant must always check that the little toe is clearly visible and is not being pressed against the plaster laterally (Fig. 6.34a). Lastly, the foam-rubber cubes are removed from between the toes and the resting position observed and adjusted if necessary (Fig. 6.34b).

The patient's leg is supported on a pillow while the cast is drying to prevent the plaster from being pushed inwards against the calf or the heel while it is still soft. The patient must not stand or even transfer himself into bed because the strain on the front of the plaster could cause it to crack. It is often better for him to remain in bed until the next day to allow the cast time to dry and harden thoroughly. Even when sitting in his wheelchair, the patient may push down against the footplates and the subsequent plantarflexion might be sufficient to break the plaster which has

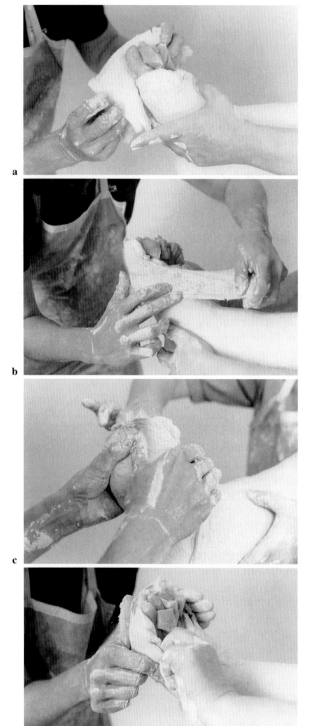

Fig. 6.33a–d. Correcting the position of the toes. **a** The moist plaster fitted beneath the toes. **b** Plastering the additional piece into place. **c** Holding the toes in extension from below. **d** Freeing the extensor tendon of the great toe

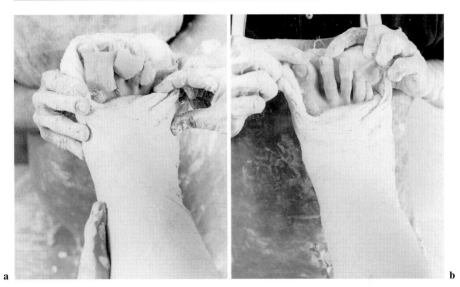

a   b

Fig. 6.34a. Pulling the plaster away from the little toe. **b** Toes have adequate space after removal of foam-rubber cubes

still not completely set. In the case of a very disabled or heavy patient, it is advisable to apply the foot cast while he is lying in his bed so that the problem of transferring him without his feet on the floor is avoided.

Preparing the Bottom of the Cast for Standing

If dorsiflexion of the foot to 90 is still not possible, the sole of the cast will not be level and when standing the patient's entire weight would be taken through the ball of his foot (Fig. 6.35a). To enable him to bear weight through the whole foot, the bottom of the cast should be levelled off. A roll of wet plaster is placed along the bottom of the cast to fill the space between the ball of the foot and the heel. The roll is pressed into shape and then plastered firmly into place with an additional plaster bandage (Fig. 6.35b). When the plaster has dried, the patient will be able to stand and weight will more likely be taken nearer to his heel (Fig. 6.35c).

Some form of sole is required for the cast to protect the plaster and to prevent the patient's foot from sliding when he is standing. or from slipping off the footrest of the wheelchair when he is sitting. The small rubber knob used for fracture casts is not satisfactory because the patient will feel insecure with such a tiny base and his foot tends to swivel outwards. Any type of rubber sole which is incorporated within the plaster has the disadvantage of not being removable when the patient goes to bed. A large size tennis shoe with its uppers cut away can be laced on over the cast to provide a flat rubber sole. Alternatively, an ingenious device is manufactured by the disabled workshop "Milchsuppe" in Basle, Switzerland, which consists of a

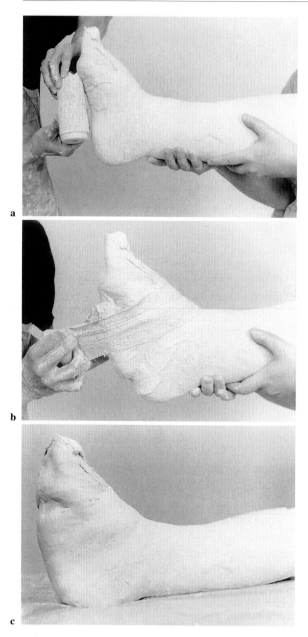

Fig. 6.35a–c. Levelling the bottom of the cast. **a** In standing, weight would pass through ball of foot. **b** Filling in the space with an extra roll of plaster. **c** Weight-bearing area extended

thick rubber sole made from a section of motor-car tyre. It is fixed in place by a broad elastic strap which passes over the top of the patient's foot and round behind his ankle, and a strong rubber lace which holds the curved sides of the sole against the cast (Fig. 6.36).

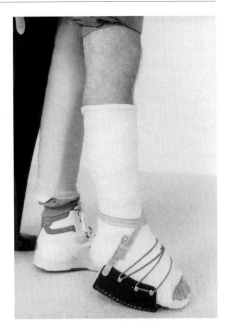

Fig. 6.36. A thick rubber sole laced on over the cast

During the period spent in a plaster cast, the patient is helped to stand daily with a knee-extension splint wide enough to fit over the foot cast if he cannot maintain knee extension. As he regains active control the therapist encourages him to extend his knee actively with his hip kept well forward (Fig. 6.37).

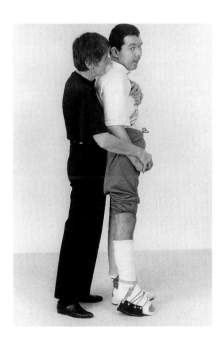

Fig. 6.37. Standing with the foot cast

Changing the Cast

After a week the plaster is renewed, and significant gain in the range of dorsiflexion is usually possible with each new cast. One of the patient's relatives or a member of staff talks to him and keeps him lying quietly on the bed while the therapist cuts through the plaster on the lateral aspect using the electric saw (Fig. 6.38a). To facilitate removing the cast, it is important to saw it open down the medial side as well so that the top section can be lifted off without the patient's foot pushing down strongly (Fig. 6.38b). The padding is then cut as well and the top section can be lifted away freely (Fig 6.39).

Before the patient's foot is lifted from the lower shell of the cast, the assistant grasps his toes and is already prepared to hold his foot in dorsiflexion (Fig. 6.40a). As the cast is taken away, the assistant increases the amount of dorsal flexion as much as she can and maintains the position so that the therapist can start to apply

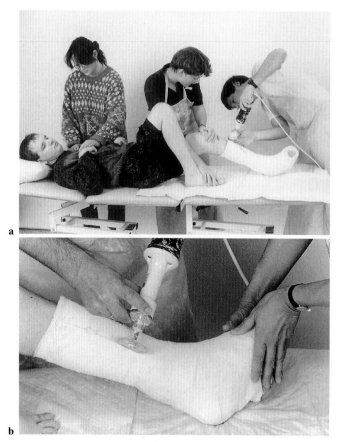

Fig. 6.38a,b. Changing the cast. **a** Cutting open the outside of the cast while a relative talks to the patient. **b** Sawing open the medial side as well facilitates removal

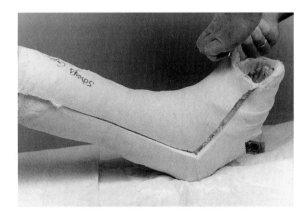

Fig. 6.39. Cutting through padding before lifting off the top section

Fig. 6.40a. Assistant's hands ready before removing cast. **b** Foot held in corrected position as cast is taken away

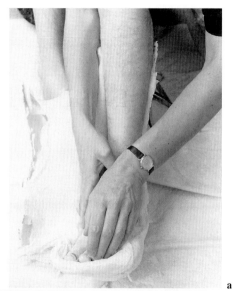

a

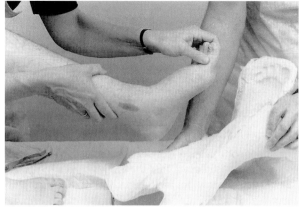

b

the new plaster without any delay (Fig. 6.40b). Maximal correction can be gained if the plaster is applied immediately before the patient's foot has a chance to push strongly into plantarflexion again. As with the first cast, the patient will need to be lifted into bed where he should stay until the next day to prevent the cast from being broken through inadvertent pressure on the footplates of his chair or while he is being transferred.

Once the contracture has been overcome and dorsiflexion regained, the lower trough of the final cast can be bandaged on to maintain the position for the first few nights. Daily standing with a knee-extension splint will ensure that the range of dorsiflexion is maintained.

Serial Plastering for the Flexed Elbow

An elbow cast is easy to apply but the thinly covered, bony prominences are most prone to develop pressure sores, particularly if the plaster slides down toward the wrist at all. For this reason as soon as the flexion contracture has been corrected to the extent that there is less than a 45 limitation of extension, the cast should be suspended to prevent any downward displacement in the way described for suspending the knee cast (see Figs. 6.23 and 6.24).

Applying the Cast

Whether the initial cast is being applied or the subsequent ones at weekly intervals, the procedure is the same. The patient lies supine and the assistant holds his arm in the air with the shoulder flexed to about 90. Once the padding material is in place, a towel is placed over the near side of the patient's head and face to protect them from drops of plaster (Fig. 6.41). The padding should reach well beyond the extent of the plaster both proximally and distally.

When the plaster has been applied but has not yet hardened, the therapist gently eases out a slight bulge behind the elbow to prevent any pressure on the bony olecranon process (Fig. 6.42). The patient's arm is maintained in elevation until the cast has dried and then lain on a pillow to prevent any indentation before the plaster has hardened.

Maintaining the Regained Elbow Extension

When full range of elbow extension has been regained the cast can be removed so that functional activity can be re-educated. If the patient is not using his arm, however, it is important that the elbow be prevented from pulling constantly into flexion as the contracture could otherwise recur. During therapy the patient is encouraged to take weight through his extended arm, perform tasks which require

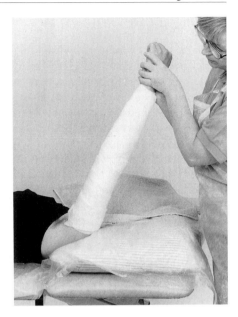

Fig. 6.41. Arm held in elevation with padding applied and a towel protecting patient's face

elbow extension with the therapist guiding his hands and learn ways in which to maintain passive range of motion for himself until he can use the arm functionally again.Until the danger of a recurrence of the contracture has passed the patient's arm is placed in a hinged splint whenever he is not being supervised and particularly during the night.

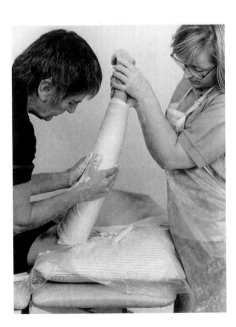

Fig. 6.42. Therapist eases out a slight bulge in the wet plaster to avoid pressure on the olecranon process

The Hinged Cast

When the elbow is fully extended a final lightweight cast is made and, before the plaster has dried completely, the therapist uses a pair of scissors or some other pointed instrument to make a row of small holes down the lateral aspect of the cast to serve as a hinge. A pencil line is drawn down the medial side of the cast diametrically opposite the row of holes (Fig. 6.43a). With the plaster saw the therapist cuts neatly through the plaster along the pencil line (Fig. 6.43b).

The spreader is used to push the edges carefully apart, and the assistant cuts through the padding with the blunt-tipped scissors (Fig. 6.44a). The therapist and her assistant ease the cast open, pressing their thumbs against the holes to ensure the correct location of the hinge mechanism until the patient's arm can be lifted out easily (Fig. 6.44b). The padding material is trimmed and held in place with a single layer of plaster.

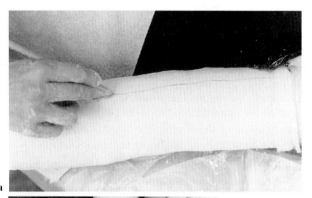

a

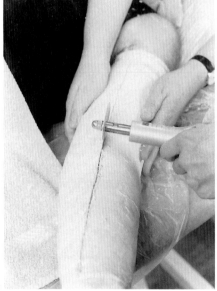

b

Fig. 6.43a,b. Hinging the elbow cast. **a** Drawing a pencil line down the medial aspect. **b** sawing along the line to open the cast

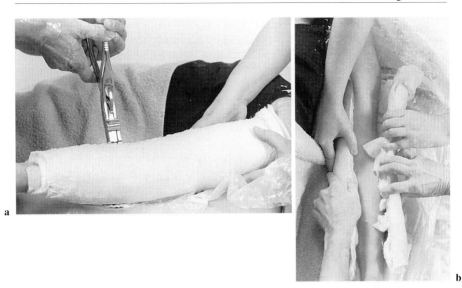

Fig. 6.44a,b. Removing the cast. **a** Prizing the cut edges apart with the spreader. **b** Opening the cast after cutting through the padding

The patient's arm is replaced in the hinged cast, which is then held in place with an elastic crepe bandage. If replacement is difficult a wooden spatula can be used to press the skin down and prevent it from being pinched while the bandage is being applied (see Fig. 6.29b). For therapy, during functional use and for washing, the cast can be easily removed and then replaced again (Fig. 6.45).

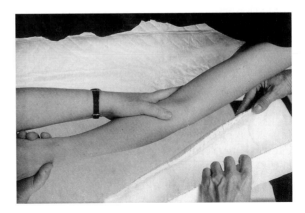

Fig. 6.45. The elbow cast can be replaced easily after therapy

During the time when the patient is in the intensive care unit and has not yet regained consciousness a circular cast can be applied to the elbow if the therapist feels that there is a resistance to full extension. After a few days the arm will have relaxed and the plaster can be hinged and removed for certain periods until it is finally left off altogether. By so doing, the danger of a contracture developing will be avoided as well as any damage to soft tissues which might precipitate the formation of HO.

Serial Plastering for the Flexed Wrist

Together with a flexion contracture of his wrist, the patient will often have shortened finger flexors as well. Serial casting of his wrist will usually suffice to overcome the problem of the flexed fingers at the same time if intensive therapy including mobilization and guiding is carried out diligently during the period of plastering and immediately thereafter. If markedly shortened finger flexors continue to be a problem, then the fingers will need to be included in a subsequent series of plasters.

Applying the Initial Cast

The patient sits with his elbow supported on a table in front of him. The assistant stands at his side and keeps his elbow on the table by pressing his shoulder forward with her body. She holds his hand in the air, adjusting her grip to allow the therapist to bandage on the padding material (Fig. 6.46a). Particular care is taken that there is sufficient padding around the base of the thumb.

The therapist applies first the 6 cm bandages, covering the metacarpophalangeal (MP) joints distally and continuing proximally with the 8 cm rolls to about three fingers below the anterior crease at the elbow so as not to impede flexion of the joint. She moulds the plaster carefully around the wrist itself and maintains the corrected position until the plaster sets, taking care not to indent the cast with her fingers or thumb (Fig. 6.46b).

Before the plaster has set completely the therapist pulls the edges away from around the base of the thumb and checks that the padding extends beyond the rim of the plaster (Fig. 6.46c). The first cast may not appear to have achieved an optimal position of the wrist, but the best correction possible at the time without causing the patient pain is accepted (Fig. 6.47). A significant improvement in range is usually obtained when the plaster is changed at the end of the first and second weeks.

Changing the Cast

In order to facilitate removal of the cast, without the patient's wrist pulling down into flexion, it is advisable to make two incisions, one laterally and one medially as in the case of the foot cast. The therapist uses the saw to cut through the plaster between the thumb and index finger before continuing up along the forearm (Fig. 6.48a). She then cuts along the length of the outside of the plaster (Fig. 6.48b).

Fig. 6.46a–c. Applying a wrist cast.
a Padding in place with wrist held in
maximal painfree extension. **b** Moulding
the plaster carefully around the wrist.
c Freeing the base of the thumb

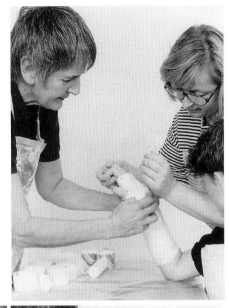

a

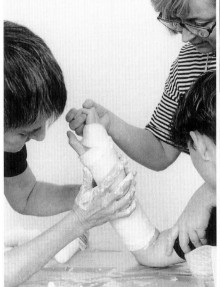

b

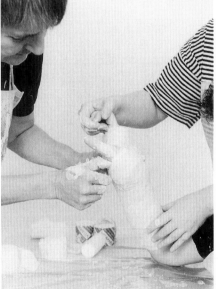

c

With the spreader, the cast is prized open and the padding cut to allow removal of the cast. The assistant holds the patient's hand so that the wrist remains dorsiflexed as the therapist opens the plaster further and draws it away (Fig. 6.49a). Immediately the cast has been taken off the therapist increases the amount of dorsal extension of the wrist by pressing her fingers down over the carpal area while at

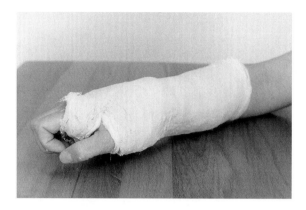

Fig. 6.47. Initial cast with thumb and elbow free to move unimpeded

the same time lifting the patient's hand upwards with her thumb in the palm (Fig. 6.49b). The assistant maintains the new position of the wrist and after a quick inspection of the skin, the therapist at once starts to apply the padding for the new cast (Fig. 6.49c). It is counterproductive to spend time washing the patient's hand or performing passive movements because within minutes the freed wrist will start to flex strongly again and the increased correction could be lost.

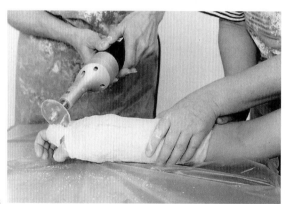

a

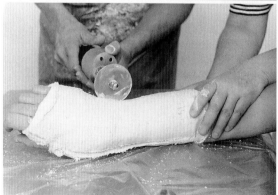

b

Fig. 6.48a,b. Changing the cast. **a** Cutting the plaster between thumb and index finger. **b** Opening the opposite side as well to allow easy removal

Fig. 6.49a. The assistant maintains wrist extension as cast is withdrawn. **b** The therapist increasing the range of extension. **c** Padding for new cast applied immediately

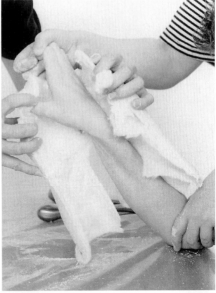

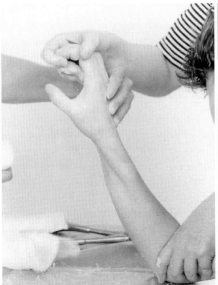

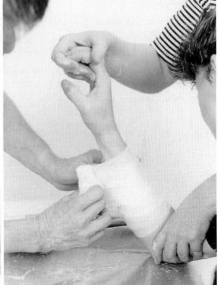

Maintaining Wrist Extension After Serial Casting

A hinged cast, made in the same way as described for the knee and the elbow, can be used after full range of wrist extension has been regained. The final cast is cut open carefully on the thumb side with the row of holes going down the ulnar side.

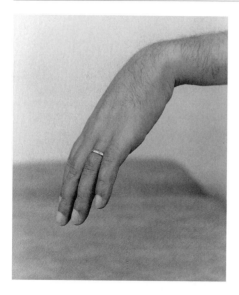

Fig. 6.50. At first the wrist needs some support after weeks of serial plastering

However, for the wrist, a small volar splint made of plaster is less cumbersome, lighter and far easier to apply. Certainly some type of support will be necessary at first until the patient has learned to extend his wrist actively or has more tone in the extensors. After the weeks of immobilization, the hand will otherwise tend to hang down with the wrist constantly in a flexed position whenever his arm is lifted off a supporting surface (Fig. 6.50).

Making the Volar Splint

A 10 cm plaster bandage is folded into about seven layers, measured to reach from the patient's MP joints to approximately 5 cm below his elbow. With the patient's elbow placed on a table in front of him, the assistant keeps his shoulder forwards and holds his hand with the wrist in extension. After soaking the folded plaster in water, the therapist kneels on the other side of the table opposite to the patient and places the wet plaster in position beneath his hand and wrist (Fig. 6.51a). The assistant leaves the patient's hand so that she can smooth the plaster on the flexor aspect of his forearm, while the therapist achieves a good position of his wrist and hand as she moulds the plaster. She presses the plaster into the palm of his hand with both her thumbs while her fingers press against its dorsal aspect to keep his wrist in extension until the plaster sets (Fig. 6.51b). Her thumbs in his palm and her fingers on the back of his hand shape the splint to form the normal contour of his hand. Once the plaster has set firmly, the splint is removed and trimmed. The inner surface can be smoothed out with the handle of a pair of scissors and a nice finish obtained by rubbing an extra piece of moistened plaster bandage over the inside.

When completely dry, the splint is positioned correctly on the palmar aspect of the patient's hand, its end just proximal to his MP joints (Fig. 6.52a). A narrow,

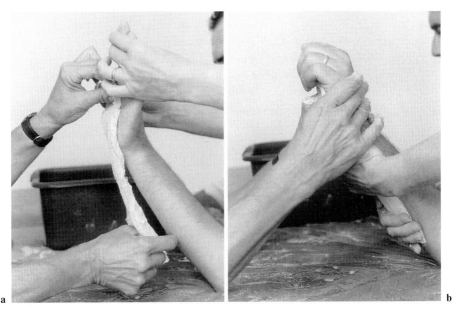

Fig. 6.51a,b. Making a volar splint. **a** Placing the layers of wet plaster in position. **b** Moulding the splint to the normal contours of the hand

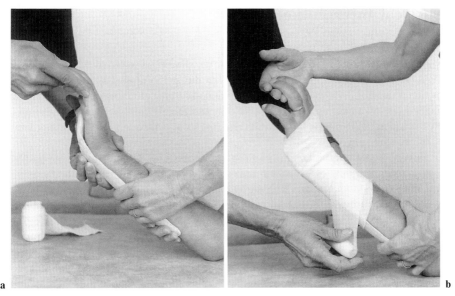

Fig. 6.52a,b. Bandaging the finished splint in position. **a** Exact positioning of the wrist in the splint. **b** Rolling the bandage on from distal to proximal

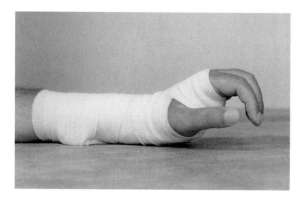

Fig. 6.53. The volar splint supports the wrist comfortably in the corrected position with the fingers free for activity

only slightly elastic crepe bandage is used to bandage the splint in place. The bandage is not pulled tightly but simply unrolled around the hand and arm to avoid uncomfortable compression (Fig. 6.52b). With the volar splint in place, no matter in what position the patient is, his hand is always comfortably supported with the wrist extended (Fig. 6.53). The crepe bandage will help to prevent any oedema from forming in the hand, which may happen after removal of the circular cast, particularly when the arm is in dependent positions such as when the patient is standing or walking. The small splint can be removed easily for therapy and active control stimulated by grasping and releasing objects with facilitation.

Surgical Intervention

Surgical procedures to overcome contractures should be avoided whenever possible because every muscle is required for the performance of normal movement. A tendon which has been lengthened, transected or transplanted can never function as perfectly as it did before, and the efficient action of other muscles which act in harmony will also be affected by any change in length, strength or balanced interplay.

For the rehabilitation team, battling unsuccessfully to prevent or overcome contractures, surgical intervention may seem a tempting alternative because of the immediate and obvious success which follows an operation. Later, however, the decision which seemed right at the time may later be regretted and adverse results are difficult if not impossible to correct. An integral part of the movement will, therefore, not be possible for the patient who later recovers functional activity. Evans (1981) emphasizes the need for caution: "The long-term implications of surgical intervention need to be considered, for example after tendon lengthening of the hamstrings some patients will experience difficulty in activities such as standing up and sitting down. These complications may eventually present more of a problem than the original contracture."

A spastic contracture may well be eliminated through the lengthening of a muscle and the pain inhibition which follows, but spasticity does not disappear into thin air. It will tend to reappear in some other part of the body and create new problems if the underlying reason for the hypertonus or extreme positions of the limbs remain unchanged. Spasticity and/or shortening of the plantar flexors of the ankle are frequently treated by surgical lengthening to enable the patient to commence standing and walking. Loss of or even weakened plantarflexion can, however, create considerable difficulties for the patient. The calf muscles provide important sensory information for balance in standing as well as contracting to prevent falling forwards. In some cases, exaggerated dorsal flexion of the feet in all positions and during all activity follows and hampers function, while in standing clawing of the toes presents problems (Fig. 6.54).

After lengthening of the Achilles tendon and resection of the toe flexors, other patients not only have little balance due to loss of active toe flexion and plantarflexion of the foot, but the whole foot may shorten due to unopposed activity in the intrinsic muscles and a fixed extension deformity of the toes develop in time (Fig. 6.55). There is no guarantee that lengthening the Achilles tendon, split anterior tibial tendon transfer (SPLATT) and toe flexor releases will "render a balanced forefoot" (Garland and Keenan 1983) although such an operation may achieve a degree of success for certain patients. Careful consideration of the following points is, therefore, essential before any irreversible surgical procedure is decided upon.

It is difficult to predict with any certainty to what extent the individual patient will eventually recover functional use of his limbs, particularly within the first years following injury. A calculated guess, based on experience and statistical likelihood can be made but surprising recovery has been known to occur in most unexpected cases. Even advocates of surgical intervention for residual limb deformity stress the need to avoid intervention too early. "Definitive surgery should

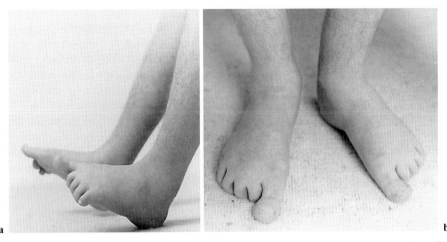

a   b

Fig. 6.54a. A patient with excessive, constant dorsal flexion of the feet after lengthening of Achilles tendons. **b** In standing his toes flex strongly

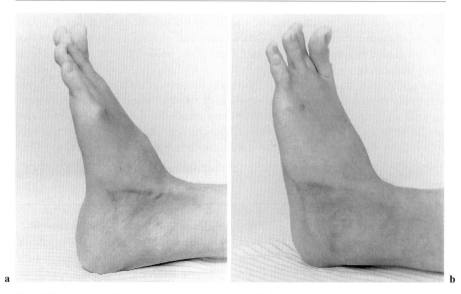

a   b

Fig. 6.55a,b. Foot problems after lengthening of Achilles tendon, release of toe flexors and split anterior tibial tendon transfer. **a** Whole foot shortened. **b** Fixed extension deformity of toes

not be performed until 1.5 years after the initial insult" (Garland and Keenan 1983). In fact nothing is lost by waiting even longer and any surgery which may ultimately prove necessary will be more likely to be successful if the patient has progressed further in his overall ability.

Frequently a contracture is wrongly thought to be the reason for a patient not being able to perform some functional activity, which leads to disappointment and frustration when the situation remains unchanged after surgery. For example, a flexion contracture of the knee, per se, is seldom the factor responsible for a patient not being able to walk. Nor is a flexed wrist or elbow the reason why he is unable to use his hand functionally as the skilled hand function of patients with rheumatoid arthritis, despite similar loss of range of motion, clearly demonstrates. Careful assessment of the patient's problems as a whole must be carried out before expensive, painful and possibly deleterious surgery is performed.

Only after every attempt has been made to overcome the contracture(s) by positioning, guiding, mobilization of adverse tension in the nervous system, active movements and of course serial casting should definitive surgery be considered, except in the cases of patients whose contractures are already too extreme to be corrected by conservative measures and surgery would be the only alternative (Fig. 6.56).

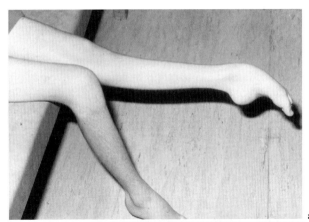

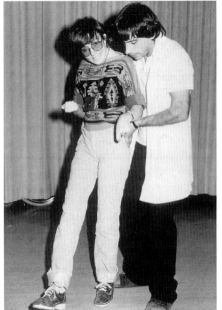

Fig. 6.56a. Foot deformity too severe for correction by conservative means.
b Patient learning to walk after surgical correction. (Archive photos from slides)

Antispastic Drugs and Nerve Blocks

For the patient with severe hypertonus and/or contractures, drugs aimed at decreasing spasticity have little to offer because of their nonspecific effect. All tend to have a generally relaxing and rather too sedative effect on the patient and, as Landau (1988) so pragmatically points out, "there are no controlled studies to show that the CNS depressants provide improved motor behaviour even when the tonic and phasic stretch reflexes are decreased. Since dantrolene weakens all the striated muscles at once, the musculature is impaired equally for purposeful behaviour as for hyperactive reflex responses. There are no controlled studies to support the idea that an afflicted patient treated with dantrolene benefits enough from weakened reflex contractions to gain a positive pay off in independent motor behaviour," and the same can be said of other antispasmolytic agents. Schlaegel (1993) reports that after complete cessation of heavy doses of all antispastic medication following admission to the centre, no patient showed a change in the degree of hypertonus, but in many there was an improvement in their level of consciousness.

Nerve and Motor Point Blocks

Landau appears to be equally unconvinced of the efficacy of differential blocks with local anaesthetic which suppress tendon jerks by raising the stretch receptor thresholds: "A similar block in patients who had both motor disability and hyperreflexia also suppressed the tendon jerks. But the impaired motor performance was *not* improved, even though hyperreflexia, the positive sign, was gone."

The use of phenol nerve and motor point blocks have become increasingly popular but should, however, be used only for specific, persistent problems which prove resistant to treatment and not as a routine procedure for all spastic symptoms. Petrillo and Knoploch (1988), for example, describe positive results after selective phenol blocks of the tibial nerve for spasticity, in a study involving 59 neurologically impaired patients: "This study demonstrates that phenol block was very effective in controlling spasticity of ankle plantar flexors, invertors and eliminating ankle clonus in all 59 patients, resulting in significant functional gains in the ambulatory as well as in the wheelchair dependent group. The procedure's effect was long-lasting in all patients and only 22 (37.2%) required a repeat block during the time of the study." The authors do not, however, specify exactly what the "significant functional gains" were, other than that surgery was prevented in 19 cases with previous indications and that gains in range of motion occurred in those patients with limitations prior to the procedure. Phenol does have the advantage of not causing permanent changes in conduction, but clinical observations have revealed untoward complications in certain cases, so that its use is not without some risk.

Because equally positive results can be gained by using the more meaningful activities described in Chaps. 3 and 4, it would seem logical to avoid measures which interfere with nerve conduction in patients who already have nervous system impairment. Irreversible resection of nerves should not be performed for the treatment of spasticity or contractures, as the procedure is unnecessary and no functional gain is achieved. The risks inherent in surgical procedures involving the stellate ganglion to overcome spastic contractures in the upper limbs as well as their destructible nature make such intervention unacceptable (Fig. 6.57).

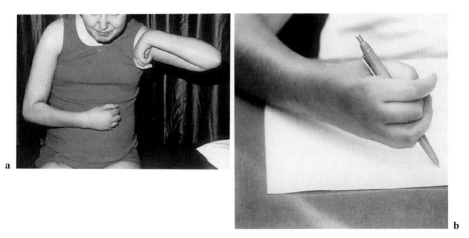

Fig. 6.57. a Shoulder abduction and elbow flexion contractures after surgical intervention to stellate ganglion for spasticity following head injury. **b** Despite good motor recovery elsewhere, upper limbs reveal spinal cord damage at C6 level. (Archive photos from slides)

Management of Fractures and Soft Tissue Injuries

Patients who have sustained a traumatic brain injury may well have sustained a fracture or some other musculoskeletal damage at the time of the accident. In combination with a brain lesion, these additional acutely painful conditions can easily lead to the development of contractures, particularly if they prevent the patient from being turned and positioned, moved and being sat out of bed or stood up with support. It is most important that they be treated with an eye to the future when it is hoped that the patient will be able to walk and use his hands functionally again.

Fractures

It is obvious that the sooner limb fractures are stabilized, the easier it will be to position and move the patient and for this reason internal fixation is the method of choice whenever possible. However, the patient's chance of a perfect end result should not be jeopardized because he is known to have a brain lesion or because routine nursing and physical therapy would be made easier. The management of the fracture should be the same as it would for any other young person who has a similar fracture but has no head injury and not be chosen solely to enable range of motion exercises to be performed. Mobilization of adverse mechanical tension in the nervous system through moving other parts of the body will help to reduce shortening of structures during the period of immobilization, and any loss of range of motion can be regained by means of intensive treatment once the fracture has united. Where internal fixation is equally appropriate, it will naturally facilitate nursing and therapeutic activities.

The fracture should never be left untreated "to heal on its own", based on the assumption that the patient is in coma and not moving anyway, or that his arm or leg is paralyzed. Subsequent nonunion can be a tremendous handicap to both early and later rehabilitation.

A Case in Point

N.N., a tall well-built 50-year-old man, suffered a severe head injury in a road traffic accident and in addition sustained a fracture of his left humerus just above the elbow joint. His right leg required amputation approximately 12 cm below the hip. While slowly regaining consciousness, N.N. fell out of bed which resulted in a fractured neck of femur on the left. Neurological symptoms were those of a severe left hemiplegia. No measures were undertaken to stabilize the humeral fracture, possibly because of its proximity to the elbow joint and possibly because N.N.'s condition was so grave that there seemed little hope of any functional recovery.

Two years later, N.N. was admitted for intensive rehabilitation. The fractures were still ununited and he had no prosthetic appliance for his right lower limb. The therapist had to stabilize the humeral fracture manually to prevent a frightening and painful slide of the lower end of the humerus just beneath the skin, which meant that any attempts to move the heavy and severely disabled patient were all but impossible. Both he and the therapist were understandably nervous, and violent outbursts occurred if the fracture moved suddenly, causing intense pain. Shortening of the wrist and finger flexors had already developed, and passive lengthening against the spastic resistance moved the ends of the fracture so that no increase in range of motion could be achieved. In fact, with so many unresolved problems no real progress could be made at all and N.N. felt helpless and frustrated, as did the rehabilitation team,

After internal fixation of the humerus had been successfully performed, N.N. was able to participate enthusiastically in the rehabilitation programme and the therapists could use their hands to facilitate movement instead of having to hold the fracture in place all the time. Unfortunately, due to the long delay, N.N.'s hand and wrist continue to cause problems. The flexion contractures have still not been overcome completely, and much therapy time is required to maintain and increase range of motion. With so little stimulation of the left upper limb having been possible during the first 2 years, integrating the arm and hand in daily life activities and regaining voluntary control have proved difficult but both are slowly improving.

With early stabilization of the fractured humerus, such as would automatically have been undertaken for a patient without a concomitant head injury, N.N. would have been able to progress far more rapidly and would certainly have suffered far less. How this indomitable patient eventually learned to walk is described in Chap. 7.

Cervical Spine Injuries

Many patients sustain some sort of cervical injury at the time of their accident because, as Jull (1986) points out, "there are very few traumatic injuries to the head which cannot involve the cervical spine." Such injuries often pass unnoticed and may cause a great variety of symptoms, the commonest being headache and facial pain in various distributions. What may be wrongly interpreted as being a prolonged "post-concussional headache" is more likely to be a misdiagnosed cervical headache (Schultz and Semmes 1950; Knight 1963). Not only can the injuries involving the cervical region give rise to pain but they can also cause other disturbing symptoms such as visual problems including nystagmus, dizziness, nausea with vomiting, voice problems, numbness of tongue and lips, lack of concentration and even ataxia (Jull 1986). Injecting procaine into the neck muscles has even been shown to produce positional nystagmus and body disorientation in normal subjects (Bower 1986).

The upper cervical spine appears to be the commonest cause of symptoms, most frequently with involvement of C2/3 but also with atlanto-occipital or atlanto-axial joints (Trott 1986). Adaptive shortening of the suboccipital muscles is present, and clinical experiments have demonstrated that the upper cervical musculature can produce referred pain in the head to the extent that saline injected into these muscles actually induced pain in the occiput and forehead (Trott 1986).

Should a patient complain of persistent headache or face pain or in fact any other unexplained symptoms such as pain in the scapular region or down his arm, his cervical spine should be examined radiologically and carefully assessed by the therapist. The same applies to other disturbing symptoms which could possibly be due to cervical spine involvement. In order for the symptoms to be successfully treated it is most important that the actual cause of the problem be differentiated. The symptoms must not be considered under the umbrella diagnostic title of "thalamic pain" or "thalamic syndrome", since this diagnosis is both misleading and erroneous and tends to lead to therapeutic nihilism. The examination, which includes palpation, assessment and treatment as described by Maitland (1986) has proved to be particularly successful for differential diagnosis and in eliminating the pain and other symptoms.

Quite apart from cervical involvement as a result of the initial trauma, referred pain can be caused by sustained head postures, particularly lower cervical flexion with upper cervical extension (Lewit 1977). "Headaches will frequently be reproduced by upper cervical extension or the upper cervical quadrant, if the position is sustained" (Magarey 1986). Patients with brain damage who lie or sit for long periods with their head in extension, particularly if it is rotated to one side, may, therefore, also suffer severe headaches. The patient who is intubated and/or has undergone cranial surgery is clearly at risk because he may well have lain or lie in such a position for some hours. Later as the patient becomes more active, he may use his neck strongly to compensate for lack of selective control when standing, walking or moving his arms and the faulty movement patterns can lead to cervical problems (Janda 1980).

Treatment

Correction of the patient's position in bed and his habitual postures when sitting or standing will help to eliminate the symptoms, as will the re-education of more normal movement patterns. Techniques of passive mobilization of the cervical spine, according to the concept of Maitland (1986) are most beneficial, mobilization which the author himself describes as "gentle coaxing of a movement by passive rhythmic oscillations performed within or at the limit of the range."

Mobilization of adverse tension in the nervous system according to Butler (1991b) is most important, and Rolf (1993) advocates mobilizing the relevant nerves at their peripheral location in the vicinity of the pain, two common examples being the great occipital nerve and the branches of the facial nerve. The nerves are located by the palpating fingers of the therapist and then literally moved transversely across the underlying tissue with a movement similar to a deep friction. Trott (1986) recommends combining "deep massage to the thickened interlaminar soft tissue and to the thickened periarticular tissues (around the affected zygapophyseal joints) with passive movement techniques."

When there is tension or shortening of the suboccipital musculature, flexion of the upper cervical spine must be performed passively to mobilize the tight structures and must also be combined with extension of the lower cervical spine. The restoration of lateral flexion of the neck has been described in Chap. 3 in conjunction with mobilization of the nervous system.

Regaining full range of movement of the cervical spine is essential, not only with regard to alleviating such symptoms as referred pain and dizziness , but also because the neck plays such a vital role in maintaining balance: the cervical vertebral column is an important source of proprioceptive information when the body moves against gravity. Tone throughout the patient's body will also be increased by tonic reflex activity with his head and neck stiffened in abnormal positions.

Other Soft Tissue Injuries

Any other soft tissue injury or joint dislocation which occurs at the time of the initial trauma must be examined and treated in the most up-to-date way possible and with the same care as it would had the patient no neurological impairment. The same applies to injuries which are sustained at a later stage through the patient falling out of bed or in some other way.

Heterotopic Ossification

A most distressing complication which may occur after brain damage is the development of ectopic bone in the muscles and other soft tissues surrounding major joints. The ossification appears to be more prevalent in muscles which originate from large areas of bone. Such pathological bone formation has been described as occurring in approximately 10%–20% of the patients and is generally known as heterotopic ossification (HO) (Garland 1991). A far higher percentage was reported by Sazbon et al. (1981). In a study of widespread periarticular new bone formation in brain-damaged patients in long-term coma, including many with coma of nontraumatic origin, 36/45 (76.8%) were found to have myositis ossificans around at least one major joint. The term "myositis ossificans", which has been loosely used to refer to ectopic bone formation in a variety of situations, literally refers to heterotopic bone formation originating in muscle (Puzas et al. 1989).

The Appearance and Development of HO

Early signs indicating the development of HO usually appear when the patient has been in coma for about 4–8 weeks, but the ossification may appear for the first time much later if the duration of the coma is of a long-term nature. "The onset of HO, regardless of the aetiology, ranges from 4–6 weeks with a peak occurrence at 2 months. Occasionally HO may be detected prior to 3 weeks or after three months." (Garland 1991). Sazbon et al. found that the onset was within 7 months of coma in 90% of their patients, the earliest evidence being obtained after 1 month in 8.6% of the group. HO can develop in patients whose coma is the result of traumatic brain injury or is of nontraumatic origin (Rothmeier et al. 1990; An et al. 1987; Sazbon et al. 1981).

Clinically, the development of HO is characterized by the following:

- An unusual, rather sudden loss of range of passive motion which is usually noted by the physiotherapist prior to any other manifestations.
- Pain on movement indicated, if the patient is not able to speak, grimacing, agitation or other signs of distress such as increased cardiac or respiratory rate.
- Typically, localized swelling is noted, possibly with other signs of intense local inflammation such as erythema and warmth. The lower extremity oedema may mimic a deep vein thrombosis or thrombophlebitis and requires careful differential diagnosis (Ragone et al. 1986; Venier and Ditunno 1971).
- Spasticity is nearly always present in the involved limb. In fact, Garland et al. (1980) state that all patients with heterotopic bone demonstrated spasticity on arrival at their unit. An increase in spasticity or muscle guarding may be felt.
- Alkaline phosphatase levels are usually, but not always raised. "The majority of the patients who develop clinically significant HO have an elevated SAP [serum alkaline phosphatase]" (Garland 1991), but it has been pointed out by the same

author that although the level of serum alkaline phosphatase will usually be elevated, it can also be elevated in patients with healing fractures (Garland et al. 1980). Significantly, even in the presence of normal levels of serum alkaline phosphatase new bone formation has been shown to occur (Grüninger 1986).

- In cases where the ossification continues to develop, joint range becomes increasingly limited and ankylosis of the involved joint may follow, resulting in a complete or almost total loss of motion (Mital et al. 1987).
- Roentgenographs are normal during the manifestation of early symptoms but 2–3 weeks later reveal the onset of ossification in the proximity of the bones (Garland 1991; Garland and Keenan 1983). Further roentgenographic examination shows the development of massive new bone formation over a period of months.
- The bone is often palpable from without at certain sites and can, for instance, be clearly felt anterior to the hip, around the elbow and in the axilla.

The loss of range of motion caused by HO can be a handicap both to the rehabilitation and can prevent full functional use of the limbs should active movement return. Because the ultimate degree of recovery cannot be predicted and has not been found to correlate with the development of HO, prevention is of the utmost importance, particularly as treatment measures to reduce existing bone which is impeding range of movement have not proved very successful. "There is no known treatment that reduces this bone mass" (Puzas et al. 1989).

Once stabilization has occurred, surgical removal may be an effective help for a limited number of selected patients but following resection many others show a marked tendency for the heterotopic tissue to form again. For example, "if spasticity remains about a joint, the recurrence rate of HO is high and a significant gain in motion is uncommon" (Garland and Keenan 1983). However, resection of bone formation posterior to the elbow causing ankylosis was claimed to have successfully restored range of motion (Garland et al. 1985; Mital et al. 1987). Mital and coauthors also describe successful excision of ectopic bone without recurrence when oral salicylates were used as a prophylactic measure starting on the day following surgery. In the light of these findings, the authors suggest in addition that, "salicylate therapy may indeed prevent the progression of ectopic bone formation when given as soon as possible after the onset of the process as this may obviate the necessity for surgery later."

Because of the risks involved in surgery and the incidence of recurrence, such intervention should not be considered too early and then only when it is certain that a functional gain will be achieved as a result. It has, therefore, been emphasized that surgery should be delayed longer than 5 years if motor recovery is prolonged (Garland 1991). The decision to operate should only be taken when all the factors involved have been seriously considered and an evaluation made as to whether the hoped-for gains outweigh the inherent risks.

To prevent ectopic bone formation altogether, or at least minimize the extent of the ossification and the number of sites, clearly becomes an important aim for all who are involved in the treatment of the patient. Likewise, treatment measures to overcome the problems associated with the loss of range due to already existing HO without surgery are infinitely preferable. Prevention is dependent upon understanding the possible cause and precipitating factors involved.

Factors Which Could Cause or Precipitate the Development of HO

Unfortunately, as has been stated, "The aetiology of heterotopic ossification remains obscure" (Ragone et al. 1986) and, "In spite of numerous clinical and experimental studies, its pathogenesis is not fully understood" (Michelsson and Rausching 1983) or been explained satisfactorily (Rothmeier et al. 1990). When the various hypotheses which have been put forward to date are considered more closely, most are contradicted by the clinical findings:

It has, for example, been proposed that there is a genetic predisposition. Because the propensity for forming HO is highly variable between individuals, it is thought that some intrinsic factor, genetic or other must be present to account for the degree of variability. One argument which goes against the possibility, however, is the high percentage of monofocal occurrence of ossification. In a review of 496 adult patients who had sustained severe injuries to the head, clinically significant heterotopic bone was identified in 57 patients involving 100 joints. Twenty-seven of the patients (approximately 50%) had monoarticular involvement (Garland et al. 1980). Mital et al. report an even higher proportion: 17 of the 22 patients had unifocal ossification and only five had multifocal occurrence.

It would not seem feasible that a predisposing factor would affect only one joint in the body. Moreover, it has also been pointed out that "there appears to be a disproportionate incidence of bone formation in the proximal as compared to the distal extremities" (Puzas et al. 1989). HO following traumatic brain injury occurs almost exclusively at the hip, shoulder, knee and elbow and only very rarely at any other sites.

The high incidence of monoarticular occurrence in bilaterally impaired patients also refutes the suggestion that immobility can induce secondary vasomotor, metabolic and trophic changes which result in metaplastic bone formation (Mielants et al. 1975). For the same reason, it would seem likely that the elevated serum alkaline phosphatase levels present in the majority of cases must be a response to the pathological bone formation per se, or to whatever factor has been responsible for provoking the ossification, rather than a cause in itself.

Another common theory postulated is that the initial trauma was responsible for precipitating the development of HO, with any additional limb fractures increasing the risk. Such a theory can no longer be accepted. Too many instances of bone formation have been observed and reported in cases where coma was not the result of violent accident but followed anoxia, thrombosis, haemorrhage, or infectious processes for example.

Spasticity in itself cannot cause HO because such ossification has been known to occur in cases of flaccid paraplegia as well.

One more plausible hypothesis deserves careful attention because, even if it is only accepted as a partial explanation, it allows steps to be taken to prevent and limit the development of HO:

Repeated traumatization of previously immobilized soft tissues, particularly muscle, can cause HO.

The possibility that minor traumas occurring during passive range of motion exercises or nursing procedures could lead to the formation of HO has been much debated by those involved in the treatment of patients with either traumatic brain damage or spinal cord injury. The following points would seem to substantiate the hypothesis and deserve consideration in relation to the prevention of HO.

Loss of Protective Pain Responses

The occurrence of neurological HO is confined to those patients who, in addition to being paralyzed, are unable to perceive pain or, if they do, are unable to protest or take evasive action. The group of patients consists, therefore, of those with complete spinal cord lesions, those who are in coma and others who, as they regain consciousness, are not able to complain verbally, scream in protest or move actively to indicate that they are experiencing pain, or use muscular contraction to resist a painful movement.

For clinical purposes, Fields (1987) defines pain in the following way: "an unpleasant sensation that is perceived as arising from a specific region of the body and is commonly produced by processes which damage or are capable of damaging body tissues." He goes on to explain that,"a major function of the pain sensory system is to prevent injury" in that "noxious stimuli elicit a variety of behaviours that all serve to protect uninjured tissues." In addition, Fields suggests that, "because of its close linkage with injury-avoiding behaviours, it is useful to think of pain as a perceptual correlate of the protective responses elicited by noxious stimuli." Without the protection of pain, the patient with spinal cord transection is not aware of the damage to tissue, while the patient in coma either does not perceive the pain or if he does is unable to react to or avoid the noxious stimuli by using any of the injury-avoiding behaviours. Evidence that the presence of pain is a protection against the formation of HO is abundant:

Patients with other severe neurological conditions, but able to perceive pain, do not develop ossification so that it is not a problem associated with multiple sclerosis or cerebral palsy. Even in hemiplegia as a result of cerebro-vascular accident, no HO develops. The stroke patient, despite the loss of other sensory modalities, will always protest strongly if pain is caused when he is being moved in bed or during therapy sessions. Only in cases where an unusually long period of unconsciousness followed the initial stroke has any ossification been known to occur.

Although patients with spinal cord lesions are particularly prone to develop HO, it always occurs below the level of the lesion (Rush 1989). The ossification is, therefore not found in the upper extremities at locations where the sensation of pain is present. The tetraplegic patient with a lesion below the level of C5 does not, for example, have ossification at the elbow or shoulder, as he complains should passive movements or stretching procedures hurt him. On the other hand, ossification may occur in the fingers where sensation is not intact.

Significantly, once the brain-damaged patient has regained consciousness to the extent that he is able to protest sufficiently, there is no longer a risk that HO will start to develop. In no case was the onset of heterotopic ossification noted after the coma had ended (Mital et al. 1987).

Repeated Minor Traumatic Injuries

In patients without neurological involvement "heterotopic bone formation at sites subjected to a minor traumatic injury is rare. However, heterotopic bone formation at sites subjected to repeated minor trauma due to occupational or recreational activities is common" (Puzas et al. 1989). Bone formation after horse-riding, rifle shooting, fencing and dancing have frequently been reported (Conner 1983), and a young, healthy individual developed extensive ossification following a marathon run (V. Kesselring, personal communication). The initiating event in such cases has been attributed to ossification of the small, repeated haematomas that must inevitably occur.

Repeated Forcible Distention of Previously Immobilized Soft Tissues

A significant contribution to understanding the reason for the occurrence of HO in brain-damaged patients has been made through a study involving 216 adult rabbits with their limbs immobilized by means of plastic splints (Michelsson and Rausching 1983). The splint was removed daily for passive movements, which were performed with force if necessary, through the maximum range. The authors state that, "within two to five weeks, heterotopic cartilage and bone formation occurred in the soft tissues around the joint and in the area of the damaged muscle." Ossification occurred especially in muscle attachments to bone and the changes which progressed during two to three months resembled morphologically and roentgenologically human myositis ossificans.

Interestingly, the animals whose joints were immobilized in extension developed ossification in the extensor muscles and those immobilized in flexion in the flexors, which correlates with the formation of HO in head-injured adults for example, at the shoulder elbow and hip (Garland 1991; Garland and Keenan 1983; Garland et al. 1980). The combination of immobilization and passive range of motion must be the salient factor, because no bone formation occurred in the rabbits who had only splinting nor in those who underwent forcible passive exercises without the splints in the experimental study. It could be argued that the patient with brain injury is not generally immobilized in splints, but due to the paralysis and coma, with the limbs in one position for prolonged periods, he is in fact virtually immobilized.

For most patients, daily passive movements are routine and particularly in the presence of spasticity, can be relatively forceful. Spasticity has been noted to be a common factor in nearly all patients who develop HO and would serve to immobilize the limbs in either flexion or extension. Although comparatively rare, ossification has been observed in flaccid paralysis of the limbs following spinal cord lesions (Hernandez et al. 1978; Hardy and Dixon 1963), and in such cases the total inactivity of the limbs would constitute the immobilization.

Muscle Injury and Soreness Are Selectively Associated with Eccentric Contractions

Closely related to the correlation between spasticity and the incidence of HO and its location is the finding that with high tensions, "numerous investigators have demonstrated that when eccentric exercise is performed, muscle damage and soreness result." (Lieber 1992). Moreover, it has been found that "in isolated skeletal muscle, a muscle that is eccentrically activated generates more tension than a muscle that is isometrically activated." and that the muscle generated relatively high tensions even if only passively stretched, certainly more than those of an isometric contraction (Lieber 1992). Skeletal muscle actions associated with lengthening (eccentric) contractions are also associated with high muscle forces.

Evans et al. (1985) demonstrated that muscle damage due to eccentric contraction is delayed and prolonged. The finding that levels of the enzyme, creatinine kinase, following intensive eccentric exercise in normal subjects were elevated a few days following the exercise bout, peaked 5 days later and remained elevated for several days thereafter suggests that, "the muscles experience some type of injury that initiates a cascade of events culminating in fiber breakage" (Lieber 1992). Lieber postulates, on the basis of further studies, that "while mechanical injury may cause the initial injury, further injury may result from subsequent tissue inflammation." Mital et al. (1987) emphasize inflammation in relation to the formation of HO: "the one common feature that was noted at all sites of heterotopic ossification whether pretraumatized or not, was the presence of intense local inflammation before the onset and during the active phase of ectopic bone formation."

The prevalence of injuries occurring during eccentric activity can be likened to minor traumas being caused during passive movements to spastic limbs and so precipitating the development of HO. Just as the rabbit limbs would have resisted the passive exercises when the splints were removed, so the spasticity in the patients' limbs either in extension or flexion would do the same. In both cases the passive movements would have to overcome an eccentric contraction.

Describing the location of HO in brain-injured patients, the relationship between the predominant direction of pull of spastic muscles and the site of the ossification has been consistently emphasized. In accordance with the spastic pattern of flexion in the upper extremity, whereby the shoulder is adducted and inwardly rotated, "in all patients the location of the bone formation was inferomedial to the glenohumeral joint" and at the elbow, "six patients had HO anterior to the joint, associated with flexor spasticity" (Garland and Keenan 1983). In contrast, HO posterior to the elbow usually occurs when there is extensor rigidity (Garland 1991).

At the hip, the commonest site for HO, the bone frequently develops in the adductor region in conjunction with adductor spasticity and in the hip flexors when a flexion pattern is present. Extensor spasticity at the knee is a common problem particularly in the acute phase and ossification can occur in the quadriceps, limiting knee flexion considerably.

HO Occurs Almost Exclusively in the Vicinity of Proximal Joints

Regardless of the aetiology, "there appears to be a disproportionate incidence of bone formation in the proximal compared to the distal extremities" (Puzas et al. 1989), a fact which has as yet not been explained. Garland (1991) asks the pertinent question, "Why are only proximal joints involved?" If repeated minor traumas are accepted as playing a major role in the development of HO, two factors could be responsible for the predominance of proximal sites of ossification in neurological patients. Firstly, the muscles acting on the proximal joints arise from large areas of bone and the extent of their bony origins and insertions could be a precipitating factor. Secondly, and perhaps the more likely reason is that the length of the lever arms of the limbs disguises the fact that a great deal of force is being applied to the joint and surrounding tissues during passive moving. The mechanical advantage created by the long lever could lead to an underestimation of the amount of leverage or power at the fulcrum.

Ossification, therefore does not occur in the gastrocnemius or soleus muscles because the short lever provided by the foot makes overstretching of spastic calf muscles all but impossible. The hip, on the other hand, with its high incidence of HO, allows a therapist or nurse to inadvertently exert great force at the fulcrum when moving the long lever of the patient's leg. The nurse, for example, in order to insert a urinary catheter may abduct the comatose patient's legs without realizing the amount of mechanical advantage she has when with her hands on his thighs she presses them apart. The therapist performing passive movements uses her body weight automatically to maintain range of abduction with her hands placed over the medial aspect of the patient's knee and ankle or when she performs a straight leg raise to lengthen his hamstrings. The shoulder may be overzealously moved in an attempt to prevent any painful stiffening, without adequate support for the glenohumeral joint or concomitant scapula rotation (Davies 1985). Tissue could be damaged in this way during physiotherapy or during nursing procedures, and the risk appears to be increased if there is hypertonus in the adductors and internal rotators of the shoulder. At the elbow, anterior ossification could be precipitated when the forearm is used as a lever. The lever effect is greater if the upper arm is supported on the bed when the therapist or nurse pushes the patient's hand down in order to straighten his elbow against the strong pull of the flexors, perhaps to maintain range of motion, measure blood pressure, or insert an intravenous drip or even when she is trying to replace the arm in a resting splint.

It is easy to imagine the minor traumas which could occur in these instances and, as has been suggested by Ragone et al. (1986), "another possible explanation for the occurrence of heterotopic ossification and haematoma could be the repeated traumatization to the same muscle groups from the aggressive physical therapy in the form of passive joint manipulation and stretching exercises against extensor spasms. In this theory trauma causes bleeding into the area, triggering post-traumatic inflammatory changes within the muscles and surrounding connective tissue and resulting in the eventual replacement by bone." The long levers of the arm and leg could easily lead to minor traumas being sustained proximally, not only during physiotherapy but also when the unconscious patient is being turned, positioned, washed or moved up and down the bed, without the protection of a pain response or active motor control.

Other Risk Factors Associated with HO

Some additional factors are said to be associated with an increased risk of HO development such as pressure sores and the open reduction and fixation of fractures, particularly of the forearm or femur. It has also been suggested that local injury sustained at the time of the initial trauma could be implicated and that forcible manipulation of the contracted elbow could initiate the process.

Considerations for the Prevention of HO

Many are still doubtful that minor traumas following immobilization can be a cause of HO, and the possibility continues to be debated: "Whether passive range of motion to the limbs acts in a prophylactic manner or increases the predisposition to the development of heterotopic ossification is debatable." (Lynch et al. 1981). In a study of widespread periarticular new bone formation in long-term comatose patients, Sazbon et al. (1981) emphatically deny that physiotherapy can be a cause but with no convincing evidence to support their claim, only stating that, "physiotherapy which included passive movements and use of the tilt board was identical for all the patients. Therefore, there was no connection between the type of physiotherapy and the development of myositis ossificans."

Such an argument cannot be accepted, however, because, although the same treatment modalities may well have been used, the physiotherapy itself could not have been identical for each patient. For instance, it seems unlikely that the same therapist treated such a large number of patients single-handed during the long period, and, even had she done so, her therapy would not have been exactly the same for each of them or even on different days. In the event that more than one therapist performed the treatment, as anyone who has personally experienced physiotherapy will agree, there is a considerable difference in the way individual therapists handle joints and limbs or apply any form of manual treatment. The "passive movements" performed by different therapists would in themselves have constituted a variable not to mention whatever activities were included within the term "use of the tilt board." Rather than denying all possibility that certain physiotherapy could precipitate or even be a cause of HO, it should at least be considered that range of motion exercises might be a contributing factor, if not necessarily a direct cause, as suggested by Stover et al. (1975).

Of all the hypotheses which have been put forward as to the cause of HO, only one makes it possible for preventative measures to be taken, namely, that minor traumas initiate the development of the ossification when the patient has no protective pain response or injury-avoiding behaviour. Although evidence in support of the hypothesis is not conclusive as yet, it appears convincing, and at least this significant risk factor can be eliminated by adapting therapeutic and nursing procedures accordingly. In view of the grave consequences of HO in addition to the neurological impairment, even minimizing its occurrence and extent or reducing its precipitation become important.

Preventative Measures

Positioning
With regular turning and correct positioning, spasticity is greatly reduced and the development of pressure sores prevented. Thus two significant, known risk factors are eliminated. Including prone lying as soon as artificial ventilation is no longer required will avoid flexion contractures of the hips, thus reducing the likelihood of HO developing on their anterior aspect. The prone position also relieves pressure from the most common sites for decubitus formation. Avoiding the supine position will help to inhibit extensor spasticity.

No force should be used to obtain the desired position. Should too much resistance be met, it is advisable to leave the limbs in a flexed position rather than to risk causing damage to tissues by forceful correction of the limb posture. Further adjustment is usually possible later when the patient has relaxed in the new position.

Sitting the patient out of bed in a wheelchair regularly reduces spasticity and thus the prolonged stereotyped postures of the limbs. It is extremely rare to find HO in patients who have been sat out of bed while still unconscious and stood early with the help of knee-extension splints.

Turning
The patient is turned every 2 h for optimal reduction of spasticity and decubitus prevention. At least two nurses are required to turn the comatose adult if all danger of traumatizing his limbs is to be eliminated. If one person attempts to carry out the change of position on her own, the patient's arm or leg may easily fall or be pulled into extreme range of motion resulting in minor trauma. It is short-sighted to try and save time or avoid disturbing others by turning the patient unaided because, although it might seem possible, at some stage an unexpected movement could suddenly occur and cause injury.

When the patient is being turned his limbs should be flexed in order to shorten the lever-arms and then gradually eased into the corrected position once he is lying on his side.

Transferring the Patient

When transferring the patient out of bed, one of the methods described in Chap. 2 is used to avoid any injury to his shoulders and elbows. If the nurse or therapist has the slightest doubt about managing on her own, an assistant should help with the transfer, or at least stand at the ready in case help is needed. On no account should the patient be lifted from beneath his shoulders or be pulled by his hands as he is moved into the wheelchair and his position corrected, or when he is being helped onto the toilet or back into bed again. The nurses back will also be protected by the use of the recommended transfers.

Other Nursing Procedures

Certain nursing procedures become particularly difficult to perform when spasticity is an added complication. Inserting a urinary catheter or cleaning the incontinent patient both require that his legs are abducted and then held in position. To avoid traumatizing the abductors, which are a common site for HO, it may be necessary for the therapist to inhibit spasticity before the legs can be safely drawn apart. Close cooperation between the nurse and therapist is essential to facilitate the timing and execution of the procedure. In the event of the patient's legs being hypotonic, extreme abduction may result if they fall apart, and pillows must be placed to avoid possible traumatization in such an end of range position.

The vulnerable, flexed elbow should be treated with the utmost care when being straightened to measure blood pressure or to be used as the site for an intravenous infusion. Whenever possible another part of the body should be chosen instead. Fluid escaping from an infusion at the elbow and causing inflammation could be an added precipitating factor for the development of HO.

Passive Movements of the Limbs

As long as the patient is in coma and unable to signify discomfort or pain, passive movements should be performed with extreme caution through a reduced range of motion. The therapist does not move the patient's limbs into extreme ranges at all but instead supports the arm or leg totally and stays well within a safe range. She repeats each movement several times to enhance circulation and maintain tissue mobility and adaptive lengthening of the nervous system. The hip, knee and shoulder are not moved into full flexion but only flexed to approximately 90 each time. The therapist can, however, strive to achieve full dorsiflexion of the foot each day, as there is not the same danger of trauma in that region.

The elbow on the other hand is extremely vulnerable and should not be forced into extension against a resistance caused either by flexor spasticity or protective holding activity on the part of the patient. Because of the elbow's peculiar susceptibility to myositis ossificans, if the therapist is experiencing too much difficulty in achieving full extension, the arm should be placed in a circular plaster cast for a few days prophylactically. HO in the vicinity of the elbow can be particularly disabling due to the loss of flexion which often follows its formation.

Dorsal extension of the wrist hand and fingers can be maintained with passive stretching, but on no account should the wrist and fingers be flexed simultaneously because the finger extensors as they cross the dorsum of the hand can easily be

traumatized. Inadvertent overstretching could be responsible for precipitating ossification at their phalangeal insertions.

The importance of performing passive movements vigorously and through a full
range of motion has been greatly emphasized in the treatment of neurological
patients, both in the literature and in physiotherapy training schools. Therapists, therefore, often feel obliged to fulfil the well-learned aim at all costs in their
efforts to help the patient. However, the premise needs to be rethought in the light
of present-day knowledge and the possible dangers involved.

A predisposing factor leading to the development of HO could well be the
genetic variation in premorbid joint range and tissue mobility, with the therapist
not able to know the patient's individual mechanical possibilities. In the absence of
any pain response, the therapist is unable to gauge the comfortable and safe range
of motion, particularly in the presence of spasticity. An explanation for monofocal
occurrence of HO could be the relative limitation of mechanical range in one location as compared to others. Multifocal sites could be the result of generalized lack
of mobility in joints and/or other tissues.

Where passive movements have been performed in a markedly reduced range in
accordance with this supposition, for example with hip flexion only to 90, a significant reduction in the incidence of HO has been noted. Interestingly, the reduced
range of passive movements did not, as had been expected, lead to an increased
danger of contractures. It should in any event be remembered that a slight loss of
mobility, should it occur, can be overcome later, but ossification can cause permanent limitation of joint range or even ankylosis.

Using the Proximal Lever Arm for Passive Movements. By using the proximal
lever-arm to perform passive movements instead of lifting the limbs from the distal
extremity, the latent force which might be exerted on the joints is reduced and the
tension within the nervous system serves as a protection. Range of motion at the
shoulder or hip can be achieved by moving the patient's trunk instead of lifting his
arm or leg, so that the joints are mobilized but the danger of trauma minimized, for
example, moving the patient's trunk forwards in long sitting rather than performing
repeated straight leg raises, or moving his trunk increasingly far backwards in side
lying with his extended arm in 90 abduction rather than lifting his hand and taking
it out sideways.

Standing the patient with his knees held in extension by back slabs will reduce
spasticity and maintain range of motion in the lower limbs and is a good starting
position, for moving his trunk proximally to mobilize distal structures. Careful
monitoring of all indications of pain and overstretching will help to guide the
therapist when she is moving the comatose patient and provide additional protection. She should be constantly on the alert for indicators such as change in blood
pressure, heart rate or respiratory rhythm as well as for increased sweating or
sudden reflex spasms.

Passive Movements After Serial Casting. With regard to passive range of motion
exercising, particular care must be taken when mobilizing the patient who has
undergone serial casting to overcome contractures. Passive movements into

flexion are avoided completely until all signs of oedema and inflammation have disappeared.

Management of Fractures and Soft Tissue Injuries

Surgical reduction and internal fixation of fractures are recognized as being increased risk factors for HO formation. Limbs which have required surgical intervention must, therefore, be handled with extreme care, with passive movements to the nearest joint(s) being omitted until postoperative swelling and acute inflammation have resolved. Similarly, inflammation due to soft tissue injuries suffered at the time of the accident should be a contraindication to full range passive movements. It is preferable to support the part in an optimal position and only commence passive movements to those joints in the immediate vicinity of the injury when signs of acute inflammation have disappeared.

In both instances, by moving the patient proximally, range of motion can be maintained and the danger of causing further inflammation avoided. The proximal movements and correct positioning combined with mobilization of adverse neural tension proximally as well as distal to the injury site will suffice to prevent serious contractures from developing.

Overcoming the Problems of Existing HO

Should HO unfortunately have developed to the extent that range of motion is markedly limited, the patient will have to contend with additional problems which the therapist must help him to overcome through appropriate treatment. The presence of HO is, however, very seldom the reason why a patient is unable to perform a task or a movement sequence, as is often automatically assumed. In reality, any such failures are more likely to be the result of disturbed perception. The rehabilitation team should always bear in mind that, even with a total loss of joint motion, an otherwise healthy individual can move and function remarkably well as the following example clearly illustrates. A postgraduate course on human kinetics was held in Switzerland for doctors, physiotherapists and occupational therapists. One of the participants, an occupational therapist, had a total arthrodesis of one hip as the result of a childhood ailment. Neither the instructor and her assistants nor the other participants noticed the therapist's disability although the course was a practical one which involved detailed observation and assessment of normal movement. It was only in the second week, when the students were required to analyze the movements involved in sitting on a gymnastic ball, that the arthrodesed hip was discovered, due to the compensatory measures adopted by the occupational therapist. The same therapist was later a participant on another course where no one knew about her hip problem. Once again she passed unnoticed until, during the analysis of gait some slight variance was noted and discussed. Knee flexion at the initiation of the swing phase appeared to be exaggerated which caused some mystification until the occupational therapist herself explained what the reason was.

As can be seen from the example above, a normal human being who was able to use alternative movements to compensate for loss of movement at a major joint could move freely and easily without being noticed, was totally independent in the activities of daily living and was capable of carrying out her duties as a practising occupational therapist. For the others on the course it turned out to be a most enlightening and learning experience, one which they will be unlikely to forget.

With the analogy born in mind, treatment of the patient with HO limiting movement at a certain joint should aim at improving cognitive function while mobilizing all other parts of his body so that he too can compensate for the restricted range of motion as the occupational therapist did.

Treatment Measures

During the active stage of HO, the therapist does not attempt to mobilize the involved joint or joints directly, since this could cause further inflammation or trauma and so increase the amount of bone formation. Instead she concentrates on attaining maximum mobility in other parts of the patient's body, especially those which he could later use to compensate for any limitation of movement resulting from the ossification. Mobilization of the lumbar spine will allow compensation for a stiffened hip, and a fully mobile thoracic spine together with a freely moving scapula enables the arm and hand to be brought into functional positions despite limited range of movement at the shoulder.

When the patient has regained consciousness sufficiently to participate more actively in the treatment, movements of his trunk in lying, sitting and standing will inhibit spasticity, mobilize soft tissues and so allow further range of motion in the part restricted by HO. Garland et al. (1983) found that, "23 of 28 joints had an increase in joint arc of motion under anaesthesia", evidence that the HO itself is not the sole reason for the loss of range. Marked adverse mechanical tension in the nervous system is one of the factors which causes the most limitation, and mobilization of both the horizontal and vertical structures of the nervous system will increase the patient's general mobility. Standing, walking and active movement will all help the patient to regain functional range of motion and sometimes even lead to diminution or disappearance of the HO. The disappearance of ossification has been reported in as many as 36% of cases studied with a long-term follow-up period (Thorndike 1940).

Perceptual disturbances, particularly those affecting the tactile/kinaesthetic systems, are the main reason for patients with traumatic brain injury being unable to perform the activities of daily life or functional movements and not the presence of HO with decreased range of motion. Typically, even without HO at the hip, patients who have severe brain damage with spastic tetraplegia will resist being brought forward in sitting and push back strongly in extension so that the difficulty should not be attributed to evidence of ossification. The same patient group has been reported as having a higher incidence of HO: "A patient with spastic quadriplegia secondary to injury to the brain stem is particularly prone to the development of heterotopic ossification and involvement of multiple joints" (Garland et al. 1985). By taking into account the perceptual disturbances and applying the principles of

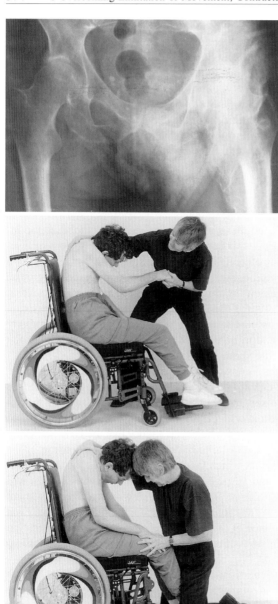

a

b

c

Fig. 6.58a–e. Perceptual problems, not HO, prevent the trunk moving forward in sitting. **a** Hip X-ray showing extensive HO. **b** Patient resisting forward flexion. Resistance decreasing steadily with. **c** Therapist kneeling in front of him. **d** A table beneath his arms. **e** A guided task

treatment described in Chap. 1, the therapist will be more successful in overcoming the problems as demonstrated in the following typical example:

A patient who had sustained a traumatic brain injury 7 months previously has extensive HO at the hip with grossly limited range of motion as a result (Fig. 6.58a). The therapist has difficulty in bringing the patient's trunk forwards in order to adjust his position in the wheelchair or in preparation for standing him up. With only an empty space in front of him, she encounters a massive resistance which she is unable to overcome (Fig. 6.58b). Because of the extensive ossification revealed on X-ray, it could easily be thought that the resultant loss of hip flexion was the cause of the problem, effectively blocking the forward movement of the trunk. When the therapist kneels in front of the patient, close up against his legs, the resistance becomes less marked and she is able to draw his trunk further forward (Fig. 6.58c). As soon as a solid table has been placed in front of him and his arms

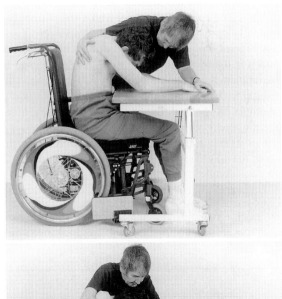

d

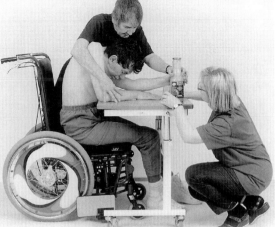

Fig. 6.58d,e

e

supported on it, the therapist can move the patient forwards without having to use any force (Fig. 6.58d). By guiding the patient's hands to perform an actual task which requires reaching forward even less resistance is felt and the strong push back into extension disappears and increased hip and trunk flexion becomes possible (Fig. 6.58e).

Bringing the patient's hands to his face and mouth with his elbows supported on the table also facilitates the movement forwards without resistance (Fig. 6.59).

If the patient lies supine in bed for long periods and sits in a wheelchair without a table in front of him he will constantly push against the supporting surface behind him and so reinforce the problem. Lying prone regularly will change the situation when he is in bed and his relatives should be taught how to achieve the forward movement and position of his trunk whenever he is sitting in a chair (Fig. 6.60a). Within a surprisingly short time the position becomes possible and can be maintained (Fig. 6.60b). While seated at the table, the patient can be guided to perform other activities which provide appropriate stimulation during therapy sessions and if his relatives do the same at other time progress will be enhanced.

The complexity of the tasks which the patient performs while being guided is gradually increased and, as cognition improves so will his ability to compensate for loss of joint mobility. Weight-bearing activities in standing should always be included in the treatment programme, as they appear to encourage resolution of the ossification and suitable problem-solving tasks can be presented with guiding being introduced while the patient is in the upright position. Because no medical treatment has been shown to remove HO or even diminish the extent of the ossification, and both manipulation under anaesthetic and surgical resection run the risk of its recurrence with a possible increase in the amount of bone, treatment along the lines described should be assiduously carried out before alternatives are considered.

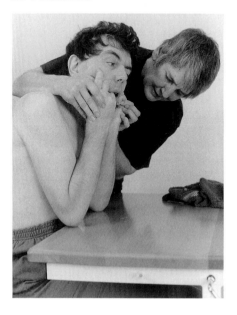

Fig. 6.59. Bringing the patient's hands to his face with his elbows supported on a table

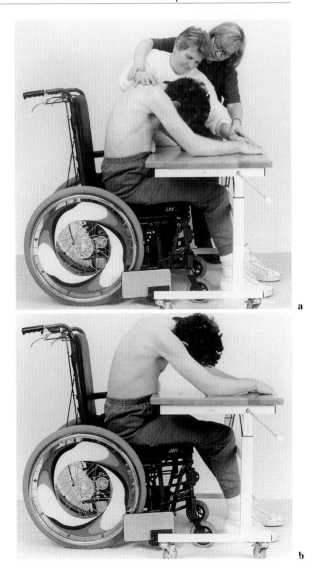

Fig. 6.60a. Patient's mother learning to assist forward movement of his trunk. **b** Able to maintain the correct position on his own

A Case in Point

F.D., a beautiful young mother of two, suffered a severe brain injury in a motor vehicle accident and was in coma for a long period. Marked monofocal HO developed at her right hip (Fig. 6.61a). Surgical resection of the bone formation did not improve function but left a distressing scar on the anterior aspect of her thigh. She continued to sit with her hips too extended and there was a marked kyphosis (Fig. 6.61b). Pressure areas could be observed over her lumbar spine, caused

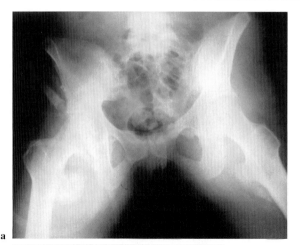

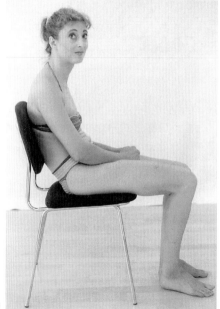

Fig. 6.61a. Monofocal HO at the right hip. **b** Patient still sitting with her hips too extended after surgical resection of HO

by her pressing against the backrest of the wheelchair. After 2 years of such sustained trunk flexion, she was unable to extend her spine actively and the compensatory extension of her neck added to both her eating problems and voice production. So strongly did F.D. push backwards in sitting, that her chair was often in danger of tipping over and had to be held in place by whoever was with her at the time. Walking was not successful, because when trying to stand up or return to sitting F.D. lost her balance completely because the strong extension of her hips and knees made it impossible for her to keep her weight forward over her

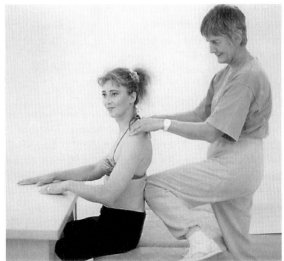

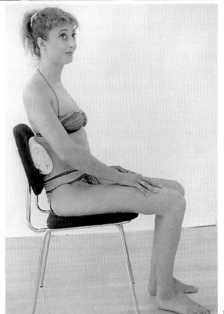

Fig. 6.62a. Posture improved with table placed in front of patient. **b** Sitting position corrected

feet. By the end of the third year, with the help of intensive therapy following the principles described, F.D. learned to extend her trunk actively and bring her weight forward in sitting and when coming to standing. Passive extension of her spine was mobilized in sitting with a table in front of her and then active, selective extension practised diligently (Fig. 6.62a). With her sitting posture able to be corrected, both her ability to produce a voice and eating improved considerably (Fig. 6.62b), F.D. learned to stand up and sit down again safely with her weight well forward and walk alone pushing a rollator. She later progressed to walking with the aid of two elbow crutches and stand-by assistance which enabled her to enjoy going out to dinner in a restaurant with her family.

HO Causing Loss of Elbow Flexion

HO at the elbow, both posteriorly and anteriorly, tends to block flexion mechanically, and thus cause particular problems. Whereas compensation for loss of range at the shoulder and hip is possible, there is no alternative movement which can be used to compensate for a total loss of flexion at the elbow. Functional use of the hand for many activities of daily living such as washing, eating, shaving or applying make-up is, therefore, impossible, except with the help of cumbersome, long-handled tools. If only one of the patient's elbows is affected, the handicap is not as great in terms of regaining independence in daily life as he can adapt to using the other hand for those activities which require flexion of the elbow beyond a right angle. (An elbow which cannot extend fully does not cause difficulties in the performance of functional activities and is in fact of little consequence to the patient except perhaps with regard to its appearance.)

Once it has been ascertained that a patient, after regaining voluntary movement in his arms and hands, is unable to perform some specific task because of the loss of elbow flexion, resection of the ossification could well be the only solution. The use of long-handled implements for tasks for which elbow flexion is essential, will help to establish whether the difficulties are due to the limitation of joint range or perceptual disorders. When only one of the patient's elbows is affected, surgical intervention is not usually essential but if he is unable to flex either elbow and could otherwise use his hands functionally, there would seem to be no alternative to resection.

Conclusion

However grave the patient's condition may appear to be, every effort must be made to prevent the development of contracture and deformity which can cause so much additional suffering and stand in the way of recovery and the attainment of independence. Although preventative measures may appear to be time-consuming, demanding and expensive, they are in no way more so than measures to overcome the problems once they have arisen.

Each and every patient deserves the chance to move freely again and without the burden of pain, so that in the event of contractures having already developed they must be overcome and a new start made. Far beyond the practical issues of rehabilitation, it would be morally untenable to leave young people imprisoned by deformity and pain, without hope of escape, and not take action because, as Maier (1988) realized, "the opposite of love isn't hate. It's indifference." Even if the

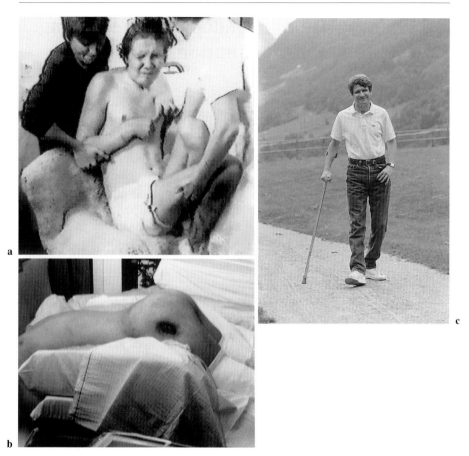

Fig. 6.63a. T.B. with all four limbs terribly contracted. **b** Prone lying commenced and serial casting of knees. (Archive photos from video films). **c** Able to enjoy walking again

contractures are long-standing and his condition appears to offer no hope of recovery, the patient must be treated in a positive way. No effort must be spared, because the results may be surprising and a fulfilling life made possible for him. T.B., whose case history is described in Chap. 2 as "*A case in point*", is just one outstanding example:

There seemed little hope that T.B. would ever be able to walk, use his hands or enjoy life again when he first arrived in a rehabilitation centre more than 9 months after his accident, still unable to move at all on his own and with all four of his limbs terribly contracted (Fig. 6.63a). After serial casting and intensive treatment such as has been described in this chapter (Fig. 6.63b) and those preceding it, T.B. not only regained his independence, but after a long and hard period of rehabilitation, was eventually able to date, dance and drive again and go for long walks in the country (Fig. 6.63c).

7 Towards Attaining Independent Walking: Preparation and Facilitation

To be able to walk again is the dream of every patient and the ability which his relatives so hope he will regain one day. Walking has been described as "the crowning glory of human bodily locomotion" (Morris 1987), a description which makes the importance of the patient's learning to walk again easy to understand. From a very early age the normal baby can be observed striving determinedly to attain the goal as he pulls himself up onto his feet continuously and demands to walk with his parents. Walking is, however, an immensely complex process and, as Morris writes, "so complicated, in fact, that muscle experts are still arguing today over the finer points of how it operates, and how we manage to stride along so successfully." Studies have shown that a child only achieves a completely adult walking pattern when it is about 7 years old (Okamato 1973), up to which time it has repeated 3 million steps to reach that level of performance (Kottke et al. 1978). It is not surprising, therefore, that for the patient with brain damage it may take a considerable time to regain the function and require long periods of intensive treatment.

Because the mechanical action is so complex, walking cannot be relearned by practising the walking itself or by the patient being marched round supported between two helpers. In the same way, playing a musical instrument cannot be improved by simply practising the set pieces day after day, but requires diligent practice of scales and various techniques for any real progress to be made.

Considerations for Treatment

For the patient to walk safely and functionally, the following will need to be made possible through appropriate treatment:

- Balance reactions
- Selective movements of the lower limbs
- Selective activity of the trunk
- Walking in conjunction with task performance

Treatment to achieve these therapeutic aims will vary according to the individual patient and his problems. Some will do better walking with facilitation at an early stage, others will require a step by step progression of specific activities while another group will need walking combined with problem-solving tasks which can be guided by the therapist. Analytical observation during actual attempts will guide the therapist as to which is the most applicable for the individual patient at his momentary stage of progression; it will also help her to decide whether the patient is ready to start walking, and what type of assistance or mechanical aid he requires.

When to Start Walking

The decision to start walking with the patient can be a difficult one for all concerned as it is so individual and depends upon a variety of factors. Certain guidelines can, however, help the therapist to make the decision and avoid unsuccessful attempts:

- Walking the patient must be possible without an excessive amount of manual support being required from those helping him. There is no point in risking injuries to either the therapist's back as she struggles to hold him upright, or to the patient should he fall because the therapist is physically unable to prevent it (Fig. 7.1). Even though a strong helper may feel capable of prevent-

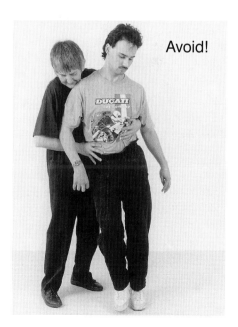

Avoid!

Fig. 7.1. Therapist scarcely able to prevent an ataxic patient from falling

ing an accident, being walked like a marionette will not enable the patient to learn to perform the movements on his own.

- The patient can be helped to walk if, with appropriate support, neither grossly abnormal movements and postures nor a marked increase in spasticity occur. Walking will then serve to stimulate normal motor activity and will also be of enormous psychological benefit to the patient who will cooperate fully as he understands the goal and what is expected of him. His relatives will be equally encouraged and, if at all feasible, should be shown how they too can facilitate walking at other times during the day.
- If the patient's knee is constantly hyperextended during the stance phase, walking should not be practised until the problem has been eliminated, either by using a different facilitation or by the retraining of selective movements (Fig. 7.2). Through walking with his knee or knees always hyperextended, an abnormal movement pattern, which will be difficult to change later, is learned by repetition and the correct muscles will not be activated (Kottke 1982a,b). As Bach-y-Rita and Balliet (1987) warn, "If unchecked, improper motor control can become a highly reinforced program". In addition the hyperextension leads to a self-reinforcing increase in plantarflexion: since the foot is never dorsiflexed during weight-bearing, the patient might require a footbrace later or even lengthening procedures for a shortened Achilles tendon. Because his knee is pushed backwards at the beginning of the stance phase, the patient's weight cannot be brought over his foot, which remains plantarflexed (Bobath

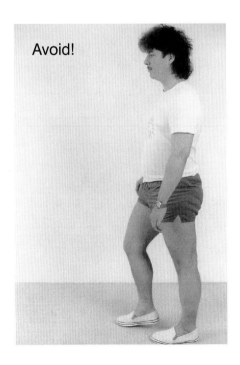

Fig. 7.2. Walking with knee constantly hyperextended

1990; Davies 1990). His hip joint moves back instead of always forwards in the direction of the movement as it would during normal gait (Klein-Vogelbach 1987). Knee flexion to initiate the subsequent swing phase is greatly hampered and the patient will tend to circumduct his stiffly extended leg with his pelvis lifted on that side in order to make a slow, effortful step. Quick automatic steps to regain balance are thus prevented, and the patient will not be able to climb stairs in a normal, economic way with only one foot on each step.

- Should a patient be thrown into panic each time walking is attempted despite the help and encouragement of the therapist, then he should not be forced to proceed or chastised for his lack of courage, even though it may appear that his motor power is adequate. Disturbed perception, which is invariably the cause of the problem, can make walking a most terrifying experience for the patient (Fig. 7.3). It could be likened to someone trying to walk across a lake covered by a thin layer of ice which is constantly shifting and in danger of breaking, or balancing on a narrow plank, ten floors above street level, in order to reach the next building. Practising walking in isolation will only reinforce the patient's panic and often lead to aggressive and possibly violent outbursts.

During walking attempts, symptoms such as bouts of dizziness and nausea may also arise as the response to the discordant motion cues (Benson 1984) received by the patient with sensory disturbances. The problems of panic or dizziness do not disappear with time alone, in fact they tend to intensify the longer the period in a wheelchair continues. The only way to help such patients to walk without being afraid is to incorporate goal-orientated activities during walking and continue to improve their perception through the treatment described in Chap. 1.

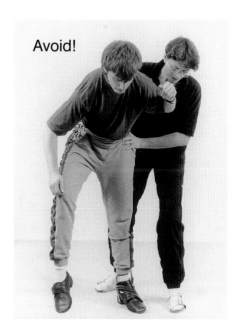

Avoid!

Fig. 7.3. With disturbed perception, walking can be a terrifying experience

A Case in Point

M.C. had received conventional rehabilitation for a period of 9 months after sustaining a traumatic brain injury in a road traffic accident. Although his condition had improved, his unsociable behaviour continued to be a grave problem, his ability to perform the activities of daily living remained limited, and it seemed that independent walking would be impossible for him to achieve. Any attempts at gait training caused total panic which resulted in either verbal obscenities or physical violence, and no progress was being made at all (see Fig. 7.3). It was decided that the only answer for M.C. was permanent placement in a long-term psychiatric institution. Fortunately for the young patient, admission to a centre specializing in the rehabilitation of severely brain damaged patients became possible at the eleventh hour and it was decided to give him a last chance. Within a relatively short time, M.C.'s condition improved remarkably after the treatment as described in Chap. 1 had been initiated to overcome his perceptual difficulties. Gait training as such was combined with problem-solving tasks which required walking for their successful resolution and any panic reactions thus avoided (see Fig. 1.21a,b).

M.C. progressed rapidly to walking independently with the aid of two elbow crutches at a reasonable pace (Fig. 7.4). He also learned to negotiate stairs without difficulty, one foot after another (Fig. 7.5) and, perhaps most important of all, his behaviour changed completely. He is now most cooperative, reasonable and willing to help in any way possible as well as able to behave appropriately in

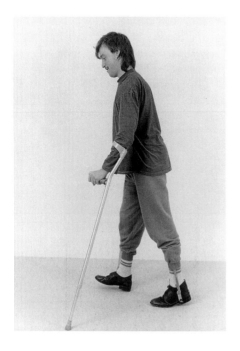

Fig. 7.4. After appropriate treatment, M.C. able to walk confidently with two crutches (Compare with Fig. 7.3)

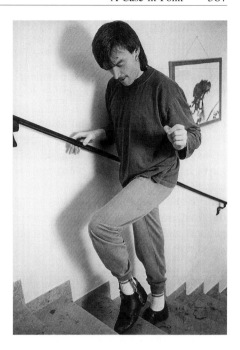

Fig. 7.5. M.C. climbing stairs in a normal pattern

most situations with charm. All members of staff enjoyed working with M.C. until his discharge from the centre to return home and hopefully to succeed in a work-retraining scheme. It would indeed have been a great pity if this hard-working and likeable young man had been transferred to a psychiatric home instead and so missed the chance to enjoy life again in a more fulfilling way (Fig. 7.6).

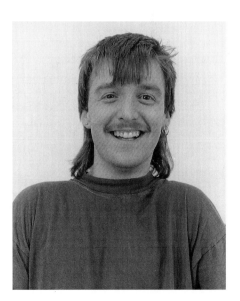

Fig. 7.6. A chance for M.C. to enjoy life again

Preparatory Activities

Appropriate activities can help patients to regain the ability to walk or improve their gait pattern if they are already walking. The therapist assesses the individual patient's ability to move actively and the movements which are still difficult or even impossible for him and decides accordingly which activities are important for the treatment at present and, as the patient makes progress, at each later stage of his rehabilitation. Many suitable activities for retraining selective control of the lower limbs and the trunk preparatory to walking or to improve its quality can be useful for patients at different stages, such as those which have been clearly described and illustrated previously by the author (Davies 1985, 1990). The following activities have been selected because they are relevant for the majority of patients and will help to provide a sound foundation for walking.

Retraining Selective Movements of the Lower Limb

Selective Hip Extension (Bridging)

As soon as the patient shows signs of regaining consciousness, he can start to lift his seat off the bed during physiotherapy and also when routine nursing tasks are being performed. When his sheet is being changed, he is being moved sideways in bed before being turned on to his side or is having his trousers pulled up, he can be asked to lift his buttocks actively. The hip extensors are activated selectively and not in a mass extension synergy because the patient's knees are flexed and his feet dorsiflexed.

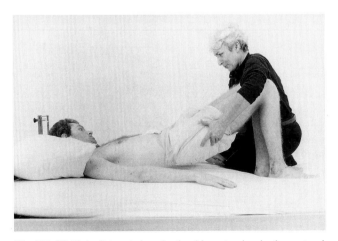

Fig. 7.7. "Bridging" to retrain selective hip extension in the acute phase

The patient lies supine with both knees flexed and his feet placed parallel to one another, his heels below his knees. The therapist or nurse places one hand on either side of the patient's pelvis to assist him as he tries to lift his bottom off the bed (Fig. 7.7). In order to move to one side of the bed, the nurse helps the patient to lift and then move his seat towards or away from her as is applicable. The shoulders are then lifted and shifted over to the same side.

Similarly, the "bridging" movement can be used when the patient is needs to be moved up or down the bed. "Bridging" is developmentally a comparatively simple movement and the patient can comprehend easily what is required of him. The normal baby at about 6 months can be seen lifting its bottom repeatedly off the floor as it too prepares for standing. As the patient's ability improves, he

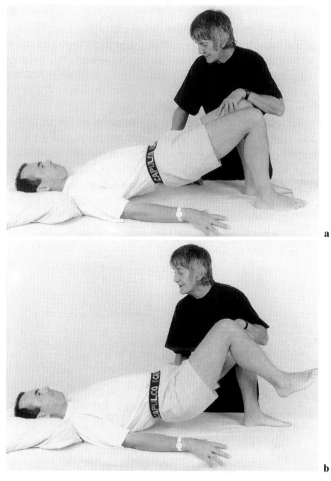

a

b

Fig. 7.8a,b. "Bridging" with one foot lifted from the bed. **a** Drawing the patient's knee over his foot. **b** Keeping the pelvis level when one foot is lifted

can practise the same movement more selectively. He first holds his seat in the air and then lifts one foot off the bed without allowing his pelvis to sink down on one side or his weight-bearing foot to slide down the bed as it will tend to do. The therapist facilitates the correct movement by placing one of her hands over the patient's knee, drawing it over his foot while at the same time pressing down so that weight is taken through his heel before he lifts the contralateral leg (Fig. 7.8a). With the extended fingers of her other hand the therapist stimulates activity in the gluteal muscles, by tapping firmly over the area, or uses the hand to help stabilize the pelvis as the patient lifts his other foot in the air (Fig. 7.8b).

Selective Knee Extension

The ability to contract the knee extensors selectively is of the utmost importance for normal walking, and isometric contractions should be carefully activated and practised. The patient must learn to tighten the extensors without his foot pushing into plantarflexion or his toes flexing as he does so. The activity is most important during the stance phase to enable the body to move forwards over the weight-bearing foot and at the end of the swing phase for a normal stride length with the heel making contact with the ground before the rest of the foot. A patient who has regained the ability to contract his quadriceps selectively will seldom need to wear a foot-brace to assist dorsiflexion later.

The patient lies supine and the therapist brings his leg slowly down into extension, maintaining full dorsiflexion of his foot against her thigh or lower abdomen. With the patient's heel supported on the bed, the therapist keeps the foot in dorsal flexion by leaning her weight forwards, as she asks him to tighten his knee actively and indicates the exact location with her finger (Fig. 7.9).

It is advisable to practise the activity first with the leg which the patient is better able to control to ensure that he knows exactly what is required of him. Usually the patient will try too hard, and the excessive effort causes simultaneous plantarflexion of his foot and activation of his hip extensors in the mass synergy of extension.

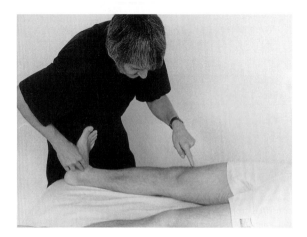

Fig. 7.9. Isometric contraction of the knee extensors with the foot held in full dorsiflexion

By choosing her words carefully and modulating her voice appropriately, the therapist can help to elicit the correct selective, isometric activity.

Selective Hip and Knee Extension During Weight-Bearing

The patient sits with his feet flat on the floor and parallel to one another. The therapist, seated on a stool directly in front of the patient, clasps one of his knees between her knees so that the medial condyles of her femur are behind his. She supports his more severely paralyzed arm by placing it under her arm and pressing it against her body with her hand beneath his elbow to maintain the position. Her other hand is placed over the patient's lower thoracic spine to draw his trunk forwards in order to bring his weight over his feet as he lifts his seat from the chair or plinth on which he is sitting (Fig. 7.10a).

Because the patient's knees will tend to move backwards as he starts to take weight through his legs due to the simultaneous plantarflexion of his feet, the therapist uses her knees to draw his knee forwards over his foot and keep his heel in contact with the floor. As the patient reaches the upright position, the therapist releases his arm and uses her hand to draw his hip forwards in extension in order to achieve a good standing position. He then can practise raising and lowering the heel of the opposite foot (Fig. 7.10b). To prevent the patient from leaning backwards to compensate for loss of active hip extensor activity, the therapist places her other hand over his lower ribs anteriorly and draws them down towards his umbilicus to facilitate the action of his abdominal muscles. If plantarflexion continues to be a problem, it can be inhibited by placing a rolled bandage beneath the patient's toes which will also prevent them from clawing or pushing down against the floor (Fig 7.10c).

Once the patient can stand confidently with his weight taken through one leg without undue effort, he can try to lift his other foot off the floor briefly at first and later hold it in the air for a few moments at a time (Fig. 7.10d). It will at first be necessary for the therapist to prevent the patient's knee from hyperextending by adducting her legs strongly, but when she feels that his knee is no longer pushing backwards, she gradually reduces the amount of assistance she is giving by moving her knees away from his. The patient learns to take weight on his leg without the knee recurvating in the total pattern of extension. When he can do so confidently, walking is facilitated at increasing speeds and with unexpected changes of direction with his leg still remaining mobile and not in a locked position.

Regaining Balance Reactions and Selective Trunk Control

In the early stages, the patient will have difficulty in maintaining his balance at all. In fact it often seems as if he is unaware that he is falling because he makes no attempt to save himself. Facilitating balance reactions as soon as the patient starts to be brought into sitting positions will activate the head and trunk righting reactions as well as stimulating muscle activity. The selective muscle control of the

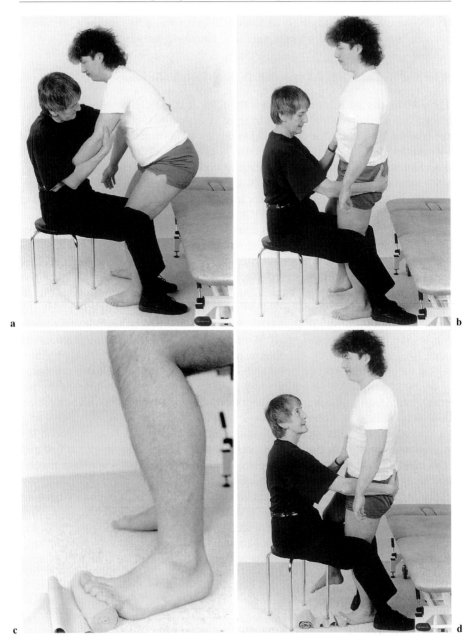

Fig. 7.10a–d. Retraining selective extension of the leg in standing. **a** Bringing the patient's weight over his feet. **b** Keeping his knee forwards. **c** A rolled bandage beneath his toes inhibits plantarflexion. **d** Maintaining hip extension while lifting the other foot off the floor

trunk and lower limbs which is necessary for walking can be promoted by the balance activities being made progressively more difficult as the patient's ability improves.

Returning to an Upright Position After Leaning Down to Either Side

Even when the patient has not yet regained consciousness, the therapist can sit him up with his legs over the edge of the bed and move him away from the vertical, either backwards or sideways, before encouraging him to return to the upright position as she facilitates the correct movement.

When the therapist has brought the patient into a sitting position with his legs over the side of the bed, she stands in front of him so that her thighs are against his knees to prevent him from sliding off the bed if his hips extend suddenly. She leans the patient's trunk over to one side until his elbow is touching the bed, her arm over his opposite shoulder supporting the weight and position of his trunk (Fig. 7.11a). She calls to the patient to sit up again, facilitating the movement by pressing her arm down firmly over his shoulder girdle. The pressure helps to elicit a head righting reaction as the patient tries to come back to a vertical position (Fig. 7.11b).

After the patient has regained the upright position, the therapist changes her hands and repeats the activity towards the other side. Frequently, after the movement has been performed a few times, the patient will start to participate actively in some way, for example his head rights towards the vertical (Fig. 7.11c). If he is able to use his arm the patient will tend to come upright by pushing down on the bed or by pulling on the therapist's hand. In order for the activity to take place in the trunk instead, the therapist holds the patient's hand lightly from above and moves with him so that no purchase is provided.

Once the patient can return to a vertical position from either side, the therapist gives less support, using only her hand on his shoulder to stimulate the righting reactions of head and trunk (Fig. 7.12). She increases the degree of difficulty by moving more quickly and by changing the direction of the movement unexpectedly, no longer always going down first to one side and then to the other.

Maintaining Balance with Weight Transferred Sideways in Sitting

Being able to balance in sitting is essential for most functional activities, but retraining the normal reactions will also improve the patient's ability to walk with regard to both the safety and the gait pattern. The therapist facilitates the correct movements with the patient sitting on his bed or on a high plinth. Until the balance reactions occur spontaneously and in a normal pattern his feet should not be touching the floor or have a support placed beneath them. The patient will otherwise block the reactions completely or cause them to be abnormal by pushing down against the floor with his foot. Later it will be necessary to practise balancing while seated on a chair as well because during the activities of daily life the feet are normally on the ground and not in the air.

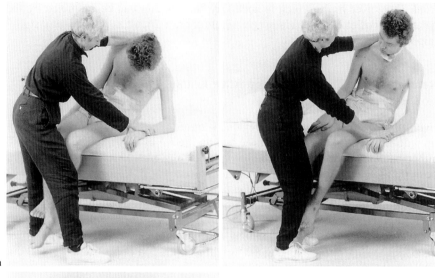

a
b

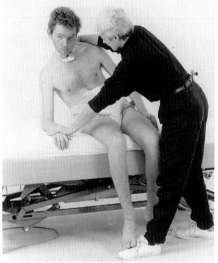

c

Fig. 7.11a–c. Returning to an upright sitting position. **a** Supporting the patient while leaning his trunk sideways. **b** Facilitation for coming upright again. **c** Head-righting reaction stimulated

Seated beside the patient, the therapist reaches round behind him to place her hand over his lower ribs on the side furthest from her. She draws the patient towards her using her other hand in his nearside axilla to support his shoulder girdle and prevent lateral flexion of his trunk. With the hand which is on his ribcage, the therapist facilitates the holding activity of his abdominal muscles by drawing his ribs downwards (Fig. 7.13a). If the patient keeps his arm in a fixed position or tries to hold on to the plinth, the therapist can take her hand from his axilla, maintain the position of his shoulder with hers, and reach across in front of him to indicate the correct, free reaction of the limb (Fig. 7.13b).

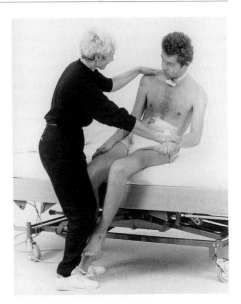

Fig. 7.12. Head and trunk righting actively as patient returns to the vertical position with less support

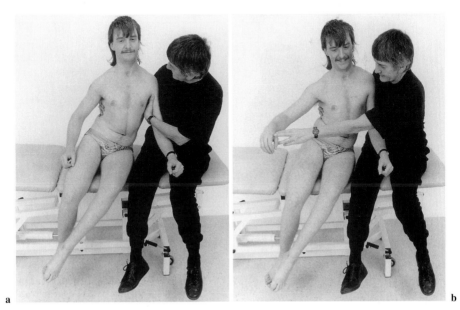

a

b

Fig. 7.13a,b. Balancing in sitting. **a** Moving the patient sideways with lateral flexion of his trunk. **b** Encouraging an arm reaction

Once the body weight has been shifted sufficiently over to one side, the further-most leg should lift reactively in abduction. If the patient's leg fails to do so auto-matically or if he is flexing it actively to hold on to the plinth, the therapist once again frees her hand to guide the leg into the air while still supporting his trunk with her body (Fig. 7.14a). The activity is continued until the patient has learned to let his leg lift in extension each time his weight has been transferred far enough side-

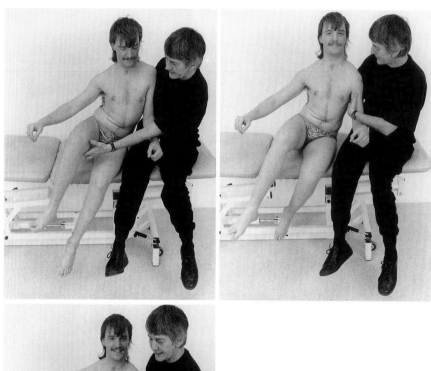

a

b

c

Fig. 7.14a–c. Facilitating normal reac-tions. **a** Helping the patient's leg to react. **b** His weight-bearing leg flexes at the knee. **c** Therapist corrects knee position with her foot under his heel

ways. As the patient's leg lifts into the air, the leg on the weight-bearing side will often flex at the knee due to a powerful contraction of the flexors which appears to be reflex in nature (Fig 7.14b). Should such flexion occur the therapist places her foot beneath the patient's heel to correct the position of his leg by extending the knee and applying a little pressure to his heel (Fig. 7.14c). In some cases the leg will not only be flexed but inwardly rotated as well, which the therapist can over-come at the same time by moving the patient's heel medially with her foot as she extends his knee. Moving the patient sideways several times with his leg in the corrected position inhibits the knee flexion and inward rotation, allowing more normal reactions to take place with less and less assistance from the therapist.

When the therapist no longer needs to correct the position of his leg with her foot, she stands in front of the patient and, holding his arm gently, draws his weight well over to the side (Fig. 7.15). She does not need to pull on his arm because the activity is only facilitated in this way once he has learned to follow the movement which she indicates and is capable of reacting adequately. Until such time, the therapist continues to move the patient from his trunk.

In order to transfer the patient's weight to the other side, the therapist can either change her position so that she can perform the facilitation as she did before while sitting beside him, or she can remain on the same side and move him away from her. Placing her hand over his ribcage on the side nearest to her, she holds his ribs down as she shifts him over towards the opposite side (Fig. 7.16). The action of the trunk side flexors is facilitated as well as lateral flexion of the lumbar spine. Should the patient's leg not lift automatically into the air, or should the motor control still be insufficient, the therapist can guide it into position with her leg and support some of its weight if it is too heavy for him to hold on his own.

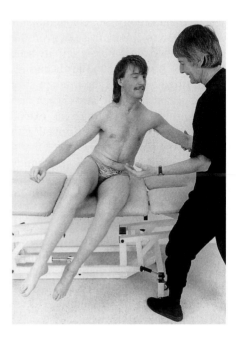

Fig. 7.15. Reacting spontaneously when moved right over to one side

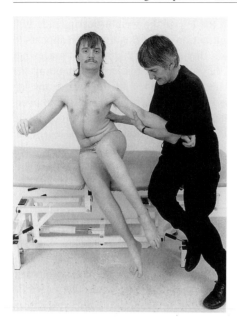

Fig. 7.16. Facilitating lateral flexion of the trunk when moving the patient towards his less affected side

Selective Lateral Flexion of the Lumbar Spine

In normal walking, the thorax is stabilized to allow the movements of the pelvis and efficient activity of the abdominal muscles. When one foot leaves the floor to make a step forwards, the pelvis on that side must be suspended from above by selective abdominal muscle activity because the leg would otherwise be too long to be able to clear the ground easily during the swing phase (Davies 1990). Practising the required control of the trunk in sitting will make it possible for the patient to take repeated rhythmic steps when he is walking instead of having to hitch his pelvis up in order to bring his extended leg forward slowly and with effort. The activity is easier if performed with the patient's feet clear of the ground at first to avoid his pressing with one foot against the floor. Any overactive extension of his leg will hamper the easy rhythmic movements of the pelvis and lumbar spine. Once the patient can move his trunk correctly, the same activity is practised while he is sitting on a low plinth or chair of the appropriate height with one of his feet flat on the floor.

The patient sits with one leg crossed over the other and the therapist stands in front of him, keeping his leg in place with her thighs. She places one of her hands over his trochanter to assist the lifting of the buttock on the side of the uppermost leg (Fig. 7.17a). The patient lifts his buttock off the plinth and then lowers it again repeating the up and down movement smoothly and rhythmically. The movement should take place in the lumbar spine and is made possible by adaptive rotation of the supporting hip as weight is transferred over that side and then back to the

Fig. 7.17a–c. Selective lateral flexion of the lumbar spine. **a** The therapist holds the patient's crossed legs in positon with her thigh. **b** Assisting elevation of the pelvis on the side of the uppermost leg. **c** Stabilizing the thoracic spine with side-flexion localized to the lumbar region

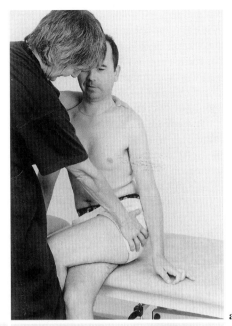

a

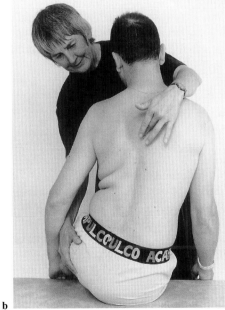

b

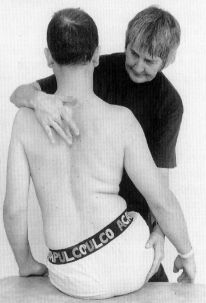

c

middle again. The therapist places her hand round over the patient's shoulder so that she can use her fingers to facilitate extension of his thoracic spine and prevent any lateral flexion from occurring in that area in conjunction with that of the lumbar spine (Fig. 7.17b). The patient's shoulders should remain level throughout the performance of the activity and his head should remain vertical with no overactive side flexion of his neck. His arms remain loosely at his sides as balance reactions should not be elicited.

To perform the activity towards the other side, the patient changes the position of his legs so that the one that is uppermost is on the side of the lifted buttock. The therapist asks the patient to make just a small movement using only the muscles in the region of his waist (Fig. 7.17c). It will usually be easier for him to localize the movement when the less involved side of his trunk is contracting but selective activity around the supporting hip naturally plays an important role as well.

Selective Flexion and Extension of the Lumbar Spine

Not only is the selective control of lateral flexion crucial for walking but also the ability to flex and extend the lumbar spine without concomitant flexion and extension of the thoracic spine. The trunk should be able to remain upright despite the activity of the lower abdominal muscles and excessive extension of the thorax and cervical spine should not accompany localized lumbar extension. A movement sequence to regain the selective flexion and extension is described in detail in Chap. 3 (see Fig. 3.34a,b). Once the patient can perform the selective movement easily in sitting, the therapist facilitates the activity while he is standing upright, with his knees remaining slightly flexed as he tilts his pelvis rhythmically anteriorly and posteriorly.

Mobilizing and Activating the Trunk

Before the activities to retrain selective movements and balance can be performed successfully, and certainly before walking is facilitated, the patient's trunk must be freely mobile and any tension or overactivity in the muscles controlling its movement must be inhibited. With the patient's trunk held stiffly in either extension or flexion to compensate for inadequate control, the tone in the muscles of the limbs will also increase and as a result of both, the free-flowing nature of walking will be rendered impossible. During her treatment the therapist, therefore, includes activities to mobilize and activate the patient's trunk in preparation for walking using different starting positions.

Flexion and Extension

The patient sits with his legs over the side of the bed or a plinth, and with his arms extended and outwardly rotated, his hands are placed flat on the supporting surface behind him. The therapist stands or kneels behind the patient and draws his shoulders backwards and towards each other with her hands as he extends his

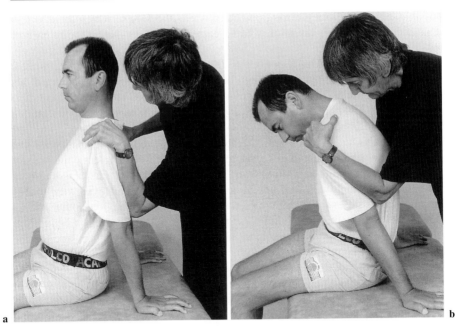

Fig. 7.18a,b. Mobilizing the trunk in sitting. **a** Therapist maintains elbow position during trunk extension. **b** Trunk flexion with scapula protraction

spine actively. With her forearm she can maintain extension of his elbow should his arm tend to flex (Fig. 7.18a). At first the patient may push his head back to assist the extension of his trunk but, once the movement is easier for him, he should try to leave his neck in a neutral position or even be asked to move it freely in different directions. His weight can also be shifted from one side to the other while the extended position is maintained.

The active extension of the trunk with adduction of the scapulae is alternated with flexion of the spine combined with protraction of the scapulae. The therapist moves the patient's shoulders as far forward as she can asking him to try not to resist the movement at all and let his head relax forwards at the same time (Fig. 7.18b). The movement from flexion to extension is repeated until it flows easily without any resistance being felt and until the arms are relaxed as well and remain in the extended position on their own.

Flexion/Rotation of the Trunk in Sitting

If the patient's trunk is held too rigidly in extension then the subtle rotation of the lower thoracic spine necessary for normal walking is prevented. The flexion/rotation of the thorax is also required for the patient to be able to use his hands for tasks which are not directly in front of him but to one or other side of the midline. The therapist will need to mobilize the patient's trunk passively before active rotation is possible. She mobilizes the rotation first towards the side to which there is less resistance, as the other direction will be easier afterwards due to the release of tension.

The patient sits with his legs over the edge of the plinth and slightly abducted. With his weight taken equally through both buttocks, he turns so that both of his hands can be placed flat on the plinth to one side of him, shoulder width apart. The therapist helps him to achieve the correct position, if necessary keeping his hand in place with her thigh resting on it.

She supports the patient's more affected arm with one of her hands placed just above his elbow from behind to keep it in extension as well as to draw the scapula and the side of his trunk forward towards her. At the same time, she presses against the patient's sternum with the back of her forearm and plantarflexed wrist to flex his thoracic spine and so enable him to keep his weight back on both buttocks (Fig. 7.19a). With her free hand the therapist moves the patient's head from one side to the other and forwards to inhibit any hypertonus and ensure that he is not holding it tensely in one fixed position. She can also reach across to abduct the leg furthest away from her should it continue to pull or fall into adduction. The therapist asks the patient to breathe out gently and relax, and try to let his hands just lie in position on the table instead of pushing down actively against it.

When rotating the patient's trunk in the other direction, the therapist can stand behind him and keep his elbow straight with one of her hands. She not only extends his elbow but at the same time gives downward pressure through the arm to keep his hand in place on the supporting surface. With her other hand placed over the patient's shoulder, the therapist draws it backwards together with that side of his trunk to facilitate the rotation while using her forearm to move his scapula downwards and medially (Fig. 7.19b). Because the patient usually has too little flexion and rotation, his buttock on the side furthest away from his hands will tend to lose contact with the plinth. The therapist sits down on the plinth behind the patient and places one arm round in front of his lower ribs and presses down to draw his chest back towards her (Fig. 7.19c). With her other hand the therapist continues to maintain extension of his elbow.

Rotation of the Lumbar Spine with the Abdominal Muscles Activated

A recommended activity for relaxed lower trunk rotation with progressively more abdominal muscle control can be practised from an early stage, and later even by the patient on his own or with the help of his relatives. The activity has the advantage that the thorax is stabilized by the bed, thus enabling the rotation to be localized to the lumbar region.

The patient lies supine with both legs flexed and his feet supported on the bed. The therapist helps him to cross one knee over the other, with the foot of the underneath leg in the midline and the heel beneath the knee. The patient's head is supported by a big pillow and his hands lie relaxed at his sides. The therapist places her

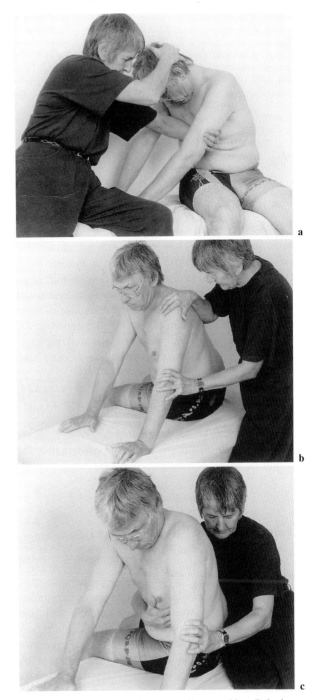

Fig. 7.19a–c. Mobilizing trunk rotation in sitting with both hands supported on one side. **a** Relaxing the patient's neck while keeping his affected arm and hand in place. **b** with rotation towards the more affected side moving his shoulder back. **c** Increasing trunk flexion

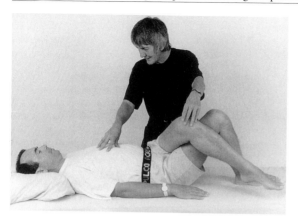

Fig. 7.20. Helping the patient to move his knees rhythmically from one side to the other

hand on the patient's knee and moves his adducted legs from one side to the other, slowly and rhythmically, asking him to try to do the movement with her (Fig. 7.20). Her other hand on his lower sternum helps him to stabilize his thorax, and he tries to keep his shoulders back on the bed as he takes over the movement more actively. The therapist gradually reduces the amount of help she is giving, guided by the harmony of the movement. Should she notice any tone increase, associated reactions or other signs that the patient is making too much effort, she immediately steps in again to allow the activity to proceed smoothly and rhythmically once again.

The patient moves his knees slowly at first and far over towards each side. As his control improves, he reduces the range of the movement and increases the tempo, both of which serve to increase the amount of muscle activity required. The aim would be for the patient to progress to moving his legs without undue effort from one side to the other at approximately the tempo of normal gait, which would be about 120 times a minute.

The Facilitation of Walking

When helping the patient to walk, the therapist should try to do so in such a way that his gait pattern is as normal as possible in order for him to experience and so learn the correct movements right from the start. She may have to try out a variety of ways in which to support him before deciding on which would be the best and the most successful for the nurses or his relatives to use when they walk with him. The type of facilitation will also vary from patient to patient and need to be adapted or changed as each improves in ability. It is often surprising what a difference the appropriate support can make to the patient's walking pattern and the ease with which he can walk. The following types of facilitation have proved most suitable for the majority of patients when they start learning to walk again.

Stabilizing the Thorax and Eliciting Reactive Steps

Many patients have difficulty in stabilizing their thoracic spine, despite having recovery of motor function in their lower limbs sufficient to permit ambulation. With inadequate balance and unsteadiness, such patients, including those with ataxia, are unable to walk on their own and will often remain wheelchair-bound if not helped to overcome the problem. Some may manage to walk with effort by keeping their weight well back, fixing their trunk in flexion to maintain their balance and hunching their shoulders with stiffly held arms to compensate for the loss of trunk control. But by continuing to walk in this manner, the return of the correct activity will be prevented (Fig. 7.21a).

A most effective way of enabling the patient to learn to walk with a more normal gait pattern is for the therapist to stabilize his thorax with her hands and move him forwards. The facilitation, as developed and demonstrated by Klein-Vogelbach (1987) originally required two assistants, one on either side of the patient, but it can be used successfully by the therapist on her own. The therapist stands beside the patient and places one of her hands over his ribcage anteriorly at about the level of the sternal angle, and her other hand on his thoracic spine below the inferior angles of his scapulae (Fig. 7.21b). With the hand in front, she draws the ribs on both sides down and towards the midline, while with both her hands she lifts the whole thorax upwards to take some of the patient's weight when he is walking. Her hand behind the patient gives counterpressure as well as maintaining the extension of the thoracic spine.

Without releasing the pressure of her hands, the therapist transports the patient's thorax forwards to initiate walking by eliciting a reactive step (Fig. 7.21c). She should not instruct the patient verbally to take a step because he will then try to lift his leg actively, leaning back as he does so. By transferring his weight slightly towards one side as well as forwards, the therapist can determine which foot will move first.

Walking at a normal speed and with her usual step length, the therapist continues to move the patient's thorax forwards through space so that repeated automatic steps are elicited. With his legs moving reactively without effort, the patient's whole walking pattern improves (Fig. 7.21d). When walking slowly and painstakingly, everybody uses very different muscle activity and requires far more balance. Adequate velocity is, therefore, an important feature of the facilitation in the truest sense of the word.

Patients, particularly if they are ataxic, who need to use crutches when walking, will tend to place them too far in front and out to either side for additional security, with the result that their trunk is inclined forwards and their hips flexed (Fig. 7.22a). Such a patient, therefore, only experiences an abnormal posture and gait pattern, which soon becomes habituated. Facilitating walking from the thorax is, therefore, most beneficial as it enables the patient to experience a more normal gait pattern in an upright posture without his crutches (Fig. 7.22b). The sensation is essential if he is to learn the correct movement sequence.

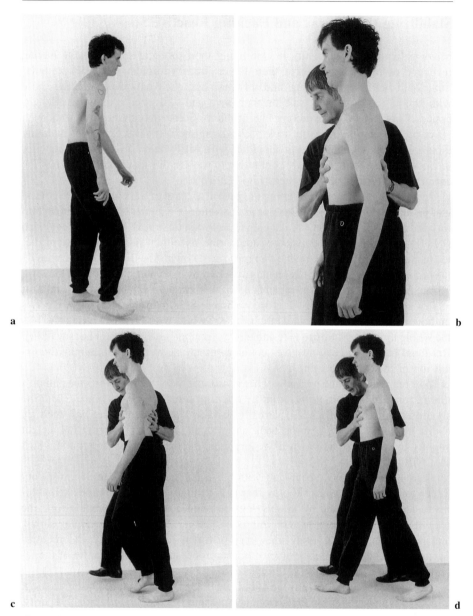

Fig. 7.21a. Ataxic patient walking with trunk and shoulders held stiffly to maintain balance. **b** Therapist stabilizes his thorax. **c** Moving the trunk forwards elicits a reactive step. **d** Walking normally with facilitation

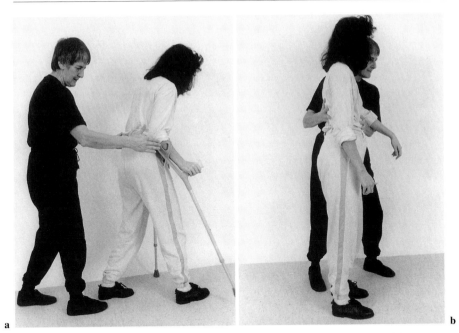

a   b

Fig. 7.22a. Walking with crutches an ataxic patient flexes her trunk and hips. **b** Upright posture experienced with thorax stabilized

Assisting Hip Extension and Avoiding a Hyperextended Knee

Many patients will have difficulty in preventing their knee from hyperextending when they start to walk again, an abnormal movement which can have serious repercussions if it is not prevented and a more normal pattern made possible. The knee hyperextends at the moment when the foot makes contact with the floor in front at the end of the swing phase, because plantarflexion occurs as the leg extends in a total synergy and pushes the tibia backwards and hence the knee into a totally extended position (Fig. 7.23a). The resistance caused by the premature action of the plantar flexors prevents the patient's weight from being brought forward over his foot to start the new stance phase. The stimulation of the ball of his foot against the floor will increase the strength of the plantarflexion with every step he takes.

During the stance phase, the hyperextension of the knee causes the hip to be pushed backwards instead of moving continuously forward as it would normally do. The knee in hyperextension at the end of the stance phase makes relaxation of the extensors to allow rapid flexion of the knee to 30 for the initiation of the swing phase difficult if not impossible (Fig. 7.23b). The patient will often have to circumduct his extended leg to bring it forward slowly and with effort or use some other compensatory movement. Careful retraining of selective hip and knee exten-

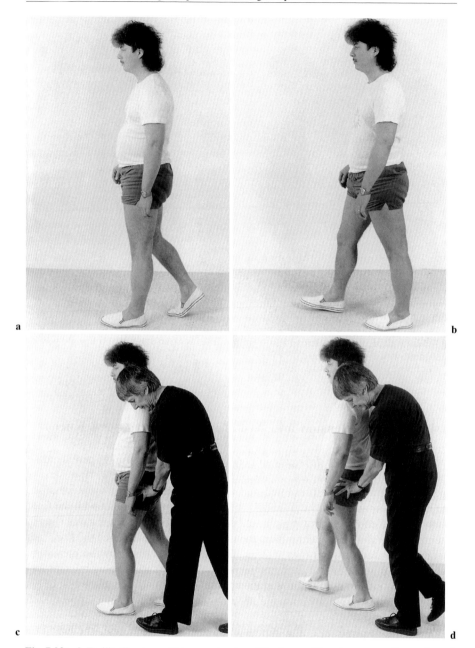

Fig. 7.23a–d. Facilitatiion to avoid hyperextension of the knee. **a** Knee hyperextending at the end of the swing phase. **b** Hip and knee moving backwards during stance phase. **c** Moving the hip forwards over the patient's foot. **d** Assisting hip extension during weight-bearing

sion in preparation for walking will make weight-bearing possible without the knee locking, and help to overcome the problem if the patient is already walking abnormally. Appropriate facilitation of walking with the hip guided forward in extension prevents hyperextension of the knee and enables the patient to learn the correct movement from the beginning or change an established, abnormal pattern.

The therapist walks next to the patient with one hand on the posterior aspect of his pelvic girdle on the side nearest to her and her other arm round behind him so that her hand rests on his lower ribs on the opposite side. As the patient's leg swings forward, the therapist moves his hip forwards as well so that, immediately his foot meets the floor in front, she can bring his pelvis and trunk diagonally forward over the foot to prevent premature plantarflexion of the ankle from pushing the knee back into hyperextension (Fig. 7.23c).

The therapist continues to guide the patient's hip forward throughout the stance phase so that the contralateral leg swings forwards reactively. Even at the end of the stance phase, the knee has not hyperextended and will be able to flex easily for the initiation of the subsequent swing phase once weight has been transferred over the foot in front. (Fig. 7.23d). For the facilitation to be successful, the position of the therapist's hands is most important and the exact way in which assistance is given with respect to the timing and direction of the movements essential.

The Hand on the Posterior Aspect of the Patient's Pelvic Girdle

- *Position*: The therapist places the hand which is furthest away from the patient so that her thumb is directly behind his hip joint pressing against the head of the femur. The dorsal extension of her wrist allows her fingers to lie on the lateral side of his pelvis (Fig. 7.24a).
- *Action*: To initiate the swing phase, knee flexion through relaxation of the extensors at the end of the stance phase is facilitated by the therapist pressing the pelvis down and forward on that side. As the leg swings forward she ensures that the hip moves forwards as well. Throughout the stance phase, from the moment when the patient's weight is taken through that leg, the therapist uses her thumb to assist hip extension by easing the femoral head forwards over his knee, thereby ensuring that the hip moves continuously forward. A slight downward pressure given at the same time will help the patient to avoid hyperextension of his knee. The continued forward pressure behind the femoral head will facilitate the reactive swing phase of the contralateral leg once the patient's body weight has been brought far enough in front of the line of gravity.

The Hand on the Far Side of the Patient's Trunk

- *Position*: The therapist's other hand is placed over the patient's lower ribs on the far side at about waist level, her flexed arm around behind him in close contact with his trunk (Fig. 7.24b).
- *Action*: During the stance phase, the therapist transfers the patient's weight towards her with her hand, to free the leg on the opposite side. At the same time she uses her arm to stabilize his trunk, take some of his weight if neces-

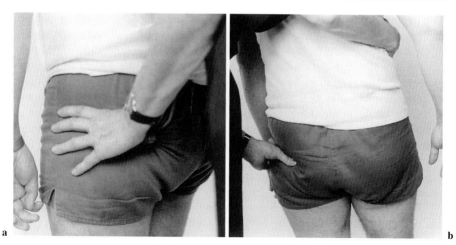

Fig. 7.24a,b. Position and action of the hands. **a** Thumb directly behind the hip presses the head of the femur forwards. **b** Hand around the patient's waist transfers his weight over the supporting leg

sary, and prevent him from leaning backwards. During the swing phase, the therapist's arm around behind him helps the patient to shift his weight diagonally forwards over the other side sufficiently far to elicit a reactive step, with the foot thus relieved of any weight. The method of facilitation is most useful for patients whose symptoms are predominantly unilateral and who have some degree of trunk control. The patient with a very unstable trunk will tend to lean too far back and his arms pull up strongly in the spastic pattern of flexion (Fig. 7.25a). The therapist, with both her hands fully occupied, can do little to control the position of the patient's arms and upper trunk. Until trunk control improves, a walking frame with adjustable armrests can be used to correct the position of his upper limbs and help him to keep his weight forward (Fig. 7.25b). Care must be taken, however, that extensor hypertonus in the lower limbs is not stimulated by using the mechanical support.

A Walking Frame with Wheels

Many therapists fear that, by using a walking frame, the patient's chances of walking unaided in the future will be jeopardized because he could become "dependent" on the frame and be disinclined to walk without its support. It is not unusual for the patient's relatives to share the opinion or even for the patient himself to refuse to use an aid for the same reason. The fear is, however, totally unfounded and could lead to the patient remaining in a wheelchair far longer than would otherwise have been necessary. In fact, walking more often, albeit with the frame, will enhance his chances of regaining the necessary activity and speed up his progress.

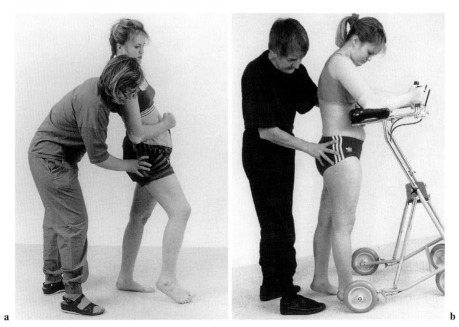

a   b

Fig. 7.25.a Patient with spasticity leans her trunk too far back and her arms pull into flexion.
b Using a walking aid corrects trunk and arm position but increases leg extension

Every normal baby learns to walk by doing so first while holding on to something or someone, be it the cot sides, furniture, its mother's hand or a toy on wheels
which it pushes. As soon as the baby's motor control has reached the right level
after such preparation, it will start to take steps without the support and soon be
walking unaided. In the same way, the patient will soon discard the walking aid
once he has sufficient motor ability to walk without it. It is the continuous sitting in
the wheelchair which hampers the patient's progress towards attaining independent
walking and not the use of a walking frame.

If it is extremely difficult for a patient to stand and walk with his body in a
vertically upright position or lift one foot off the floor to take a step, he will have
little opportunity to practise walking at all (Fig. 7.26a,b). Those who would otherwise be more than willing to help him walk are loath to do so for fear of letting him
fall or sustaining injuries themselves. An immediate difference is frequently observed when the patient uses a walking frame for support (Fig. 7.26c). He feels less
insecure because of the orientation it affords him, his weight is brought forwards
and his trunk remains upright in the midline. A walking frame which has wheels is
recommended because it does not interrupt the continuous forward motion of normal gait. If when using the frame the patient requires much less assistance or only
stand-by help because he can even take a few steps unaided then the nursing staff or
his relatives will be prepared to walk with him far more often. Because the therapist
no longer needs to support the patient totally, she can use her hands to facilitate a

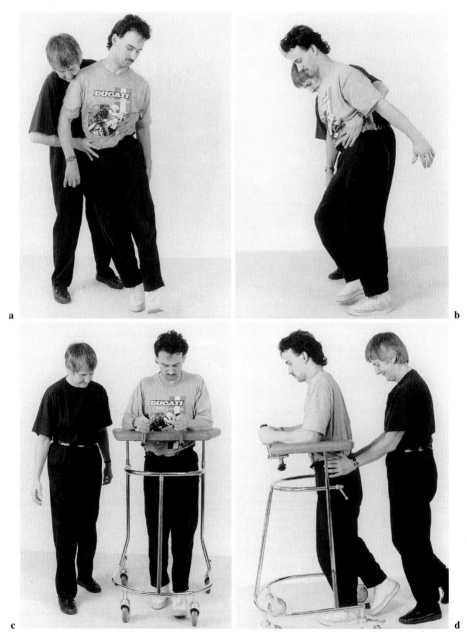

Fig. 7.26a–d. Using a walking frame on wheels to overcome difficulties. **a** Extreme difficulty in walking upright. **b** Unable to take a step despite facilitation. **c** Walking vertically upright with the frame. **d** Able to take steps easily

more normal walking pattern instead, for instance, by correcting hip adduction or a lateral shift of his pelvis (Fig. 7.26d).

Another advantage of using a walking frame is that it can help the patient to stand up from a chair and sit down again in such a way that he learns the normal movement sequence. He is encouraged to push the frame well forwards before lifting his seat off the chair as he comes to standing so that his head is well over his knees and feet and his back extended (Fig. 7.27a). After standing up correctly his first steps will be more normal as well (Fig. 7.27b). In order to sit down in a normal way, the patient should turn so that the chair is immediately behind him, place his feet in line with one another and then lower his bottom far back in the chair without pulling the walking frame towards him (Fig. 7.28). The therapist has a hand on his back to help him maintain trunk extension and to guide the speed of the downward movement.

Adapting the Walking Frame for Functional Tasks

In order for the patient to use the frame for carrying out functional activities, it will need to have a tray and some sort of container attached to it if these are not a standard fitting. The adaptation makes it possible for the patient to carry objects from one place to another which he will need to do when performing most tasks. Before getting dressed he will need to take his clothes from the cupboard to his bed

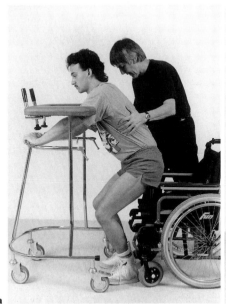
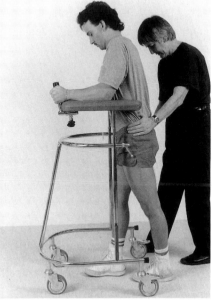

a
b

Fig. 7.27.a Pushing the walking frame forwards when coming to standing. **b** Initial steps more normal after standing up correctly

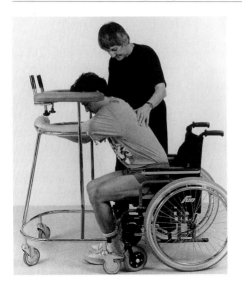

Fig. 7.28. When sitting down the frame facilitates a normal pattern of movement by keeping the patient's weight forward

or chair, and after selecting a drink from the machine must carry it to sit down at a table. If the patient helps to put fresh linen on his bed or goes to take a shower armed with his soap, towel and clothes, the same applies. A tray and a basket or plastic basin can be easily attached to most types of walking frame (Fig. 7.29a).

Therapeutic guiding during the activities of daily life is made possible in standing positions by the adaptation, and the therapist or nurse will find many opportunities to guide the patient spontaneously as he performs actual tasks which incorporate standing and walking (Fig. 7.29b).

Using Other Walking Aids

There are many and varied types of walking aid available and the therapist should be well informed in order to choose the most appropriate for each patient should some form of support be necessary.

- *Shoes.* It should not be forgotten that shoes in themselves can make a remarkable difference to the patient's walking ability and gait pattern. Some patient's may walk better in a sports shoe with a thick rubber sole, while for others considerable improvement is noted when shoes which have a firm leather sole and a slight heel are worn. Before deciding on a specific walking aid, the therapist should first try to find out which shoes are most suitable for the individual patient because the need for an additional aid may even be obviated altogether.
- *Crutches.* If the patient's difficulty is mainly one of balance, elbow crutches may enable him to walk safely on his own and can be particularly helpful when he leaves the confines of his room. The disadvantage of using crutches is that he

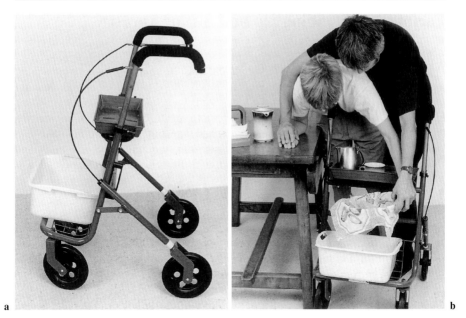

Fig. 7.29.a A tray and container can be attached to a standard walking frame. **b** The attachments enable the therapist to guide the patient spontaneously in real life situations

cannot carry anything in his hands. It is usually not advisable to use only one crutch as almost inevitably an asymmetrical posture and walking pattern result. The same applies to using a cane.

- *Foot braces.* A brace to hold the patient's foot in position will seldom be required if the standing activities described in Chap. 4 are diligently carried out from the beginning. If his foot supinates strongly, however, his ankle will need to be protected from injury and, in the presence of marked plantarflexion, a brace is usually required to assist dorsal flexion. Whichever type of brace is chosen, it should be as light and as malleable as is possible without loss of supportive function. Because the patient's ability often improves rapidly once he starts walking, the decision to order a definitive brace can be delayed by holding his foot firmly in position with an elastic crepe bandage which is bandaged on over his shoe in way similar to that used to support a lateral sprain of the ankle (Davies 1985).

Facilitating Standing Up and Sitting Down

For walking to be truly functional, the patient must be able to stand up from a chair and sit down again safely and without too much effort. If he does not take weight through both his legs or pushes back into extension he will be in danger of losing his balance and falling. The therapist will need to spend considerable time teaching the patient to stand up and sit down in a normal way, but it will be time well spent because the movements also serve to retrain selective activity of the trunk and lower limbs. Whether he is being helped to rise from his bed, a chair or the toilet, the facilitation remains the same.

The person who is assisting stands at the patient's side with one hand on either side of his pelvis and encourages him to lean well forward before lifting his seat. The assistant uses her shoulder to prevent him from pushing his trunk backwards as he comes upright. Her hands on his pelvis assist hip extension as he reaches the upright position and ensure that his weight is over both feet. As soon as he is standing she moves even closer to him and helps to maintain balance.

The same method in reverse enables him to return to sitting in a controlled way, the helper guiding the patient's trunk well forwards with her shoulder just before and while he lowers his bottom slowly back onto the chair behind him. Simultaneously her hands facilitate hip flexion and prevent any lateral deviation of the pelvis which could cause the patient to sit down too close to one side of the chair.

The therapist or whoever else may be helping the patient to stand up should not stand in front of him to give assistance because by doing so an abnormal pattern is encouraged which can easily become a habit. The patient will tend either to pull himself up by holding on to the helper or by pushing back in extension against the stable support provided by her hands regardless of where she places them. In both cases his legs will extend in a total synergy with his knees and trunk moving backwards instead of forwards.

PROBLEM SOLVING

It can be extremely difficult to support a patient who has difficulty in finding the midline, particularly if he pushes strongly to one side when he stands up from sitting. The difficulty is further increased if the patient is also very tall. Placing a stool or chair in front of him can help to provide him with more information as to where the middle is.

While the patient is still seated, a firm stool or chair is placed directly in front of the him at exactly the right distance away so that his head will be over his feet when he puts his hands flat on top of it with his arms extended. The therapist stands beside him as before and, with one hand on the far side of his pelvis, she places her other over his knee on the side nearest to her. The patient is asked to lift his bottom into the air without letting his hands move out of position. The therapist draws his knee forwards over his foot and keeps his trunk well forwards and in line by pressing her shoulder against him from behind (Fig. 7.30a). With her hip poster-

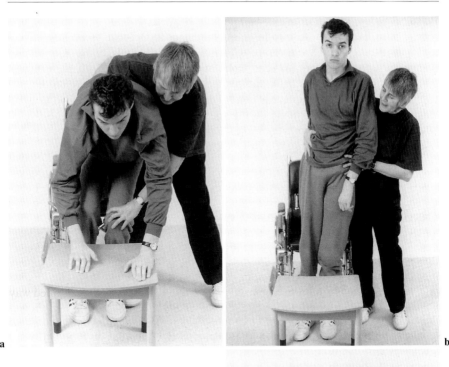

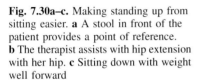

Fig. 7.30a–c. Making standing up from sitting easier. **a** A stool in front of the patient provides a point of reference. **b** The therapist assists with hip extension with her hip. **c** Sitting down with weight well forward

ior to his hip, she assists the extensor activity required to reach the erect position (Fig. 7.30b). Her body close to his makes it easier for balance to be maintained.

In order to sit down, the patient once again places his hands on the stool in front of him and slowly lowers his seat to the middle of the chair. With her shoulder pressing down against his back and one hand beneath his trochanter on the side furthest from her, the therapist can control the speed of the movement and keep his trunk forwards. Her other hand on his knee enables her to draw it forwards and outwards over his foot to prevent his leg from extending and adducting as it would otherwise do in the mass synergy of extension (Fig. 7.30c).

Dealing with Additional Problems Which Prevent Walking

Because walking plays such a vital role in the total rehabilitation of the patient, every effort must be made to overcome any problems which are standing in the way of his getting back on his feet. Should contractures of his feet or knees have developed and be preventing him from standing they can be treated successfully in the ways described in Chap. 6. In addition to such conditions directly related to the brain lesion, traumatic injuries sustained at the time of the original accident or later through falls may also prevent the patient from starting to stand and walk if they are not dealt with appropriately. The condition which most frequently prevents the patient from walking after such an injury is that of an ununited lower limb fracture. In the acute stage, the patient with a severe head injury may not always receive the same meticulous treatment of a femoral or tibial fracture as would his nonbrain-damaged counterpart. In fact, in some instances the fracture may even be overlooked, and in both instances nonunion could result. Internal fixation or whatever other type of management is deemed optimal should be considered, regardless of the patient's brain lesion, although it may be thought at the time that the patient will in any event never recover sufficiently to walk again. The same principle applies to the patient who falls out of bed or from his wheelchair and sustains a fractured neck of femur. He, too, must receive optimal treatment, including a total hip replacement if necessary, and should not be left lying in bed in the hope that the fracture will heal on its own simply because he is not able to move actively. Any patient who has the misfortune to have a lower limb amputation in addition to a traumatic brain injury must certainly have the very best type of prosthesis available if he is to learn to walk at all.

It should always be remembered that, although for some reason completely independent walking may not be achieved and the patient be unable to walk fast or cover long distances despite appropriate support and intensive training, the ability to stand up and walk even a little way can make a big difference to his life and that of those who care for him. Standing and walking will also lead to a noticeable improvement in many other areas as well.

A Case in Point

Two years after sustaining a severe head injury in a road traffic accident N.N. was finally admitted to a rehabilitation centre specializing in the treatment of brain-damaged patients. The many additional problems with which he and the rehabilitation team had to contend have been described in Chap. 6 (see "A case in point").

Two main problems still stood firmly in the way of N.N. being helped to stand and learn to walk again, namely the ununited fracture of his left femur and the high amputation of the right leg for which no prosthesis had been provided. Surgery was undertaken but was unfortunately not the hoped for success, as the hip replacement dislocated as a result of marked adductor spasticity. A second operation with the adductors inhibited by phenol blocks solved the problem satisfactorily and weight-bearing on the left leg could commence with a back slab supporting the knee in extension. The first artificial limb was a grave disappointment and caused endless frustration in that it either pinched painfully or the tiny stump popped out of the socket whenever N.N. moved actively or was helped to stand. Eventually, with the help of many people, an orthopaedic technician was found who with patience and determination was able to construct a well-fitting, modern prosthesis which made all the difference. After 3 years in sitting, N.N. could at last stand on two feet again and be congratulated (Fig. 7.31a). The technician had not only provided an artificial limb which stayed firmly in place and could flex at the knee during the swing phase, but had also taken the trouble to make it look as much like the other leg as possible (Fig. 7.31b). Because of the close fit of the prosthesis, N.N. can take all his weight on that leg confidently and also make a controlled step forwards with it despite a rather short stump (Fig. 7.31c). He is at present also learning to balance without the aid of a crutch (Fig. 7.32a). Although he still requires an elbow crutch for support and the help of another person, he is able to rise from sitting and manage limited distances on foot (Fig. 7.32b).

N.N. continues to improve slowly but surely which means progressively less physical strain for his wife. Being able to walk and climb stairs, even though he still needs considerable help and cannot cover long distances, has made a big difference to the quality of N.N.'s life. His dream house in which he has lived so happily for years, is built on three levels and without being able to manage stairs he would have been forced to move to other accommodation. On a recent holiday with his wife he could rent the apartment of his choice despite a passage too narrow for his wheelchair and a difficult entrance with a high step (Fig. 7.33). To his great joy, N.N. can go swimming every week with the aid of a light, water-resistant prosthesis which enables him to walk to the poolside.

Such accomplishments and many others like them have only been possible for N.N. because such determined efforts were made to overcome the seemingly insuperable problems which stood in his way.

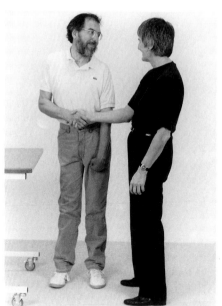

Fig. 7.31.a N.N. standing upright after 3 years in sitting. **b** An artificial limb carefully formed to look like his other leg. **c** A secure fit despite the high amputation

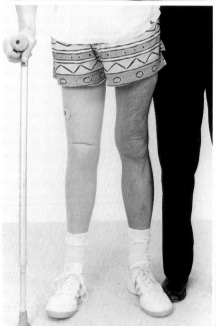

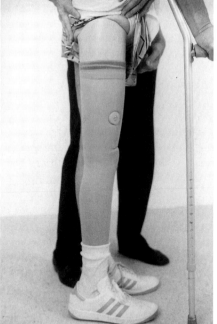

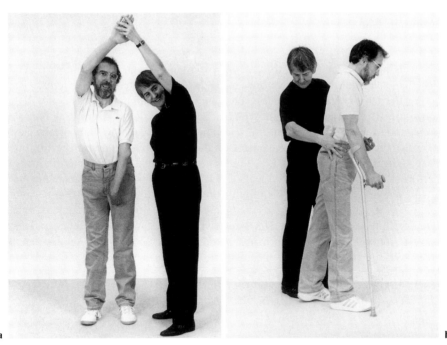

Fig. 7.32.a N.N. learning to balance without a crutch. **b** Able to walk short distances with a crutch and the help of another person

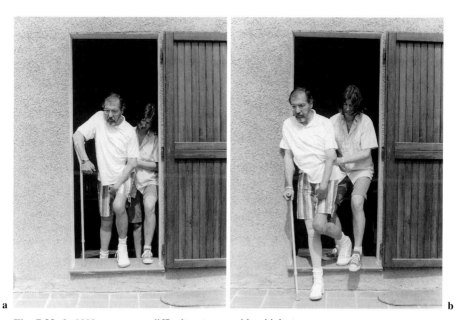

Fig. 7.33a,b. N.N. manages a difficult entrance with a high step

Learning to Go Up and Down Stairs

For walking to be functional, the patient will often be required to negotiate stairs once he leaves the sheltered confines of the hospital or rehabilitation centre. The sooner the activity is included in his rehabilitation programme, the easier it will be for him to climb stairs confidently and in a normal pattern. As well as being a preparation for future functional use, ascending and descending stairs can be used to retrain the many selective movements of the lower limbs inherent in performing the activity. Because the action is so familiar to the patient, it is far easier for him to perform than if he were to try to learn the separate components by practising isolated exercises on his bed or the plinth. Ritchie Russell (1975) rightly points out that the mechanism of forming a new memory must be inherently more complex than recalling an old one. The stairs themselves together with the adjacent wall and banisters provide plenty of information for the patient so that he is not dependent solely on his own feedback mechanisms to ascertain whether the task is being performed correctly or not. The patient does not need to be able to walk well before stair climbing is commenced. On the contrary, his walking will improve as a result of the motor control he regains while practising going up and down stairs.

Going Up Stairs

The therapist stands beside the patient at the foot of the stairs and facilitates the necessary movements as required, for instance by lifting one of his feet on to the first step while helping him to maintain his balance with her arm around his trunk. She may need to support his knee as he steps up with the other foot on to the step above. When going up or down stairs, the patient should not be told verbally exactly which movements to perform but be asked simply to go upstairs and the repeated flowing movements facilitated by the therapist's hands and body. At first the patient should hold on to the side rail and, if his foot tends to supinate, it can be bandaged securely in place, the bandage being applied over the outside of his shoe. For the initial attempt, if the therapist feels unsure as to how the patient will manage, she can ask an assistant to stand behind him to help her should anything untoward occur and she be unable to support him on her own.

Going Down Stairs

Descending the stairs tends to be more difficult for the majority of patients so that the same precautions must be taken when it is first attempted. As was the case when going up stairs, only one foot is placed on each step in the normal way and the therapist uses her hands to facilitate any movement component which is still difficult for the patient or even impossible for him without her help. Succeeding in reaching the next floor by way of the staircase is an enormous psychological boost for the patient regardless of how much help he received. It is an achievement that he can really understand and he will often be unaware that the therapist is supporting him at all.

Recreational Activities Which Encourage Active Movement

The patient who is not yet able to walk independently has little chance to move on his own and as a result spends many hours sitting immobile in his wheelchair. It is important that activities be found that he can not only enjoy with the help of his relatives outside of therapy times, but will also help to stimulate the return of active function in the most normal movement patterns possible. Depending upon the patient's abilities and the availability of the necessary equipment, there is a wide range of possibilities from which to select, ranging from table tennis and archery to pony-riding for the disabled. Some are more expensive and time-consuming than others and require expert supervision but two activities which have proved beneficial and enjoyable for many patients, without much additional expense, are swimming and cycling. Both of these activities allow the patient to move more freely and share a pleasurable experience with able-bodied relatives and friends.

Swimming

For teaching the patient to swim, the Halliwick method is recommended because it takes into account the need to avoid increased tone and associated reactions, facilitates normal movement patterns, and aims to make swimming without aids possible. Many courses on the method are offered, or the therapist can seek the help of someone who is already trained and has experience in working with neurologically impaired patients. An excellent book on teaching patients to swim has recently been published which includes the Halliwick principles as well as many other helpful hints and invaluable information. At present only available in German, the book is well-illustrated with numerous photographs of patients in action and gives concise descriptions of therapeutic possibilities in water (Weber 1993). Being able to swim provides an opportunity for the patient to move freely without the fear of falling and without having to contend with the pull of gravity, an experience which most will enjoy very much.

Cycling

A patient who can only walk very slowly and with great effort or uses a wheelchair when outside may be able to cycle instead on a bicycle or tricycle which is appropriately adapted to meet his special needs. He will be better able to keep pace with his companions, look less obviously disabled and enjoy the active movement.

- *Adult tricycles.* There are a number of modern, sporting tricycles available for adults in a variety of attractive colours with a choice of saddles or seats to suit the individual patient as well as special fittings for the pedals. Such three-wheelers eliminate the need for balance, regardless of whether two wheels are situated at the back or, as is sometimes advocated, at the front, as is the case, for example, with the "Trike" by Freewiel Techniek (DE Eersel, Holland).
- *A coupled-bike system.* An ingenious way of coupling two standard bicycles together simply and inexpensively enables "disabled and able-bodied to ride together" side by side (Nava 1986). The bicycles are joined together by rigid upper and lower transverse bars attached fore and aft, a procedure which can easily be carried out by a friend or member of the family. If required, an adapted saddle or seat can be incorporated. Balance is no longer a problem and the person accompanying the patient can guide the steering as much as is necessary, so that even with a severe spastic tetraplegia, cycling may be possible.
- *A tandem.* Riding tandem may be the answer for the patient with sufficient voluntary control and balance, with a member of his family or a friend taking over the steering from the front seat. Two standard bicycles may be fitted to one another or a special tandem purchased.
- *The handbike.* A single rider, arm-powered bicycle, called the Handbike, has been developed for patients with more marked lower limb involvement (Schwandt et al. 1984). If a patient is not able to manage entirely on his own, however, the Handbike can be fitted to the front of a standard bicycle to form a tandem.

Being able to ride some type of cycle can make it possible for the patient to move about more freely in the world outside long before he is able to walk safely on his own. The activity involved may also help him to attain the ultimate goal of walking independently.

Conclusion

In most hospitals and rehabilitation centres, considerable emphasis is placed on the patient's ability to walk or the progress he is making towards achieving independent walking. The doctor, for one, will often ask the therapist repeatedly how the patient is getting on with walking. The question is understandable because the activity is one which is actually measurable and thus provides him with more objective information than the therapist telling him, for example, that balance and muscle tone are "a little better this week". The patient's relatives eagerly await each walking attempt because they tend to relate walking with independence, although the two are not necessarily inter-related. At least they can see that the patient is making some progress as they count the number of steps he can take and compare the distance he covers with that which he could the previous week. The patient himself may keep asking the therapist to let him walk instead of performing other exercises because it is an activity that he really understands and a goal which he yearns to achieve.

Such constant emphasis on walking can even be a source of irritation for the therapist if she considers that, from a motor point of view, it is far too early for the patient to attempt such a complex activity. However, she is usually well-advised to adapt to the situation without any sign of impatience and leave enough time at the end of each treatment session to walk with the patient because the many advantages to be gained far outweigh any disadvantages. Psychologically walking can be of great benefit to the patient because it gives him the feeling that he is really making progress and, by the same token, his family will certainly be encouraged. Because he understands the aim of the activity the patient will usually cooperate fully and as a result, be prepared to work harder at other tasks as well. When walking, every muscle in his body is activated which can serve to counteract the detrimental effects of long term immobility. If the patient can walk with help in such a way that nothing goes terribly wrong with regard to increased tone or the reinforcement of abnormal motor patterns then he will benefit from the activity. Waiting too long before commencing walking can lead to the patient becoming increasingly afraid to move freely in an upright position and voluntary control of his legs will be further delayed by his not using them. As is the case when someone is learning to speak a foreign language, waiting for the performance to be perfect could well mean never starting at all. It is far better for the patient to walk with assistance even though his gait still reveals certain abnormalities than for him to sit flexed in his wheelchair all day without taking weight through his legs.

Whenever possible, the patient should be helped to walk when carrying out those daily life activities that he previously performed in the upright position. He can walk to the bathroom, stand while brushing his teeth or combing his hair, walk to fetch his clothes from the cupboard each morning and walk into the dining-room to sit at table, leaving his wheelchair outside in the passage. The occupational therapy kitchen with its many supporting surfaces offers ideal opportunities for standing and walking while preparing meals and washing-up afterwards. In order for such goal-orientated walking to be practicable, not only the different therapists but also the nurses and the patient's relatives will need to know how to facilitate his standing up from sitting and how to support the patient correctly when he is walking. By incorporating walking with real functional activities, there will be many more opportunities for the patient to walk during the day, instead of only the short practice which forms part of a therapy session. His walking will become a part of his everyday life and not be just an exercise which he carries out in the physiotherapy department.

For each patient such functional walking will surely be synonymous with starting again on the long road to regaining lost independence and being able to lead a fuller and more normal life.

References

Ackerman S (1992) Discovering the brain. National Academic Press, Washington

Affolter F (1981) Perceptual processes as prerequisites for complex human behaviour. Int Rehabil Med 3(1):3–9

Affolter F (1991) Perception, interaction and language. Springer, Berlin Heidelberg New York

Affolter F, Bischofberger W (1993) Wenn die Organisation des zentralen Nervensytems zerfällt und es an gespürter Information mangelt. Neckar-Verlag, Villingen-Schwenningen

Affolter F, Stricker E (eds) (1980) Perceptual processes as prerequisites for complex human behaviour. A theoretical model and its application to therapy. Huber, Bern

Agnew D S Shetter AG, Segall HD, Flom RA (1983) Thalamic pain. In: Bonica JJ, Lindblom U, Iggo A (eds) Advances in pain research and therapy, vol 5. Raven, New York, pp 941–946

American Academy of Paediatrics (1983) The Doman-Delecato treatment of neurologically handicapped children. The Exceptional Parent (October)

American Academy of Physical Medicine and Rehabilitation (1968) Doman-Delecato treatment of neurologically handicapped children, 1967. Arch Phys Med Rehabil 49:4

An HS, Ebraheim N, Kim K, Jackson WT, Kane JT (1987) Heterotopic ossification and pseudoarthrosis in the shoulder following encephalitis: a case report and review of the literature. Clin Orthop 219:291

Arbib MA (1981) Perceptual structures and distributed motor control. In: Brooks VB (ed) Motor control, part 2. Williams and Wilkins, Baltimore, pp 1449–1480 (Handbook of physiology, sect 1; the nervous system, vol 2)

Armstrong KK, Saghal V, Block R, Armstrong KJ, Heinemann A (1990) Rehabilitation outcome in patients with posttraumatic epilepsy. Arch Phys Med Rehabil 71:156–160

Atkinson HW (1986) Principles of assessment (chapter 6). Principles of treatment (chapter 7). In: Downie PA (ed) Cash's textbook of neurology for physiotherapists. 4th edn. Faber and Faber, London

Bach-y-Rita P (1981) Central nervous system lesions: sprouting and unmasking in rehabilitation. Arch Phys Med Rehabil 62:413–417

Bach-y-Rita P, Balliet R (1987) Recovery from stroke. In: Duncan P, Badke M (eds) Stroke rehabilitation: the recovery of motor control. Year Book Medical, Chicago, pp 81–82

Baker LL, Parker K, Sanderson D (1983) Neuromuscular electrical stimulation for the head-injured patient. Phys Ther 63(12):1967–1974

Bannister D (1974) Personal construct theory and psychotherapy. In: Bannister D (ed) Issues and approaches in psychotherapy. Wiley, New York

Basmajian J (1979) Muscles alive. Their functions revealed by electromyography, 4th edn. Williams and Wilkins, Baltimore

Basmajian J (1980) Biofeedback in clinical practice. Unpublished lecture given during a course on EMG-Biofeedback, University Hospital Geneva

Basmajian J (1981) Biofeed-back in rehabilitation: a review of principles and practices. Arch Phys Med Rehabil 62:469–475

Bass NH (1988) Neurogenic dysphagia: Diagnostic assessment and rehabilitation of feeding disorders in the neurologically impaired. In: Eisenberg MG (ed) Advances in clinical rehabilitation, vol 2. Springer, New York, Berlin, Heidelberg, pp 186–228

Bass NH (1990) Clinical signs, symptoms and treatment of dysphagia in the neurologically disabled. J Neuro Rehab 4:227–235

Bass NH Morrell MM (1984) The neurology of swallowing. In: Groher ME (ed) Dysphagia — diagnosis and management, 2nd edn. Butterworth, Boston, pp 1–29

Benson AJ (1984) Motion sickness. In: Dix MR (ed) Vertigo. Wiley, Chichester, pp 391–426

Bentham J (1789) Introduction to principles of morals and legislation. London

Beukelmann DR, Traynor C, Poblete M, Warren G (1984) Microcomputer-based communication augmentation systems for two non-speaking, physically handicapped persons with severe visual impairment. Arch Phys Med Rehabil 65: 89–91

Biquer B, Donaldson IML, Hein A, Jeannerod M (1986) La vibration des muscles de la nuque modifie la position apparente d'une cible visuelle. Acad Sci Paris, series 111, p 303

Biquer B, Donaldson IML, Hein A, Jeannerod M (1988) Neck muscle vibration modifies the representation of visual motion and detection in man. Brain 111:1405–1424

Bobath B (1968) Abnorme Haltungsreflexe bei Hirnschäden. Thieme, Stuttgart

Bobath B (1971) Abnormal postural reflex activity caused by brain lesions. Heinemann, London

Bobath B (1978) Adult hemiplegia: evaluation and treatment. 2nd edn. Heinemann, London

Bobath B (1990) Adult hemiplegia. Evaluation and treatment, 3rd edn. Heinemann, London

Bobath K (1966) Motor deficit in patients with cerebral palsy. Clinics in Developmental Medicine, No. 23. William Heinemann Medical Books, London

Bobath K (1988) Neurophysiology 11. Unpublished lecture given during a course on the treatment of adult hemiplegia. Post-graduate Study Centre Hermitage, Bad Ragaz

Boivie J, Leijon G (1991) Clinical findings in patients with central poststroke pain. In: KL Casey (ed) Pain and central nervous system disease: the central pain syndromes. Raven, New York

Booth BJ, Doyle M, Montgomery J (1983) Serial casting for the management of spasticity in the head-injured adult. Phys Ther 63(12):1960–1965

Bourgeois BFD, Prensky AL, Palkes HS, Talent BK (1983) Intelligence in epilepsy: a prospective study in children. Ann Neurol 14:438–444

Bower KD (1986)The patho-physiology and symptomology of the whiplash syndrome. In: GP Grieve (ed) Modern manual therapy of the vertebral column. Churchill Livingstone, Edinburgh

Bowsher D (1991) Neurogenic pain syndromes and their management. In: Wells JCD, Woolf CJ (eds) Pain mechanisms and management. Churchill Livingstone, Edinburgh (British Medical Bulletin Series, vol 47, no. 3)

Bowsher D, Lahuerta J, Brock L (1984) Twelve cases of central pain, only three with thalamic lesion. Pain Suppl 2: 83

Breig A (1978) Adverse mechanical tension in the central nervous system. Almqvist and Wiksell, Stockholm

Brodal A (1973) Self-observations and neuro-anatomical considerations after a stroke. Brain 96:675–694

Bromley I (1976) Tetraplegia and paraplegia. Churchill Livingstone, Edinburgh

Buchholz DW (1987) Neurologic evaluation of dysphagia. Dysphagia 1:187–192

Burghart W, Schepach W, Hofmann K, Weingartner P, Kleine B, Ptok M, Kasper H (1989) Perkutane endoskopische Gastrostomie: Erfahrungen mit 124 Patienten. Akt Ernähr 14:179–184

Butler D (1991a) The component concept. Lecture given during a course on abnormal neural tension. Postgraduate Study Centre Hermitage, Bad Ragaz

Butler DS (1991b) Mobilisation of the nervous system. Churchill Livingstone, Melbourne

Butler D, Gifford L (1989) The concept of adverse mechanical tension in the nervous system. Physiotherapy 75(11):622–636

Charlton JE (1991) Management of sympathetic pain. In: Wells JCD, Woolf CJ (eds) Pain mechanisms and management. Churchill Livingstone, Edinburgh (British Medical Bulletin Series, vol 47, no. 3)

Conner JM (1983) Soft tissue ossification. Springer, Berlin Heidelberg New York

Coombes K (1995) Rehabilitation of the face and oral tract. Springer, Berlin Heidelberg New York, (to be published)

Cope DN, Hall K (1982) Head injury rehabilitation: benefit of early intervention. Arch.Phys Med Rehabil 63:433–437

Creech R (1980) Do you like your larynx? Communication Outlook 2(4):l, 10 ff

Damasio A (1992) Mapping the brain. Newsweek CXIX (16):April 20

Damasio A, Damasio H (1992) Brain and language. Sci Amer 267(3) September

Davies PM (1985) Steps to follow. A guide to the treatment of adult hemiplegia. Springer, Berlin Heidelberg New York

Davies PM (1990) Right in the middle. Selective trunk activity in the treatment of adult hemiplegia. Springer, Berlin Heidelberg New York

Dennet D C (1991) Consciousness explained. Penguin, Allen Lane

Dikmen S, Reitan RM (1978) Neuro-psychological performance in posttraumatic epilepsy. Epilepsia 19:177–183

Donner MW (1986) The evaluation of dysphagia by radiography and other methods of imaging. Dysphagia 1:49–50

Donner MW, Bosma J, Robertson D (1985) Anatomy and physiology of the pharynx. Gastrointest Radiol 10:196–212

Downing AR (1985) Eye controlled and other fast communicators for speech and physically handicapped persons. Australas Phys Eng Sci Med 8(1):17–21

Espinola D (1986) Radionuclide evaluation of pulmonary aspiration: Four birds with one stone — esophageal transit, gastroesophageal reflux, gastric emptying and bronchoopulmonary aspiration. Dysphagia 1:101–104

Evans CD (1981) Rehabilitation after severe head injury. Churchill Livingstone, Edinburgh

Evans WJ, Meredith CN, Cannon JG, Dinareilo CA, Frontera WR, Hughes VA, Jones BH, Knuttgen HG (1985) Metabolic changes following eccentric exercise in trained and untrained men. J Appl Physiol 61:1864–1868

Fields H L (1987) Pain. McGraw-Hill, New York

Foutch PG, Haynes WC, Bellapravalu S, Sanowski RA (1986) Percutaneous endoscopic gastrostomy (PEG). A new procedure comes of age. J Clin Gastroenterol 8(1):10–15

Franz SI (1902) On the functions of the cerebrum: the frontal lobes in relation to the production and retention of simple sensory-motor habits. Am J Physiol 8:1–22

Friday N (1981) My mother my self. Dell, New York

Garcin R (1968) Thalamic syndrome and pain of central origin. In: Soulairac A, Cahn J, Charpentier J (eds) Pain. Academic, London, pp 521–541

Garland DE (1991) A clinical perspective on common forms of acquired heterotopic ossification. Clin Orthop Related Res 263:13–29

Garland DE, Blum CE, Waters RL (1980) Periarticular heterotopic ossification in head-injured adults: incidence and location. J Bone Joint Surg [Am] 62(7):1143–1146

Garland DE, Keenan MAE (1983) Orthopedic strategies in the management of the adult head-injured patient. Phys Ther 63(12):2004–2009

Garland DE, Hanscom DA, Keenan MA, Smith C, Moore T (1985) Resection of heterotopic ossification in the adult with head trauma. J Bone Joint Surg [Am] 67:1261–1269

Gibson JJ (1966) The senses considered as perceptual systems. Houghton, Boston

Giles GM, Clark-Wilson J (1993) Brain injury rehabilitation. A neurofunctional approach. Chapman and Hall, London

Gold L (1990) Improving communication in the medical team. Lecture during a course organised by the Post-graduate Study Centre Hermitage, Bad Ragaz

Goldman A, Lloyd-Thomas AR (1991) Pain management in children. In: Wells JCD, Woolf CJ (eds) Pain mechanisms and management. Churchill Livingstone, Edinburgh (British Medical Bulletin Series, vol 47, no. 3) pp 676–689

Goldsmith E, Golding RM, Garstang RA, Macrae AW (1992) A technique to measure windswept deformity. Physiotherapy 78(4):235–242

Grosswasser Z, Stern MJ(1989) Dynamic cognitive and behavioral changes during the rehabilitation process of traumatic brain injury. International Rehabilitation Medicine Association Monograph Series April

Grüninger W (1986) Die Rehabilitation bei Querschnittlähmung. In: Schirmer M (ed) Querschnittlähmungen. Springer, Berlin Heidelberg New York, pp 538–547

Guttmann L (1948) Bedsores. Br Surg Practice 2:65

Guttmann Sir L (1973) Spinal cord injuries: comprehensive management and research. Blackwell, London

Hagen C, Malkmus D, Durham P (1972) Levels of cognitive functioning. Rancho Los Amigos Hospital, Los Angeles

Hardy AG, Dixon JW (1963) Pathological ossification in traumatic paraplegia. J Bone Joint Surg [Br] 45:76–87

Heimlich HJ (1978) The Heimlich maneuver. Emergency Med 10:89–101

Heimlich HJ (1983) Rehabilitation of swallowing after stroke. Ann Otol Rhinol Laryngol 92:357–359

Hernandez AM, Forner JV, De La Fuente T, et al (1978) The para-articular ossifications in our paraplegics and tetraplegics: a study of 704 patients. Paraplegia 16:272–275

Hobson EPG (1956) Physiotherapy in paraplegia. Churchill, London

Horner J (1984) Communication for the speechless patient. N C Med J 45(8):505–509

Ideström C, Schalling D, Carlquist U, Sjöqvist F (1972) Acute effects of diphenylhydantoin in relation to plasma levels. Psychol Med 2:111–120

Ignazzi V, Ramsden VS (1984) Eye operated keyboard. Australas Phys Eng Sci Med 7(2):58–62

Jacobs HE (1988) Yes, behaviour analysis can help but do you know how to harness it? Brain Inj 2(4):339–346

Janda V (1980) Muscles as a pathogenic factor in back pain. Proceedings of the International Fedration of Orthopaedic Manipulative Therapists, 4th Conference. Christchurch, New Zealand, pp 1–23

Jeannerod (1990) The neural and behavioural organisation of goal-directed movements. Clarendon, Oxford, (Oxford Psychology Series No. 15)

Jennet B (1979) Post-traumatic epilepsy. Adv Neurol 22:137–147

Jennet B (1987) Epilepsy after head injury and intracranial surgery. In: Hopkins A (ed) Epilepsy. Chapman and Hall, London, pp 401–441

Jennet B, Teasdale G, Galbraith S, Braakman R, Avezaat C, Minderhoud J, Heiden J, Kurze T, Murray G, Parker L (1979) Prognosis in patients with severe head injury. Acta Neurochir Suppl 28:149–152

Jennet B, Snoek J, Bond MR, Brooks N (1981) Disability after severe head injury: observations on the use of the Glasgow Outcome Scale. J Neurol Neurosurg Psychiatr 44:285–293

Johnson JR, Higgins L (1987) Integration of family dynamics into the rehabilitation of the brain-injured adult. Rehab Nurs 12(6)

Jull GA (1986) Headaches associated with the cervical spine — a clinical review. In: Grieve GP (ed) Modern manual therapy of the vertebral column. Churchill Livingstone, Edinburgh

Karbowski K (1985) Epileptische Anfälle. Phänomenologie, Differentialdiagnose und Therapie. Springer, Berlin Heidelberg New York

Kesselring J (1992a) Wandel der Physiotherapie in der Neurorehabilitation — ein ABC der Neurorehabilitation. Unpublished lecture given at the farewell ceremony for Dr Busch, Gailingen, March 21

Kesselring J (1992b) Eine neurologie des Verhaltens als Grundlage der Neurorehabilitation. Schweiz Med Wochenschr 122(33):1197–205

Kesselring J (1993) Taktil-Kinästhetische Wahrnehmung und die Organisation des Zentralen Nervensystems. In: Affolter F, Bischofberger W (ed) Wenn die Organisation des zentralen Nervensystems zerfällt und es an gespürter Information mangelt. Neckar-Verlag, Villingen-Schwenningen

Kirby DF, Craig RM, Tsang T-K, and Plotnick BH (1986) Percutaneous endoscopic gastrostomies: a prospective evaluation and review of the literature. J Parenter Enter Nutr 10(2):155–159

Klein-Vogelbach S (1987) Functional kinetics. Lecture for the 3rd meeting of IBITAH in the Postgraduate Study Centre, Hermitage, Bad Ragaz

Klein-Vogelbach (1990) Functional kinetics. Observing analysing and teaching human movement. Springer, Berlin Heidelberg New York

Knight G (1963) Post-traumatic occipital headache. Lancet 1:6–8

Knott M (1970) Treatment of the face and mouth. Lecture during the PNF course held from July-December. Vallejo, California

Knott M, Voss DE (1968) Proprioceptive neuromuscular facilitation. Harper, New York

Kottke FJ (ed) (1982a) The neurophysiology of motor function. Saunders, Philadelphia, pp 218–252 (Krusen's handbook of physical medicine and rehabilitation)

Kottke FJ (ed) (1982b) Therapeutic exercise to develop neuromuscular coordination. Saunders, Philadelphia, pp 403–426 (Krusen's handbook of physical medicine and rehabilitation)

Kottke FJ, Halpern D, Easton JKM, Ozel AT, Burril CAV (1978) The training of coordination. Arch Phys Med Rehabil 59:567–572

Landau WM (1988) Clinical neuromythology 11. Parables of palsy pills and PT pedagogy: a spastic dialect. Neurology 38:1496–1499

Larson DE, Burton DD, Schroeder KW, DiMagno EP (1987) Percutaneous endoscopic gastrostomy. Indications, success, complications and mortality in 314 consecutive patients. Gastroenterology 93(1):48–52

Lazzarra G deL, Lazarus C, Logemann JA (1986) Impact of thermal stimulation on the triggering of the swallowing reflex. Dysphagia 1:73–77

Lewin W, Roberts AH (1979) Long.term prognosis after severe head injury. Acta Neurochir Suppl 28:128–133

Lewit K (1977) Pain arising in the posterior arch of the atlas. Eur Neurol 16:263–269

Lezac MD (1988) Brain damage is a family affair. J Clin Exp Neuropsychol 10(1):111–123

Lieber R (1992) Skeletal muscle structure and function. Implications for rehabilitation and sports medicine. Williams and Wilkins, Baltimore

Logemann JA (1988) The role of the speech language pathologist in the management of dysphagia. Otolaryngol Clin N Am 21(4):783–788

Logemann JA (1983) Evaluation and treatment of swallowing disorders. College Hill Press, San Diego

Logemann JA (1985) The relationship between speech and swallowing in head and neck surgical patients. Semin Speech Lang 6(4):351–359

Loiseau P Strube E Signoret J-L (1988) Memory and epilepsy. In: Trimble MR, Reynolds EH (eds) Epilepsy, behaviour and cognitive function. Wiley, Chichester

Long CG, Moore JR (1979) Parental expectations for their epileptic children. J Child Psychol Psychiatr 20:299–312

Louis R (1981) Vertebroradicular and vertebromedullar dynamics. Anat Clin 3:1–11

Luria AR (1978) The working brain. Penguin, Allen Lane

Lynch M, Grisogno V (1991) Strokes and head injuries. Murray, London

Lynch C, Pont A, Weingarden SI (1981) Hetroectopic ossification in hand of patient with spinal cord injury. Arch Phys Med Rehabil 62:291–293

McMahon SB (1991) Mechanisms of sympathetic pain. In: Wells JCD, Woolf CJ (eds) Pain mechanisms and management. Churchill Livingstone, Edinburgh (British Medical Bulletin Series, vol 47, no. 3), pp 584–600

MacPhee GJA, Goldie C, Roulston D et al (1986) Effects of carbamazepine on psychomotor performance in naive subjects. Eur J Clin Pharmacol 30:37–42

Magarey M (1986) Examinaton of the cervical spine. In: Grieve GP (ed) Modern manual therapy of the vertebral column. Churchill Livingstone, Edinburgh

Magnus R (1926) Some results of studies in the physiology of posture. Lancet, September 11, 1926: 531–536

Maier F (1988) A second chance at life. Newsweek CXII: September 12

Maisel AQ (1964) Hope for brain-injured children. Reader's Digest, (October), pp 134–140

Maitland GD (1986) Vertebral manipulation, 5th edn. Butterworths, London

Meinck HM, Benecke R, Meyer W, Hohne J, Conrad B (1984) Human ballistic finger flexion; uncoupling of the three-burst pattern. Exp Brain Res 55:127–133

Melzack R (1991) Central pain syndromes and theories of pain. In: Casey KL (ed) Pain and central nervous system disease: the central pain syndromes. Raven, New York

Michelsson J-E, Rausching W (1983) Pathogenesis of experimental heterotopic bone formation following temporary forcible exercising of immobilized limbs. Clin Orthop Rel Res 176:265–272

Mielants H, Vanhove E, De Neels J, Veys E (1975) Clinical survey of and pathogenic approach to para-articular ossifications in long-term coma. Acta Orthop Scand 46:190–198

Miller AJ (1986) Neurophysiological basis of swallowing. Dysphagia 1:91–100

Millesi H (1986) The nerve gap. Hand Clin 2:651–663

Mital MA, Garber JE, Stinson JT (1987) Ectopic bone formation in children and adolescents with head injuries: its management. J Pediatr Orthop 7:83–90

Molcho S (1983) Körper-Sprache. Mosaik, Munich

Moore J (1980) Neuroanatomical considerations relating to recovery of function following brain injury. In: Bach-y-Rita P (ed) Recovery of function: theoretical considerations for brain injury recovery. Huber, Bern

Moran BJ, Frost RA (1992) Percutaneous endoscopic gastrostomy in 41 patients: indications and outcome. J R Soc Med 85(June):320–321

Moran B, Taylor M, Johnson C (1990) Percutaneous endoscopic gastrostomy: a review. Br J Surg 77:858–862

Morris D (1987) Manwatching. A field guide to human behaviour. Grafton, London

Mouritzen Dam A (1980) Epilepsy and neuron loss in the hippocampus. Epilepsia 21:617–629

Nava LC (1986) Coupled bicycles for disabled and able-bodied to ride together. Prosthetics Orthotics Int 10:103–104

Nehen H-G (1988) Gute Erfahrung mit der PEG. Altenpflege 10:644–646

Okamato T (1973) Electromyographic study of the learning process of walking in 1-and 2 year-old infants. Med Sport 8:328–333

Ossetin J (1988) Methods and problems in the assessment of cognitive function in epileptic patients. In: Trimble MR, Reynolds EH (eds) Epilepsy, behaviour and cognitive function. Wiley, Chichester

Peschl L, Zeilinger M, Munda W, Prem H, Schragel D (1988) Perkutane endoskopische Gastrostomie — eine Möglichkeit der enteralen Ernährung von Patienten mit schweren zerebralen Funktionsstörungen. Wien Klin Wochenschr 10(Mai 13):314–318

Petrillo CL, Knoploch S (1988) Phenol block of the tibial nerve for spasticity: a long term follow-up study. Int Disability Studies 10(3):97–100

Pfaltz CR (1987) Pathophysiological aspects of vestibular disorders. Adv Otorhinolaryngol 39/4

Plaget J (1969) Das erwachen der Intelligenz beim Kinde. Klett, Stuttgart, pp 39–51

Ponsky JL, Gauderer MWL (1989) Percutaneous endoscopic gastrostomy: indications, limitations, techniques and results. World J Surg 13:165–170

Puzas JE, Miller MD, Rosier RN (1989) Pathalogic bone formation. Clin Orthop Related Res 245:269-281

Ragone DJ, Kellerman WC, Bonner FJ(1986) Heterotopic ossification masquerading as deep vein thrombosis in head-injured adult: complications of anticoagulation. Arch Phys Med Rehabil 67:339–341

Reason JT (1978) Motion sickness adaptation. A neural mismatch model. J R Soc Med 71:819–829

Riddoch G (1938) The clinical features of central pain. Lancet 234: 1093–1098, 1150–1156, 1205–1209

Ritchie Russell W (1975) Explaining the brain. Oxford University Press, London

Rodin EA, Schmaltz S, Tuitly G (1986) Intellectual functions of patients with childhood-onset epilepsy. Dev Med Child Neurol 28:25–33

Rolf G (1993) Neurale Gegenspannung in der Befundaufnahme und in der Behandlung von Patienten mit einer Läsion des zentralen Nervensystems. Lecture given at the congress of the Schweizerischer Verband für Manipulative Physiotherapie. Zurich, November 1993

Rosenzweig M (1980) Animal models for effects of brain lesions and for rehabilitation. In: Bach-y-Rita P (ed) Recovery of function: theoretical considerations for brain injury rehabilitation. University Park Press, Baltimore, pp 127–172

Rosenzweig M, Bennet EL, Diamond MC et al (1969) Influences of environmental complexity and visual stimulation on development of occipital cortex in rats. Brain Res 14:427–445

Rothmeier J, Schreiber H, Fröscher W (1990) Myositis ossificans circumscripta nach ungewöhnlichem Hirntrauma. Fortschr Med 108(21):415/31–32/416

Ruch, Patton (1970) Physiology and biophysics, vol 2. Saunders, Philadelphia

Rush PJ (1989) The rheumatic manifestations of traumatic spinal cord injury. Semin Arthritis Rheuma 19(2) (October):77–89

Sazbon L, Najenson T, Tartovsky M, Becker E, Grosswaser Z (1981) Widespread periarticular new-bone formation in long-term comatose patients. J Bone Joint Surg [Br] 63(1):120–125

Scherzer BP (1988) Rehabilitation following severe head trauma: results of a three-year program. Arch Phys Med Rehabil 67:366–374

Schlaegel W (1993) Was geschiet mit den Patienten im Koma?. In: Affolter F, Bischofberger W (ed) Wenn die Organisation des zentralen Nervensystems zerfällt - und es an gespürter Information mangelt. Neckar-Verlag, Villingen-Schwenningen

Schlee P, Keymling M, Wörner W (1987) Die perkutane, endoskopisch kontrollierte Gastrostomie (PEG) bei neurologischen Krankheiten und in der Geriatrie. Medwelt 38:45–47

Schmidbauer W (1978) Die hilflosen Helfer. Über die seelische Problematik der helfenden Berufe. Rowohlt, Reinbek

Schultz EC, Semmes RE (1950) Head and neck pain of cervical disc origin. Laryngoscope 60: 338–343

Schwandt D, Leifer L, Axelson P, Gaines R, Wong F (1984) Arm-powered tandem for disabled and able-bodied to ride together. Rehabilitation Research and Development Centre, Veteran's Administration Medical Centre, Palo Alto, CA. pp 1–2

Schwartz S (1964) Effect on neonatal corical lesions and early environmental factors on adult rat behaviour. J Comp Physiol Psychol 57:72–77

Searle J (1984) Minds, brains and science. BBC Publications, London

Sherrington C (1947) The integrative action of the nervous system 2nd edn. Yale University Press, New Haven

Siebens AA, Linden P (1985) Dynamic imaging for swallowing reeducation. Gastrointest Radiol 10:251–253

Shorvon SD (1988) Late onset seizures and dementia: a review of epidemiology and aetiology. In: Trimble MR, Reynolds EH (eds) Epilepsy, behaviour and cognitive function. Wiley, Chichester

Shorvon S, Reynolds EH (1979) Reduction in polypharmacy for epilepsy. Br Med J 2:1023–1025

Smith CG (1956) Changes in length and posture of the segments of the spinal cord with changes in posture in the monkey. Radiology 66:259–265

Sonderegger H (1993) The treatment of perceptual disturbances. Lecture during a course on the treatment of traumatic brain injury in St José, California

Stover SL, Hataway CJ, Zieger HE (1975) Hetrotopic ossification in spinal cord-injured patients. Arch Phys Med Rehabil 56:159-204

Teasdale G, Jennet B (1974) Assessment of coma and impaired consciousness: a practical scale. Lancet 2:81–84

Teasdale G, Parker L, Muray G, Knill-Jines R, Jennet B (1979) Predicting the outcome of individual patients in the first week after severe head injury. Acta Neurochir Suppl 28:161–164

ten Kate JH, Verbeek DGF, Hogervorst R, Duyvis JD (1985) Discrete eye-position for alternative communication. Med Progr Technol 10:201–211

Thornedike A (1940) Myositis ossificans traumatica. J Bone Joint Surg 22:315

Travis AM, Woolsey CN (1956) Motor perfomance of monkeys after bilateral partial and total cerebral decortication. Am Phys Med 35:273–310

Trimble M R (1988) Anticonvulsant drugs: mood and cognitive function. In: Trimble MR, Reynolds EH (eds) Epilepsy, behaviour and cognitive function. Wiley, Chichester

Trott PH (1986) Tension headache. In: Grieve GP (ed) Modern manual therapy of the vertebral column. Churchill Livingstone, Edinburgh

Tuchmann-Duplessis H, Auroux M, Haegel P (1975) Nervous system and endocrine glands. Springer, Berlin Heidelberg New York (Illustrated human embryology, vol 3)

Venier LH, Ditunno JF (1971) Heterotopic ossification in the paraplegic patient. Arch Phys Med Rehabil 52:475

Vojta V, Peters A (1992) Das Vojta-Prinzip. Springer, Berlin Heidelberg New York

Von Randow G (1991) Die Erfindung der Hand. Geo 11/21.10 1991

Wall PD (1987) Foreword. In: Fields HL (ed) Pain. McGraw-Hill, New York

Wall PD (1991) Neurogenic pain and injured nerve: central mechanisms. In: Wells JCD, Woolf CJ (eds) Pain mechanisms and management. Churchill Livingstone, Edinburgh (British Medical Bulletin Series, vol 47, no. 3)

Weber H (1993) Erlebnis Wasser. Springer, Berlin Heidelberg New York

Winstein CJ (1983) Neurogenic dysphagia. Frequency, progression and outcome in adults following head injury. Phys Ther 63(12):1992–1996

Woodworth CN (1899) The accuracy of voluntary movements. Psychol Rev Monogr Suppl 3

Woolf CJ (1991) Generation of acute pain: central mechanisms. In: Wells JCD, Woolf CJ (eds) Pain mechanisms and management. Churchill Livingstone, Edinburgh (British Medical Bulletin Series, vol 47, no. 3) pp 523–533

Zablotny C, Andric MF, Gowland C (1987) Serial casting: clinical applications for the adult head-injured patient. J Head Trauma Rehabil 2(2):46–52

Zekir S (1992) The visual image in mind and brain. Sci Amer (September) 267(3)

Subject Index